Diagnosis and Management of Headache Disorder

Diagnosis and Management of Headache Disorder

Editor: Sienna West

AMERICAN
MEDICAL PUBLISHERS
www.americanmedicalpublishers.com

AMERICAN
MEDICAL PUBLISHERS
www.americanmedicalpublishers.com

Cataloging-in-Publication Data

Diagnosis and management of headache disorder / edited by Sienna West.
p. cm.
Includes bibliographical references and index.
ISBN 978-1-63927-288-4
1. Headache. 2. Headache--Diagnosis. 3. Headache--Treatment. 4. Head--Diseases.
5. Pain. I. West, Sienna.
RC392 .D53 2022
616.849 1--dc23

American Medical Publishers,
41 Flatbush Avenue,
1st Floor, New York,
NY 11217, USA

ISBN 978-1-63927-288-4 (Hardback)

Contents

Preface ... IX

Chapter 1 **The burden of headache disorders in Nepal: estimates from a population-based survey** ... 1
Kedar Manandhar, Ajay Risal, Mattias Linde and Timothy J. Steiner

Chapter 2 **Altered serum levels of kynurenine metabolites in patients affected by cluster headache** ... 11
Martina Curto, Luana Lionetto, Andrea Negro, Matilde Capi, Francesca Perugino, Francesco Fazio, Maria Adele Giamberardino, Maurizio Simmaco, Ferdinando Nicoletti and Paolo Martelletti

Chapter 3 **Headaches attributed to airplane travel: a Danish survey** ... 17
Sebastian Bao Dinh Bui, Torben Petersen, Jeppe Nørgaard Poulsen and Parisa Gazerani

Chapter 4 **Comorbidities of psychiatric and headache disorders in Nepal: implications from a nationwide population-based study** ... 22
Ajay Risal, Kedar Manandhar, Are Holen, Timothy J. Steiner and Mattias Linde

Chapter 5 **Headache: an important factor associated with muscle soreness/pain at the two-year follow-up point among patients with major depressive disorder** ... 31
Ching-I Hung, Chia-Yih Liu, Ching-Hui Yang and Shuu-Jiun Wang

Chapter 6 **Post procedure headache in patients treated for neurovascular arteriovenous malformations and aneurysms using endovascular therapy** ... 39
Sabrina Khan, Faisal Mohammad Amin, John Hauerberg, Markus Holtmannspötter, Julie Falkenberg Petersen, Zainab Fakhril-Din, David Gaist and Messoud Ashina

Chapter 7 **Headache yesterday in Karnataka state, India: prevalence, impact and cost** ... 47
Timothy J. Steiner, Girish N. Rao, Girish B. Kulkarni, Gopalkrishna Gururaj and Lars J. Stovner

Chapter 8 **The prevalence of primary headache disorders in Ethiopia** ... 53
Mehila Zebenigus, Redda Tekle-Haimanot, Dawit K. Worku, Hallie Thomas and Timothy J. Steiner

Chapter 9 **The association of headache frequency with pain interference and the burden of disease is mediated by depression and sleep quality, but not anxiety, in chronic tension type headache** ... 62
María Palacios-Ceña, Juan J. Fernández-Muñoz, Matteo Castaldo, Kelun Wang, Ángel Guerrero-Peral, Lars Arendt-Nielsen and César Fernández-de-las-Peñas

Chapter 10 **Copeptin for risk stratification in non-traumatic headache in the emergency setting** 70
Claudine Angela Blum, Bettina Winzeler, Nicole Nigro, Philipp Schuetz, Silke Biethahn, Timo Kahles, Cornelia Mueller, Katharina Timper, Katharina Haaf, Janina Tepperberg, Margareth Amort, Andreas Huber, Roland Bingisser, Peter Stephan Sándor, Krassen Nedeltchev, Beat Müller, Mira Katan and Mirjam Christ-Crain

Chapter 11 **Primary headache disorders in the adult general population of Pakistan** 81
A. A. Herekar, A. Ahmad, U. L. Uqaili, B. Ahmed, J. Effendi, S. Z. Alvi, M. A. Shahab, U. Javed, A. D. Herekar, Rafiq Khanani and T. J. Steiner

Chapter 12 **Clinical patterns of primary stabbing headache** 90
Dong Yeop Kim, Mi Ji Lee, Hyun Ah Choi, Hanna Choi and Chin-Sang Chung

Chapter 13 **Identification of subgroups of patients with tension type headache with higher widespread pressure pain hyperalgesia** 99
César Fernández-de-las-Peñas, Elena Benito-González, María Palacios-Ceña, Kelun Wang, Matteo Castaldo and Lars Arendt-Nielsen

Chapter 14 **Restless legs syndrome and tension-type headache** 106
Pil-Wook Chung, Soo-Jin Cho, Won-Joo Kim, Kwang Ik Yang, Chang-Ho Yun and Min Kyung Chu

Chapter 15 **The course of headache in patients with moderate-to-severe headache due to mild traumatic brain injury** 114
Chang-Ki Hong, Jin-Yang Joo, Yu Shik Shim, Sook Young Sim, Min A Kwon, Yong Bae Kim and Joonho Chung

Chapter 16 **Prevalence and burden of headache disorders in Lithuania and their public-health and policy implications: a population-based study within the Eurolight Project** 121
Daiva Rastenytė, Dalia Mickevičienė, Lars Jacob Stovner, Hallie Thomas, Colette Andrée and Timothy J Steiner

Chapter 17 **Post-traumatic headache in patients with minimal traumatic intracranial hemorrhage after traumatic brain injury** 131
Chang-Ki Hong, Yu Shik Shim, Sook Young Sim, Jin-Yang Joo, Min A Kwon, Yong Bae Kim and Joonho Chung

Chapter 18 **Insomnia in tension-type headache** 139
Jiyoung Kim, Soo-Jin Cho, Won-Joo Kim, Kwang Ik Yang, Chang-Ho Yun and Min Kyung Chu

Chapter 19 **Sphenopalatine ganglion stimulation for cluster headache, results from a large, open-label European registry** 148
Mads Barloese, Anja Petersen, Philipp Stude, Tim Jürgens, Rigmor Højland Jensen and Arne May

Chapter 20 **The burden of headache is associated to pain interference, depression and headache duration in chronic tension type headache** 155
Stella Fuensalida-Novo, Maria Palacios-Ceña, Juan J. Fernández-Muñoz, Matteo Castaldo, Kelun Wang, Antonella Catena, Lars Arendt-Nielsen and César Fernández-de-las-Peñas

Chapter 21 **Headache following head injury: a population-based longitudinal cohort study (HUNT)** 163
Lena Hoem Nordhaug, Knut Hagen, Anne Vik, Lars Jacob Stovner, Turid Follestad, Torunn Pedersen, Gøril Bruvik Gravdahl and Mattias Linde

Chapter 22 **Vitamin D deficiency in patients with cluster headache** 172
Jong-Hee Sohn, Min-Kyung Chu, Kwang-Yeol Park, Hong-Yup Ahn and Soo-Jin Cho

Chapter 23 **Pre-treatment with sumatriptan for cilostazol induced headache in healthy volunteers** 179
Katrine Falkenberg and Jes Olesen

Chapter 24 **Headache attributed to aeroplane travel: the first multicentric survey in a paediatric population affected by primary headaches** 184
Debora De Carlo, Irene Toldo, Agnese Maria Tamborino, Barbara Bolzonella, Maria Giuseppina Ledda, Lucia Margari, Vincenzo Raieli, Margherita Santucci, Vittorio Sciruicchio, Angelo Vecchio, Sergio Zanini, Stefano Sartori, Michela Gatta, Alberto Verrotti and Pier Antonio Battistella

Chapter 25 **Field testing primary stabbing headache criteria according to the 3rd beta edition of International Classification of Headache Disorders** 190
Minwoo Lee, Min Kyung Chu, Juyoung Lee, Jinhyuk Yoo and Hong Ki Song

Chapter 26 **Chronic cluster headache and the pituitary gland** 197
Annelien De Pue, Bart Lutin and Koen Paemeleire

Chapter 27 **Medication overuse headache in Europe and Latin America: general demographic and clinical characteristics, referral pathways and national distribution of painkillers in a descriptive, multinational, multicenter study** 201
Ninett Louise Find, Rossana Terlizzi, Signe Bruun Munksgaard, Lars Bendtsen, Cristina Tassorelli, Giuseppe Nappi, Zaza Katsarava, Miguel Lainez, Maria Teresa Goicochea, Beatriz Shand, Ricardo Fadic, Santiago Spadafora, Marco Pagani and Rigmor Jensen

Chapter 28 **Assessment of headache characteristics in a general adolescent population: a comparison between retrospective interviews and prospective diary recordings** 213
Anne-Berit Krogh, Bo Larsson, Øyvind Salvesen and Mattias Linde

Permissions

List of Contributors

Index

Preface

This book aims to highlight the current researches and provides a platform to further the scope of innovations in this area. This book is a product of the combined efforts of many researchers and scientists, after going through thorough studies and analysis from different parts of the world. The objective of this book is to provide the readers with the latest information of the field.

Headaches occur as a symptom of pain in the head or neck region. The three main types of headache disorders are migraines, cluster headaches and tension-type headaches. Migraines generally affect one half of the head and are pulsating in nature. Cluster headaches are severe and recurring in nature. They can be accompanied by pain around the eye, eye watering, swelling around the eye and nasal congestion. Tension-type headaches affect the lower back of the head, neck, eyes and both sides of the brain. Frequent occurring of severe headaches can also cause depression. Headache disorder occurs due to various causes. The most common of them are medication effects, sleep deprivation, the effects of recreational drugs, head injury, loud noises and dental issues. The treatment of the headache depends on its cause but the most common treatment is pain medication. This book provides comprehensive insights into headache disorder. It consists of contributions made by international experts. The book is meant for students who are looking for an elaborate reference text on headache disorder.

I would like to express my sincere thanks to the authors for their dedicated efforts in the completion of this book. I acknowledge the efforts of the publisher for providing constant support. Lastly, I would like to thank my family for their support in all academic endeavors.

Editor

The burden of headache disorders in Nepal: estimates from a population-based survey

Kedar Manandhar[1,2], Ajay Risal[1,2], Mattias Linde[1,3] and Timothy J. Steiner[1,4*]

Abstract

Background: Headache disorders, particularly migraine and tension-type headache (TTH), are among the most prevalent global public-health problems. Medication-overuse headache (MOH) is a common sequela of mismanagement of these. Migraine and MOH are highly disabling. Formulation of responsive health policy requires reliable, locally-derived, population-based data describing both individual and societal impact of headache disorders. South-East Asia is the only one of WHO's six world regions in which no such national data have yet been gathered.

Methods: In a nationwide population-based cross-sectional study, a representative sample of Nepalese-speaking adults (18–65 years) were randomly selected by stratified multistage cluster sampling. Trained interviewers made unannounced door-to-door visits and enquired into headache and its attributable burden using a culturally-adapted and validated Nepalese translation of the Headache-Attributed Restriction, Disability, Social Handicap and Impaired Participation (HARDSHIP) questionnaire.

Results: Among 2100 participants, 1794 (85.4 %) reported headache during the preceding year (male: 689 [38.4 %], female 1105 [61.6 %]; mean age 36.1 ± 12.6 years). Mean headache frequency was 3.8 ± 6.2 days/month, mean headache intensity 2.1 ± 0.7 on a 0–3 scale, and mean attack duration 41.9 ± 108.5 h. All aspects of symptom burden (frequency, intensity and duration) were greater among females ($p < 0.001$). Participants with headache had poorer quality of life (QoL) than those without ($p < 0.001$); QoL was worst among those with probable MOH (pMOH). Mean proportions of total available time spent in the ictal state were 5.4 % among participants with migraine, 3.9 % among those with TTH and 44.7 % among those with pMOH, with headache-related disabilities of 2.4, 0.15 and 9.7 % respectively. At population level, these disorders were responsible for reduced functional capacities of 0.81, 0.06 and 0.20 %. Total lost productive time due to headache was 6.8 % for the 85 % of the population with headache. Males lost more paid worktime than females ($p < 0.001$); the reverse was so for household worktime ($p < 0.001$).

Conclusions: Headache disorders, very common in Nepal, are also highly burdensome at both individual and population levels. There is a substantial penalty in lost production. The remedy lies in better health care for headache; structured headache-care services are urgently needed in the country, and likely to be cost-saving.

Keywords: Migraine, Tension-type headache, Medication-overuse headache, Public health, Population-based study, Burden of disease, Disability, Nepal, South-East Asia region, Global campaign against headache

* Correspondence: t.steiner@imperial.ac.uk
[1]Department of Neuroscience, Norwegian University of Science and Technology, Edvard Griegs Gate, Trondheim, NO 7489, Norway
[4]Division of Brain Sciences, Imperial College London, London, UK
Full list of author information is available at the end of the article

Background

Primary headache disorders – migraine and tension-type headache (TTH) – are among the most prevalent diseases in the world [1–3]. These disorders, together with their major sequela, medication-overuse headache (MOH), are of substantial importance to public health nationally and globally because they lead to widespread ill health and impaired quality of life (QoL) and are disabling [4] The Global Burden of Disease Study 2013 (GBD2013) found migraine to be the sixth highest cause of disability worldwide, and MOH the 18th, measured in years of life lost to disability (YLDs) [3]. Collectively, headache disorders are the third highest cause of disability in the world [5]. The economic consequences through productivity losses are substantial [6].

Mitigating action is required, a message strongly endorsed by the World Health Organization (WHO) [4, 7]. But decisions about the allocation of national health-care resources are best informed by reliable, locally-derived, population-based data. This is especially important in developing countries such as Nepal, which have very constrained health budgets and a clear imperative to maximise health gain from them. In the case of headache care, this means data on the burden attributable to headache disorders harvested from the population of Nepal as the basis of needs assessment. Recent population-based studies in other developing countries [8–10] have shown high headache prevalences and heavy headache-attributable burden, but these factors remain poorly described in many large and populous areas of the world [2, 4] – nowhere more obviously than in the South-East Asia Region (SEAR). In fact, SEAR, in which Nepal lies, is the only one of WHO's six world regions for which no national data of this type have yet been gathered in any country [4].

Nepal is one of the poorest countries within SEAR [11], but with great geographic and cultural diversity. Its location in the Himalayas, and their foothills and plains beyond, includes eight of the world's ten highest peaks, among them Mount Everest, the highest point on Earth [11]. Its population is approximately 30 million [12], with a rather unequal distribution of wealth so that about one quarter live below the international poverty line [11]. The majority of Nepalese engage in agriculture [13]. More than 70 ethnic groups maintain different cultures and spoken languages [13].

We earlier reported headache prevalence data from our adult population-based study in Nepal [14]. The 1-year prevalence of migraine in this country (34.1 %) was uniquely high, while the point prevalence of probable MOH (pMOH) (2.1 %) was towards the upper end of the range for most countries studied [15]. The 1-year prevalence of TTH (44.1 %) was in line with the global average [2, 3]. Here, with the specific purpose of informing health policy, and as a study conducted within the Global Campaign against Headache, we report the estimates of burden attributable to these disorders in Nepal.

Methods

Ethics

The Nepal Health Research Council, the Institutional Review Committee of Kathmandu University School of Medical Sciences, Dhulikhel Hospital, and the Regional Committee for Health and Research Ethics in Central Norway all approved the study protocol.

All participants were informed about the nature and purpose of the study and this was documented in accordance with requirements of the three committees.

Study design and sampling

The study design, sampling and data collection procedures have been reported in detail previously [16]. In summary, this was a cross-sectional survey using structured interviews administered by trained health workers making unannounced door-to-door visits during May, 2013. To obtain a nationally representative sample, we used multistage stratified cluster sampling in all three physiographic divisions of the country and, within each division, all five development regions (Far-Western, Midwestern, Western, Central and Eastern). We randomly selected one eligible adult (aged 18–65 years, Nepalese-speaking and living in Nepal) from each household.

Instruments

We used the Headache-Attributed Restriction, Disability, Social Handicap and Impaired Participation (HARDSHIP) questionnaire developed by *Lifting The Burden* (LTB) for population-based studies [17]. The original English-language version was translated into Nepalese according to LTB's translation protocol for hybrid documents [18] and modified according to Nepalese culture [19]. The questionnaire consisted of four parts relevant to this report. For all participants there were (i) personal and demographic enquiry and (ii) a neutral headache screening question ("Have you had a headache during the last 12 months?"). Those who answered "no" to the latter were classified as headache-free. Those who answered "yes" were asked whether their headaches were of one or more types and, if more than one, to focus only on the most bothersome type. Only those who answered positively to the screening question were also asked (iii) diagnostic questions in line with the International Classification of Headache Disorders (ICHD-3 beta) [20], and (iv) questions ascertaining various aspects of headache burden.

We measured symptom burden in terms of frequency (days/month), intensity (with response options "not bad", "quite bad" and "very bad", which we interpreted as mild, moderate and severe) and duration (hours).

We enquired into willingness to pay (WTP) as an overall measure of burden [17] using a bidding game method [21]. We asked how much participants would be willing to pay per month for an effective treatment such that their headaches would no longer bother them. Bidding began at NPR 100/month (at the time of the survey, NPR 100 ≈ USD 1): was the respondent willing to pay this amount? If "yes", the interviewer incremented the bidding stepwise (NPR 200, 400, 1000 and 2000) until the answer was "no", or it was clear that the participant would pay > NPR 2000. If the opening bid of NPR 100 was declined, the interviewer instead reduced stepwise (NPR 40 and 20) until the participant said "yes", or it became clear that nothing would be paid. Finally, in every case, an exact amount was agreed upon as the individual's WTP-value.

We assessed QoL using the World Health Organization Quality of Life-8 (WHOQOL-8) questionnaire [22]. Its eight items addressed subjective wellbeing and satisfaction in four domains (two in each): psychological, physical, social and environmental [17]. Each item was graded on a scale of 1–5, with a higher score indicating better QoL.

We estimated lost time due to headache during the preceding 3 months using the Headache-Attributed Lost Time (HALT) questionnaire [23]. Its first two questions asked for the numbers of days in that period (i) completely missed from paid work and (ii) with <50 % productivity because of headache while at work; the next two asked for numbers of days of household work (iii) completely missed and (iv) with <50 % productivity; the last enquired into (v) the number of days on which family, social or leisure activities were missed because of headache.

Headache diagnosis

The diagnostic method has been described previously [14]. Diagnoses were not made during the interviews but later according to an algorithm. Participants reporting headache on ≥15 days/month were first separated as a distinct group because they cannot be fully diagnosed by questionnaire. Those who in addition were overusing acute medication were considered to have pMOH [24]; the remainder were categorised as "other headache on ≥15 days/month". To all others, reporting headache on ≤14 days/month, the algorithm applied modified ICHD-3 beta criteria [20] in the following order: definite migraine, definite TTH, probable migraine and probable TTH. Definite and probable migraine were subsequently considered together, and likewise definite and probable TTH, for attribution of burden. The few remaining cases were unclassifiable.

Statistics

Categorical variables are presented as numbers and percentages. Continuous variables are presented as means with standard deviations (SDs) and/or medians with interquartile ranges (IQRs).

We transformed the categorical variable for headache intensity (mild, moderate, and severe) into a numerical scale 0–3 (0 being no pain), and treated these results as continuous data.

We summed responses to the first four items (i-iv) of HALT to estimate total productivity loss. These scores were treated as continuous variables. We separately summed the first and second items (i, ii) to estimate lost paid worktime, and the third and fourth (iii, iv) to estimate lost household worktime.

We estimated individual and population-level disability attributable to migraine, TTH and pMOH using the disability weights (DWs) from GBD2013 [3] for the ictal states of each. We calculated the mean absolute time spent in the ictal state (T_{abs}) as the product of mean attack frequency (AF) and mean attack duration (D). For migraine, because headache frequency (HF) had been recorded as days/month, we assumed participants with attacks lasting >24 h had counted days affected rather than number of attacks per month. Therefore, to calculate mean AF we made separate computations for those with attack durations of ≥24 h and <24 h, using the formula AF = HF/D in the former group. We then took the weighted mean of the two groups. We did not need to perform the same manipulation for TTH, because the mean duration of headache was <24 h (Table 1). For pMOH, we made separate calculations for those describing durations of <24 h and those asserting pain "never goes away", for whom we assumed AF = 30 and D = 24; there were no respondents in between. Again we took the weighted mean. From T_{abs} (in hours/year) we calculated the proportion of total available time that was spent in the ictal state (T_{pro}) by dividing by (24*365). We multiplied this proportion by the DW for the disorder in question to calculate individual disability (DIS_{per}), and then by the prevalence of the disorder to arrive at population-level disability (DIS_{pop}).

We used Student's *t*-test for significance of differences between means of two groups and one-way analysis of variance (ANOVA) for more than two groups. Since most of the continuous variables were skewed in distribution, we also used the non-parametric Mann–Whitney *U*-test or Kruskal-Wallis test to examine differences between groups. We considered $p < 0.05$ as statistically significant. All data were analysed with SPSS 21.0 software (SPSS Inc., Chicago, IL, USA).

Results

We interviewed 2100 participants aged 18–65 years (participation rate >99 % [16]), of whom 1794 (85.4 %) reported headache during the preceding year (male: 689 [38.4 %], female 1105 [61.6 %]; mean age 36.1 ± 12.6 years;

Table 1 Symptom burden: frequency, intensity and duration of headache for all headache and each headache type, by gender

	All	Male	Female	p^a
All headache (*N* = 1794 [males 689; females 1105])				
Headache frequency (days/month)				
Mean ± SD	3.8 ± 6.2	2.9 ± 4.8	4.3 ± 6.9	<0.001
Median [IQR]	2.0 [0.4–3.0]	1.0 [0.3–3.0]	2.0 [0.5–4.0]	<0.001
Headache intensity				
Not bad	373 (20.8)	184 (26.7)	189 (17.1)	
Quite bad	901 (50.2)	344 (49.9)	557 (50.4)	
Very bad	520 (29.0)	161 (23.4)	359 (32.5)	
Mean[b] ± SD	2.1 ± 0.7	2.0 ± 0.7	2.2 ± 0.7	<0.001
Median[b] [IQR]	2 [2, 3]	2 [1, 2]	2 [2, 3]	<0.001
Headache duration (hours)				
Mean ± SD	41.9 ± 108.5	23.3 ± 46.8	53.4 ± 131.9	<0.001
Median [IQR]	8.0 [2.0–45.0]	6.0 [1.3–24.0]	10.0 [2.3–48.0]	<0.001
Migraine (*N* = 728 [males 249; females 479])				
Headache frequency (days/month)				
Mean ± SD	2.3 ± 0.6	2.2 ± 2.3	2.4 ± 2.3	0.46
Median [IQR]	2.0 [0.4–3.0]	2.0 [0.3–3.0]	2.4 [0.6–3.0]	0.29
Headache intensity				
Not bad	60 (8.2)	21 (8.4)	39 (8.1)	
Quite bad	354 (48.6)	123 (49.4)	231 (48.2)	
Very bad	314 (43.1)	105 (42.2)	209 (43.6)	
Mean[b] ± SD	2.3 ± 0.6	2.2 ± 0.6	2.4 ± 0.6	0.72
Median[b] [IQR]	2 [2, 3]	2 [2, 3]	2 [2, 3]	0.71
Headache duration				
Mean ± SD	33.6 ± 47.9	29.7 ± 43.3	35.7 ± 50.0	0.093
Median [IQR]	12.0 [4.0–48.0]	10.0 [4.0–48.0]	14.0 [4.0–48.0]	0.084
Tension-type headache (*N* = 863 [males 384; females 479])				
Headache frequency (days/month)				
Mean ± SD	1.8 ± 0.6	1.6 ± 1.9	2.0 ± 2.3	0.009
Median [IQR]	1.0 [0.3–2.0]	1.0 [0.2–2.0]	1.0 [0.3–3.0]	0.011
Headache intensity				
Not bad	292 (33.8)	154 (40.1)	138 (28.8)	
Quite bad	477 (53.3)	198 (51.6)	279 (58.2)	
Very bad	94 (10.9)	32 (8.3)	62 (12.2)	
Mean[b] ± SD	1.8 ± 0.6	1.7 ± 0.6	1.9 ± 0.6	<0.001
Median[b] [IQR]	2 [1–3]	2 [1–2]	2 [1–2]	<0.001
Headache duration				
Mean ± SD	16.0 ± 31.0	14.0 ± 27.1	18.0 ± 33.6	0.043
Median [IQR]	4.0 [0.8–15.0]	4.0 [0.8–20.0]	4.0 [0.8–20.0]	0.030
Probable medication-overuse headache (*N* = 46 [males 11; females 35])				
Headache frequency (days/month)				
Mean ± SD	23.1 ± 6.2	19.4 ± 4.4	24.0 ± 6.3	0.010
Median [IQR]	20.0 [16.7–30.0]	17.0 [16.0–20.0]	30.0 [19.0–30.0]	0.063

Table 1 Symptom burden: frequency, intensity and duration of headache for all headache and each headache type, by gender *(Continued)*

Headache intensity				
Not bad	1 (2.2)	0 (0.0)	1 (2.9)	
Quite bad	15 (32.6)	6 (54.5)	9 (25.7)	
Very bad	30 (65.2)	5 (45.5)	25 (71.4)	
Mean[b] ± SD	2.6 ± 0.5	2.5 ± 0.5	2.7 ± 0.5	0.65
Median[b] [IQR]	3 [2–3]	2 [2–3]	3 [2–3]	0.23
Headache duration				
Mean ± SD	318.9 ± 309.6	91.0 ± 82.8	390.5 ± 320.6	0.21
Median [IQR]	176.0 [40.0–720.0]	48.0 [32.0–200.0]	375.0 [45.0–720.0]	0.020

Values (if not otherwise stated) are n (%); *SD* standard deviation, *IQR* interquartile range; [a]comparing genders using Student's *t*-test for difference between means and Mann–Whitney *U*-test for medians; [b]mean and median on a scale of 0–3

686 [38.2 %] rural; 949 [52.9 %] living at altitude ≥1000 m). These 1794 were included in the analysis of burden; 728 [40.5 %] reported migraine, 863 [48.1 %] TTH, 46 [2.6 %] pMOH and 115 [6.4 %] other headache on ≥15 days/month.

Symptom burden

Symptom burden is presented in Table 1 by headache type and gender. From a public-health perspective it was substantial: the mean overall reported headache frequency was 3.8 days/month – 1 day in every eight – and mean overall reported intensity was 2.1. Half of all participants with headache (901; 50.2 %) reported moderate headache and another nearly one third (520; 29.0 %) reported severe headache. By headache type, pMOH was of course the most frequent headache; it was followed by migraine, then TTH. The same rank order was seen for both headache intensity and duration. On every measure, females were worse affected than males with regard to all headache and TTH, but not significantly so with regard to migraine or (taking both means and medians into account) pMOH.

Quality of life and willingness to pay

Participants without headache had significantly higher (*ie*, better) WHOQOL-8 scores than those with headache (median 29.0 [IQR: 27.0–31.0] *vs* 28.0 [25.0–30]; $p < 0.001$). WHOQOL-8 scores differed significantly between headache types ($p < 0.001$), being lowest among people with pMOH closely followed by those with migraine (Table 2). However, WHOQOL scores were negatively associated with frequency and intensity of headache (both $p < 0.001$); accordingly, among participants with headache, QoL was best in those with TTH (Table 2).

Participants with headache were willing to pay on average NPR 1134 ± 2760 (median 250 [IQR: 100–1000]) per month for effective headache care. WTP differed significantly ($p = 0.013$) between headache types, being highest among those with pMOH. WTP was positively associated

Table 2 Quality of life (WHOQOL-8 score) and willingness to pay according to headache type, frequency and intensity

	WHOQOL-8 score			Willingness to pay (NPR/month)		
	Mean ± SD	Median [IQR]	p^a	Mean ± SD	Median [IQR]	p^a
Headache type						
Migraine	26.7 ± 3.9	27.0 [24.0–29.0]	<0.001	1144 ± 2755	250 [100–250]	0.013
Tension-type headache	28.2 ± 3.7	28.0 [26.0–30.0]		1074 ± 2673	200 [60–200]	
Probable medication-overuse headache	25.7 ± 4.2	26.0 [23.0–29.0]		2031 ± 3960	500 [150–2000]	
Headache frequency (days/month)						
1–3	27.7 ± 3.9	28.0 [25.0–30.0]	<0.001	1056 ± 2760	200 [80–800]	<0.001
4–14	26.8 ± 3.7	27.0 (24.0–27.0)		1301 ± 2273	300 [150–1500)	
≥ 15	25.8 ± 4.0	26.0 (23.0–26.0)		1493 ± 3428	300 [150–1050)	
Headache intensity						
Not bad	28.7 ± 4.0	29.0 [26.0–32.0]	<0.001	1252 ± 4084	200 [50–900]	<0.001
Quite bad	27.6 ± 3.5	28.0 [26.0–30.0]		977 ± 2013	250 [100–800]	
Very bad	26.1 ± 4.1	26.0 [23.0–29.0]		1.322 ± 2690	300 [110–1200]	

IQR interquartile range, *NPR* Nepalese rupee; [a]Kruskal-Wallis test

with both frequency and intensity of headache ($p < 0.001$), and therefore least in TTH (Table 2).

Disability

Among the 728 participants with migraine, 289 reported attacks of ≥24 h' duration, with a mean of 57.1 h (D1) and a headache frequency of 2.38 days/month (HF1) (Table 3). Using the formula AF = HF/D (see Methods), we calculated AF for this group as AF1 = 2.38/(57.1/24), which we took to be 1. Among the 46 with pMOH, 17 reported headache that "never goes away". We took their attack frequency (AF1) as 30, and duration (D1) as 24. All other calculations of disability are explained in the Methods section and set out in Table 3.

Mean DIS_{per} for migraine was 2.4 %; DIS_{pop} was 0.81 %. The corresponding values for TTH were substantially lower (0.15 and 0.06 %). For pMOH, however, DIS_{per} was very much higher, at 9.7 %, while DIS_{pop} was only 0.20 % because of the low prevalence.

Headache-attributed lost time

Headache-attributed lost time in the preceding 3 months is presented by headache type in Table 4. All summed scores (total lost productive time, lost paid worktime and lost household worktime) had much higher means for pMOH than for migraine, which itself had means more than double those of TTH. However, it should be noted that, for all five individual items and all headache types, including pMOH, most medians were zero; this meant not only that distributions were very highly skewed, but also that at least half of respondents in most groups lost no time at all.

More household worktime (2.7 ± 5.9 days) was lost than paid worktime (1.7 ± 5.1 days), this difference being largely but not entirely attributable to migraine (Table 4). Regardless of headache type, males lost more paid worktime than females and the reverse was the case with household worktime.

From policy and economic perspectives, attention might focus on total lost productive time (4.4 days in 3 months) from all headache, since this was the mean loss for 85.4 % of the population. Assuming there were 13*5 working days in 3 months, this was a loss of 6.8 % for those affected, or 5.8 % for the population generally. However, 5.4 days lost in 3 months represented an 8.3 % individual loss for those with migraine. As they were 34.1 % of the population [14], this was a 2.8 % loss for the population generally.

Discussion

This is the first nationwide population-based survey to estimate the burden of headaches disorders in Nepal, or in any country within the South-East Asia Region. The survey covered the whole country, recruiting a large representative sample through careful random selection and minimizing participation bias by achieving a very high participation rate (>99 %).

As is the case elsewhere in the world, we found burden levels were high in Nepal, on both individual and population levels. The symptom burden was itself large,

Table 3 Population-level disability (adults aged 18–65 years), by headache type

	Migraine $n = 728$ ≥ 24 h' duration: $n = 289$; <24 h' duration: $n = 439$	Tension-type headache $n = 863$	Probable medication-overuse headache $n = 46$ "never goes away": $n = 17$; other: $n = 29$
Reported mean headache frequency [HF] (d/m)	2.3 (HF1 = 2.38, HF2 = 2.27)	1.8	23.1 (HF1 = 30, HF2 = 19.1)
Reported mean attack duration [D] (h)	33.6 (D1 = 57.1, D2 = 12.2)	16.0	12.1 (D1 = 24.0, D2 = 5.04)
Mean attack frequency [AF] (per month) (see text for explanation)	AF1 = 1, AF2 = 2.27	1.8	AF1 = 30, AF2 = 19.1
Mean absolute time in ictal state [T_{abs} = AF*D] (h/m)	Weighted mean of AF1*D1 and AF2*D2 = 39.36	AF*D = 28.8	Weighted mean of AF1*D1 and AF2*D2 = 326.8
Mean time in ictal state as proportion of total time $T_{pro} = (T_{abs}*12)/(365*24)$] (%)	5.4	3.9	44.7
Disability weight [DW] (from GBD 2013 [3]	0.441	0.037	0.217
Mean disability per person with headache $DIS_{per} = T_{pro}*DW$] (%)	2.4	0.15	9.7
Prevalence in adults aged 18–65 years [P] (%)	34.1	41.5	2.1
Disability in population [$DIS_{pop} = DIS_{per} * P$] (%)	0.81	0.06	0.20

For migraine, HF1, D1 and AF1 refer to those with attacks of ≥24 h' duration, HF2, D2 and AF2 to those with attacks of <24 h' duration; for probable medication-overuse headache, HF1, D1 and AF1 refer to those who report headache that never goes away, HF2, D2 and AF2 to those with headache of determinable duration; *D* days, *m* month, *h* hours

Table 4 Headache-attributed lost time in preceding 3 months for all headache and each headache type, by gender

	Total lost productive time		Lost paid worktime		Lost household worktime		Missed social and leisure activities	
	Mean ± SD	Median [IQR]	Mean ± SD	Median [IQR]	Mean ± SD	Median [IQR]	Mean ± SD	Median [IQR]
All headache								
all (*n* = 1794)	4.4 ± 9.2	1 [0–5]	1.7 ± 5.1	0 [0–0]	2.7 ± 5.9	0 [0–3]	0.5 ± 2.8	0 [0–0]
male (*n* = 689)	4.5 ± 9.6	0 [0–5]	2.5 ± 5.6	0 [0–3]	2.0 ± 5.9	0 [0–2]	0.7 ± 4.1	0 [0–0]
female (*n* =1105)	4.4 ± 9.0	1 [0–5]	1.2 ± 4.8	0 [0–0]	3.2 ± 5.9	0 [0–4]	0.4 ± 1.4	0 [0–0]
p[a]	0.91	0.034	<0.001	<0.001	<0.001	<0.001	0.046	0.10
Migraine								
all (*n* = 728)	5.4 ± 8.9	3 [0–7]	1.9 ± 4.6	0 [0–1]	3.5 ± 6.5	1 [0–5]	0.8 ± 4.1	0 [0–0]
male (*n* = 249)	7.1 ± 12.0	3 [0–9]	3.7 ± 6.3	0 [0–5]	3.4 ± 8.8	0 [0–3]	1.3 ± 6.5	0 [0–1]
female (*n* = 479)	4.5 ± 6.6	2 [0–6]	0.9 ± 3.0	0 [0–0]	3.5 ± 5.2	1 [0–5]	0.5 ± 1.7	0 [0–0]
p[a]	0.001	0.023	<0.001	<0.001	0.89	0.002	0.039	0.002
Tension-type headache								
all (*n* = 863)	2.2 ± 4.7	0 [0–3]	0.9 ± 3.1	0 [0–0]	1.3 ± 2.8	0 [0–1]	0.2 ± 0.9	0 [0–0]
male (*n* = 384)	2.0 ± 5.0	0 [0–2]	1.2 ± 3.6	0 [0–1]	0.8 ± 2.1	0 [0–0]	0.2 ± 0.8	0 [0–0]
female (*n* = 479)	2.3 ± 4.3	0 [0–2]	0.7 ± 2.5	0 [0–0]	1.6 ± 3.2	0 [0–2]	0.2 ± 0.9	0 [0–0]
p[a]	0.31	0.009	0.010	<0.001	<0.001	<0.001	0.76	0.94
Probable medication-overuse headache								
all (*n* = 46)	16.9 ± 25.9	6.5 [0–25.5]	8.0 ± 16.4	0 [0–6.2]	8.9 ± 13.6	0.5 [0–15]	1.2 ± 2.9	0 [0–7.3]
male (*n* = 11)	13.1 ± 14.7	7 [0–24]	10.2 ± 15.6	3 [0–24]	2.9 ± 6.2	0 [0–10]	2.8 ± 5.0	0 [0–2]
female (*n* = 35)	18.1 ± 28.1	6 [0–27]	7.3 ± 16.9	0 [0–5]	10.9 ± 14.7	5 [0–17]	0.7 ± 1.6	0 [0–0]
p[a]	0.44	0.87	0.60	0.23	0.015	0.089	0.18	0.17

SD standard deviation, *IQR* interquartile range; [a]p was estimated using Student's *t*-test for differences between means and Mann–Whitney *U*-test for medians

carried by females more than males. On all measures, migraine imposed the greatest burden at population level while pMOH did so on affected individuals. This was reflected in impact on QoL. Participants with migraine spent, on average, 5.4 % of their time (equivalent to 20 days/year) in the ictal state, with headache of mean intensity 2.3, which would certainly be disabling. However, this 5.4 % is less than the 8.3 % lost productive time attributed to migraine, which says something about the relationship between these. Lost paid worktime was higher among males than females, but the reverse was true of lost household worktime.

Headache-attributed lost productive time is a well-validated measure of headache burden [17, 23, 25], yet it is not clear exactly what its determinants may be. It reflects not so much disability as behavioural response to impairment since, except in extreme cases, there is a degree of choice in either continuing or abandoning work when affected by headache [17]. In India, time spent by those with migraine in the ictal state (4.2 %) was also lower than the proportion of lost productive time (5.8 %) [26]. Rao et al. observed that it is in the nature of migraine that motivation and energy are lost, and that these symptoms, likely also to contribute to lost productivity, may for some time outlast what is described as the ictal state [26]. Additionally, our method of calculating time in ictal state for migraine was perhaps conservative in cases when attack duration was >24 h. In calculating lost productive time our assumption might also be questioned that there were only 65 working days in 3 months, especially for household work, but on the other hand this made no allowance for "holiday" time. It has also to be said that the high symptom burden of migraine in Nepal was not reflected in lost productive time to the extent that might be anticipated: lost paid and household worktime were both lower than in China [27], Georgia [28] and Zambia [8], although higher than in India [26] and much the same as in Russia [29].

In Nepal there are particular considerations that may be relevant. The proportion of people in paid employment is very low [13, 30]. This is especially true for women, who are predominantly engaged in agriculture; few have skilled manual jobs, and they are much less likely than men to be employed in professional, technical or managerial fields [30]. The work of many women in Nepal requires carriage of heavy loads by tumpline, weight-bearing on head and neck – not easy with any type of headache. Further, our enquiry might not have been clear that time spent, for example, in producing goods for home consumption, such as growing vegetables, should have counted in the context of the Nepalese economy as paid ("income"-generating) rather than household work. Therefore it is likely that lost productive worktime was underestimated, especially among women. The finding of greater lost productivity among males than females should be interpreted with caution in view of this and since the symptom burden was actually higher among females.

At population level, migraine caused most disability (0.81 %). We might compare this with 0.46 % in neighbouring India, where the survey used very similar methods but was conducted only in the southern State of Karnataka [26]. The difference approximately reflects the lower prevalence of migraine in India (25.2 %) [9]. The 0.81 % implies a reduction by this amount of population functional capacity. Whereas above we noted a 1.5-fold discrepancy between time spent in the ictal state of migraine and lost productive time, here there is much greater disparity: at population level, lost productive time due to migraine was 2.8 %, or 3.5 times the disability. Very similar disparities were found in India (3.3 times) [26] and in Zambia (also 3.3 times, despite a higher disability of 0.98 %) [8]. The determinants of lost productive time due to migraine may be unclear and probably complex, but we see evidence here, nonetheless, of constancy in its relationship to disability, which survives the influences of different behaviours among peoples from different cultures.

Information on WTP can, in theory, be used to estimate reasonable pricings and make economic forecasts before introducing new health-care services [31, 32]. We doubt its reliability for this purpose when gathered in surveys of this type, but see it more as a measure of overall burden [17]. As judged from the median WTP (in view of the skewed distribution), participants with headache were willing to pay NPR 250 (USD 2.50) per month for effective headache care, the amount correlating with headache type (pMOH > migraine > TTH), frequency and intensity. The absolute monetary value of this might be lower than has been reported from other, even low-income countries [28] but, put into local context, it would be a day's earnings for an average Nepalese citizen [33]. As a measure of burden, this suggests heavy burden. As a reflection of what people with headache might be willing to invest in headache services, it signals need but probably not sufficient willingness (or ability) to pay.

Like all cross-sectional surveys, this study had limitations. Most importantly it relied on retrospective enquiry over 3 months, and therefore participants' recall, to estimate impact of headache on work absence and productivity. The effect of recall error is uncertain, but it is more likely to have introduced random degrees of over- and underestimation than systematic error [24]. We focused on the most bothersome headache type in participants identifying more than one. In fact this avoided double-counting: although it might be possible in such a survey to diagnose multiple headache types, correctly attributing burden between them is not a realistic proposition. Among those with both migraine and TTH, the former would usually be the more bothersome [34]; this meant that some part of the burden of TTH was instead attributed to migraine, but from a public-health perspective this would have little consequence.

Implications for Nepal

Headache disorders are not only common in Nepal but also highly burdensome: symptom burden is heavy, there is much consequential disability and substantial lost productivity. The economic cost is certain to be high. The remedy lies in better health care for headache; structured headache-care services are urgently needed in the country. However, Nepal is among the least developed countries in the world, with uneven distribution of its limited resources [11]. Government allocation to the health sector is also scarce; gaps in specialized health care exist at all levels [35]. Furthermore, Nepal's rural hilly/mountainous geography poses great challenges to community health services. Creating new headache care services would certainly demand investment of additional financial and human resources in the health sector; on the other hand, refraining from doing so will leave undiminished the burden of these highly prevalent but cost-effectively treatable brain disorders [36]. Structured headache services based in primary care [37] would be an efficient, effective, affordable and equitable model for Nepal, likely to be cost-saving [4]. Such services, appropriately adapted, could be implemented within the existing health-service structure of Nepal. This potential solution requires further research in order to inform political decision-makers. Doing nothing is almost certainly a more costly option.

Conclusions

Headache disorders, very common in Nepal, are also highly burdensome at both individual and population levels. They cause disability and reduced functional capacity, with a substantial penalty in lost production. The remedy lies in better health care for headache; structured headache-care services are urgently needed in the country, and likely to be cost-saving.

Abbreviations

ANOVA: Analysis of variance; DW: Disability weight; GBD: Global burden of disease; HALT: Headache-attributed lost time; HARDSHIP: Headache-attributed restriction, disability, social handicap and impaired participation; ICHD: International classification of headache disorders; IQR: Interquartile range; LTB: *Lifting the burden*; MOH: Medication-overuse headache; NPR: Nepalese rupee; pMOH: probable MOH; QoL: Quality of life; SD: Standard deviation; SEAR: South-East Asia Region; SPSS: Statistical package for social sciences; TTH: Tension-type headache; USD: United States dollar; WHOQOL-8: World Health Organization quality of life-8; WTP: Willingness to pay; YLD: Year of life lost to disability.

Competing interests
TJS is a Director and Trustee of *Lifting The Burden*.

Authors' contributions
All authors were involved in conception and design of the project. KM, AR, ML and TJS took part in acquisition, analysis and interpretation of the data. KM drafted the manuscript. All authors reviewed it critically for intellectual content and approved the final version of the manuscript.

Acknowledgements
This project was funded by grants from Samarbeidsorganet, the Liaison Committee between the Central Norway Regional Health Authority and the Norwegian University of Science and Technology (NTNU). It was conducted within the Global Campaign against Headache, led by the nongovernmental organization *Lifting The Burden* in official relations with the World Health Organization, and with the support of Dhulikhel Hospital, Kathmandu University Hospital, Dhulikhel, Kavre, Nepal.
We are grateful to Professor Grethe Albrektsen, Professor in Medical Statistics, Faculty of Medicine Department of Public Health and General Practice, NTNU, for advice in statistical analysis.

Author details
[1]Department of Neuroscience, Norwegian University of Science and Technology, Edvard Griegs Gate, Trondheim, NO 7489, Norway. [2]Dhulikhel Hospital, Kathmandu University Hospital, Kavre, Dhulikhel, Nepal. [3]Norwegian Advisory Unit on Headache, St Olavs University Hospital, Trondheim, Norway. [4]Division of Brain Sciences, Imperial College London, London, UK.

References

1. Jensen R, Stovner LJ (2008) Epidemiology and comorbidity of headache. Lancet Neurol 7(4):354–361. doi:10.1016/s1474-4422(08)70062-0
2. Stovner L, Hagen K, Jensen R, Katsarava Z, Lipton R, Scher A, Steiner TJ, Zwart JA (2007) The global burden of headache: a documentation of headache prevalence and disability worldwide. Cephalalgia 27(3):193–210. doi:10.1111/j.1468-2982.2007.01288.x
3. Vos T, Barber RM, Bell B, Bertozzi-Villa A, Biryukov S, Bolliger I, Charlson F, Davis A, Degenhardt L, Dicker D, Duan L, Erskine H, Feigin VL, Ferrari AJ, Fitzmaurice C, Fleming T, Graetz N, Guinovart C, Haagsma J, Hansen GM, Hanson SW, Heuton KR, Higashi H, Kassebaum N, Kyu H, Laurie E, Liang X, Lofgren K, Lozano R, MacIntyre MF et al (2015) Global, regional, and national incidence, prevalence, and years lived with disability for 301 acute and chronic diseases and injuries in 188 countries, 1990–2013: a systematic analysis for the global burden of disease study 2013. Lancet 386:743–800. doi:10.1016/s0140-6736(15)60692-4
4. World Health Organization and Lifting The Burden (2011) Atlas of headache disorders and resources in the world 2011. WHO, Geneva
5. Steiner TJ, Birbeck GL, Jensen RH, Katsarava Z, Stovner LJ, Martelletti P (2015) Headache disorders are third cause of disability worldwide. J Headache Pain 16:58. doi:10.1186/s10194-015-0544-2
6. Linde M, Gustavsson A, Stovner LJ, Steiner TJ, Barré J, Katsarava Z, Lainez JM, Lampl C, Lantéri-Minet M, Rastenyte D, Ruiz de la Torre E, Tassorelli C, Andrée C (2012) The cost of headache disorders in Europe: the eurolight project. Eur J Neurol 19(5):703–711. doi:10.1111/j.1468-1331.2011.03612.x
7. Steiner TJ, Stovner LJ, Dua T, Birbeck GL, Jensen R, Katsarava Z, Martelletti P, Saxena S (2011) Time to act on headache disorders. J Headache Pain 12(5):501–503. doi:10.1007/s10194-011-0368-7
8. Mbewe E, Zairemthiama P, Paul R, Birbeck GL, Steiner TJ (2015) The burden of primary headache disorders in Zambia: national estimates from a population-based door-to-door survey. J Headache Pain 16:36. doi:10.1186/s10194-015-0513-9
9. Kulkarni GB, Rao GN, Gururaj G, Stovner LJ, Steiner TJ (2015) Headache disorders and public ill-health in India: prevalence estimates in Karnataka State. J Headache Pain 16:67. doi:10.1186/s10194-015-0549-x
10. Mbewe E, Zairemthiama P, Yeh HH, Paul R, Birbeck GL, Steiner TJ (2015) The epidemiology of primary headache disorders in Zambia: a population-based door-to-door survey. J Headache Pain 16:30. doi:10.1186/s10194-015-0515-7
11. United States Central Intelligence Agency, Office of Public Affairs. The World Factbook. https://www.cia.gov/library/publications/the-world-factbook/geos/np.html. Accessed 19 Sep 2015
12. Government of Nepal, National Planning Commission Secretariate (2012) Population and housing census 2011. Central Bureau of Statistics, Kathmandu, Nepal
13. Government of Nepal, National Planning Commission Secretariate (2014) Population monograph of Nepal, vol I. Central Bureau of Statistics, Kathmandu, Nepal
14. Manandhar K, Risal A, Steiner TJ, Holen A, Linde M (2015) The prevalence of primary headache disorders in Nepal: a nationwide population-based study. J Headache Pain 16:95. doi:10.1186/s10194-015-0580-y
15. Westergaard ML, Hansen EH, Glumer C, Olesen J, Jensen RH (2014) Definitions of medication-overuse headache in population-based studies and their implications on prevalence estimates: a systematic review. Cephalalgia 34(6):409–425. doi:10.1177/0333102413512033
16. Manandhar K, Risal A, Steiner TJ, Holen A, Koju R, Linde M (2014) Estimating the prevalence and burden of major disorders of the brain in Nepal: methodology of a nationwide population-based study. J Headache Pain 15: 52. doi:10.1186/1129-2377-15-52
17. Steiner TJ, Gururaj G, Andrée C, Katsarava Z, Ayzenberg I, Yu SY, Al Jumah M, Tekle-Haimanot R, Birbeck GL, Herekar A, Linde M, Mbewe E, Manandhar K, Risal A, Jensen R, Queiroz LP, Scher AI, Wang SJ, Stovner LJ (2014) Diagnosis, prevalence estimation and burden measurement in population surveys of headache: presenting the HARDSHIP questionnaire. J Headache Pain 15(1):3. doi:10.1186/1129-2377-15-3
18. Peters M, Bertolote JM, Houchin C, Kandoura T, Steiner TJ (2007) Translation protocol for hybrid documents. J Headache Pain 8(Suppl 1):S40–S47
19. Risal A, Manandhar K, Steiner TJ, Holen A, Koju R, Linde M (2014) Estimating prevalence and burden of major disorders of the brain in Nepal: cultural, geographic, logistic and philosophical issues of methodology. J Headache Pain 15:51. doi:10.1186/1129-2377-15-51
20. International Headache Society Classification Comittee (2013) The international classification of headache disorders, 3rd edition (beta version). Cephalalgia 33(9):629–808. doi:10.1177/0333102413485658
21. Dong H, Kouyate B, Cairns J, Sauerborn R (2005) Inequality in willingness-to-pay for community-based health insurance. Health Policy 72(2):149–156. doi:10.1016/j.healthpol.2004.02.014
22. Schmidt S, Muhlan H, Power M (2006) The EUROHIS-QOL 8-item index: psychometric results of a cross-cultural field study. Eur J Public Health 16(4):420–428. doi:10.1093/eurpub/cki155
23. Steiner TJ (2007) The HALT and HART indices. J Headache Pain 8(Suppl 1):S22–S25
24. Stovner LJ, Al Jumah M, Birbeck GL, Gururaj G, Jensen R, Katsarava Z, Queiroz LP, Scher AI, Tekle-Haimanot R, Wang SJ, Steiner TJ (2014) The methodology of population surveys of headache prevalence, burden and cost: Principles and recommendations from the Global Campaign against Headache. J Headache Pain 15(1):5. doi:10.1186/1129-2377-15-5
25. Stewart WF, Lipton RB, Kolodner KB, Sawyer J, Lee C, Liberman JN (2000) Validity of the migraine disability assessment (MIDAS) score in comparison to a diary-based measure in a population sample of migraine sufferers. Pain 88(1):41–52
26. Rao GN, Kulkarni GB, Gururaj G, Stovner LJ, Steiner TJ (2015) The burden attributable to headache disorders in India: estimates from a community-based study in Karnataka State. J Headache Pain 16(1):94. doi:10.1186/s10194-015-0574-9
27. Yu S, Liu R, Zhao G, Yang X, Qiao X, Feng J, Fang Y, Cao X, He M, Steiner T (2012) The prevalence and burden of primary headaches in China: a population-based door-to-door survey. Headache 52(4):582–591
28. Lampl C, Steiner TJ, Mueller T, Mirvelashvili E, Djibuti M, Kukava M, Dzagnidze A, Jensen R, Stovner LJ, Katsarava Z (2012) Will (or can) people pay for headache care in a poor country? J Headache Pain 13(1):67–74. doi:10.1007/s10194-011-0398-1
29. Ayzenberg I, Katsarava Z, Sborowski A, Chernysh M, Osipova V, Tabeeva G, Steiner TJ (2014) Headache-attributed burden and its impact on productivity and quality of life in Russia: structured healthcare for headache is urgently needed. Eur J Neurol 21(5):758–765. doi:10.1111/ene.12380
30. Ministry of Health and Population (MOHP) [Nepal], New ERA, and ICF International Inc (2012) Nepal demographic and health survey 2011. Ministry of health and population. New ERA, and ICF International, Kathmandu, Nepal
31. Shono A, Kondo M, Ohmae H, Okubo I (2014) Willingness to pay for public health services in rural central java, Indonesia: methodological

considerations when using the contingent valuation method. Soc Sci Med 110:31–40. doi:10.1016/j.socscimed.2014.03.025
32. Yasunaga H, Ide H, Imamura T, Ohe K (2006) Willingness to pay for health care services in common cold, retinal detachment, and myocardiac infarction: an internet survey in Japan. BMC Health Serv Res 6:12. doi:10.1186/1472-6963-6-12
33. Government of Nepal, National Planning Commission Secretariate (2011) Nepal living standards survey 2010/11, vol II. Central Bureau of Statistics, Kathmandu, Nepal
34. Krogh AB, Larsson B, Linde M (2015) Prevalence and disability of headache among Norwegian adolescents: a cross-sectional school-based study. Cephalalgia 35(13):1181–1191. doi:10.1177/0333102415573512
35. Karkee R, Jha N (2010) Primary health care development: where is Nepal after 30 years of Alma Ata declaration? J Nepal Med Assoc 49(178):178–184
36. Linde M, Steiner TJ, Chisholm D (2015) Cost-effectiveness analysis of interventions for migraine in four low- and middle-income countries. J Headache Pain 16:15. doi:10.1186/s10194-015-0496-6
37. Steiner TJ, Antonaci F, Jensen R, Lainez MJ, Lantéri-Minet M, Valade D (2011) Recommendations for headache service organisation and delivery in Europe. J Headache Pain 12(4):419–426. doi:10.1007/s10194-011-0320-x

2

Altered serum levels of kynurenine metabolites in patients affected by cluster headache

Martina Curto[1,2,4*], Luana Lionetto[3], Andrea Negro[2,3], Matilde Capi[3], Francesca Perugino[2], Francesco Fazio[5], Maria Adele Giamberardino[6], Maurizio Simmaco[3], Ferdinando Nicoletti[5,7] and Paolo Martelletti[2,4]

Abstract

Background: The reported efficacy of memantine in the treatment of patients with cluster headache (CH) suggests that NMDA receptors are involved in mechanisms of nociceptive sensitization within the trigeminal system associated with CH. NMDA receptors are activated or inhibited by neuroactive compounds generated by tryptophan metabolism through the kynurenine pathway. In the accompanying manuscript, we have found that serum levels of all kynurenine metabolites are altered in patients with chronic migraine. Here, we have extended the study to patients affected by episodic or chronic CH as compared to healthy controls.

Method: We assessed serum levels of kynurenine (KYN), kynurenic Acid (KYNA), anthranilic acid (ANA), 3-hydroxy-anthranilic acid (3-HANA), 3-hydroxykynurenine (3-HK), xanthurenic acid (XA), quinolinic acid (QUINA), tryptophan (Trp) and 5-hydroxyindolacetic acid (5-HIAA) by means of a liquid chromatography/tandem mass spectrometry (LC/MS-MS) method in 21 patients affected by CH (15 with episodic and 6 with chronic CH), and 35 age-matched healthy subjects. Patients with psychiatric co-morbidities, systemic inflammatory, endocrine or neurological disorders, and mental retardation were excluded.

Results: LC/MS-MS analysis of kynurenine metabolites showed significant reductions in the levels of KYN (-36 %), KYNA (-34 %), 3-HK (-51 %), 3-HANA (-54 %), XA (-25 %), 5-HIAA (-39 %) and QUINA (-43 %) in the serum of the overall population of patients affected by CH, as compared to healthy controls. Serum levels of Trp and ANA were instead significantly increased in CH patients (+18 % and +54 %, respectively). There was no difference in levels of any metabolite between patients affected by episodic and chronic CH, with the exception of KYN levels, which were higher in patients with chronic CH.

Conclusion: The reduced levels of KYNA (an NMDA receptor antagonist) support the hypothesis that NMDA receptors are overactive in CH. A similar reduction in KYNA levels was shown in the accompanying manuscript in patients affected by chronic migraine. The reduced levels of XA, a putative analgesic compound, may contribute to explain the severity of pain attacks in CH. These data, associated with the data reported in the accompanying manuscript, supports a role for the kynurenine pathway in the pathophysiology of chronic headache disorders.

Keywords: Kynurenine, Cluster headache, Glutamate, Pain, NMDA receptors

* Correspondence: martina.curto@uniroma1.it
[1]Department of Psychiatry, Harvard Medical School, Boston, MA, USA
[2]Department of Molecular Medicine, Sant'Andrea Medical Center, Sapienza University of Rome, Via di Grottarossa 1035-1039, Rome 00189, Italy
Full list of author information is available at the end of the article

Background

Cluster headache (CH), the most frequent primary headache disorder among the trigeminal autonomic cephalalgias, can be chronic or episodic depending on the presence of remission periods between the headache bouts [1–5]. The molecular events underlying the pathophysiology of CH are unknown because of the lack of valuable experimental animal model, and, therefore the treatment is largely based on empirical evidence [6]. It is intuitive that the hypothalamus and the trigeminal system are involved in the pathophysiology of CH. The involvement of the hypothalamus is suggested by the circannual and circadian periodicity of headache and by the prevalence of CH in males. In addition, changes in the secretion of hormones regulated by the hypothalamus, such as prolactin, growth hormone and cortisol are found in patients affected by CH [7–9], and functional imaging studies showed the activation of hypothalamic gray matter during headache attacks [6, 10]. Headache pain of CH is conveyed to the CNS *via* the ophthalmic branch of the trigeminal system, and, similarly to migraine, activation of the trigeminovascular system has been demonstrated during CH attacks [11]. Mechanisms of nociceptive sensitization developing at the synapses between primary afferent fibers and secondary order neurons of the caudal trigeminal nucleus, and in upper regions of the pain neuraxis likely contribute to the development of the typical unilateral attacks of pain associated with CH. Glutamate acting at N-methyl-D-aspartate (NMDA) receptors plays a key role in the induction of nociceptive sensitization [12], and this suggests that alterations in NMDA receptor signaling or in the endogenous machinery that activates NMDA receptors may be relevant to the pathophysiology of CH. It is consistent with this hypothesis that memantine, a fast off-rate NMDA-gated ion channel blocker, has shown efficacy in reducing CH attacks in resistant patients, even if clinical studies are still limited [13].

The kynurenine pathway of tryptophan metabolism generates neuroactive metabolites that influence the activity of NMDA receptors as well as other glutamate receptor types [14, 15]. In this pathway, L-tryptophan is first metabolized into N-formyl-kynurenine, which is then converted into L-kynurenine (KYN). KYN is then transaminated into KYNA by kynurenine aminotransferases (KATs), or, alternatively, converted into 3-hydroxykynurenine (3-HK) by kynurenine monoxygenase or transformed into anthranilic acid (ANA) by kynureninase. 3-HK is the precursor of 3-hydroxyanthranilic acid (3-HANA), quinolinic acid (QUINA), and xanthurenic acid (XA) (reviwed by Schwarcz et al. 2012) [16]. QUINA is an NMDA receptor agonist, whereas KYNA blocks the action of the co-agonist, glycine, at the GluN1 subunit of NMDA receptors (reviewed by Schwarcz et al. 2012) [16]. XA activates mGlu2 and mGlu3 metabotropic glutamate receptors, although its precise mechanism of action is unknown [17]. In the accompanying manuscript we showed for the first time that chronic migraine is associated with alterations in serum levels of kynurenine metabolites, which are in line with the hypothesis of a hyperactivity of NMDA receptors in migraine. Since hyperactive NMDA receptors play a role in nociceptive sensitization, we hypothesized that kynurenine glutamatergic metabolites might be altered in CH and extended the analysis to patients affected by episodic or chronic CH as compared to age-matched healthy controls.

Methods

Patients

The protocol was carried out in accordance with the declaration of Helsinki and the study design was reviewed and approved by the Ethical Committee at Sapienza, University of Rome, Sant'Andrea Hospital. All subjects signed free informed consent for participation in the study. All subjects were enrolled by the Regional Referral Headache Center of S. Andrea Hospital and evaluated by two experts in headache disorders (A.N. and P.M.). 21 patients met the ICHD-3beta criteria [1] for cluster headache, chronic or episodic, and were included in the CH group and 35 healthy volunteers, recruited among the Hospital and University employees, were included in the age-matched control group. Inclusion criteria for CH patients were: (i) age between 18 and 65 years; (ii) patients affected by CH during the active phase (ICHD-3beta criteria) [1]; (iii) patients treated with verapamil (120–480 mg) for prophylactic therapy and sumatriptan (oral 50 mg, subcutaneous 6 mg) as the acute pain medication.

Exclusion criteria for both patients and controls were: (i) the presence of psychiatric co-morbidities, systemic inflammatory disorders, endocrine disorders, neurological disorders, and mental retardation; (ii) lifetime history of cluster headache (for healthy volunteers); and (iii) the use of any drug of abuse in the last 3 months (except cigarette smoking).

A detailed medical anamnesis was obtained from patients and controls, and the daily frequency of cluster headache attacks was recorded for each patient. Patients were sampled during the CH active phase, independently of the presence of an ongoing attack. Sumatriptan intake was allowed until 12 h before the blood sample.

Blood collection and KP measurement

Serum samples from patients and controls with empty stomach were collected between 10 am and 12 am. Blood (5 ml) was sampled in anticoagulant-free tubes and kept at room temperature for 1 h before the serum was isolated (centrifugation at 2000 g for 10 min at 20 °C). Aliquots of serum were stored at -80 °C until analysis.

We developed a reliable liquid chromatography/tandem mass spectrometry (LC/MS-MS) method for the assay of serum levels of all kynurenine metabolites. The method allowed a reliable detection of KYN, KYNA, ANA, 3-HANA, 3- HK, XA, and QUINA. Levels of tryptophan (Trp) and 5-hydroxyindolacetic acid (5-HIAA) were also detected. Details on sample preparation, reagents, standard solutions, chromatographic conditions, mass spectrometry conditions, and validation parameters are reported in Tables S1-S3 of Fazio et al. 2015 [17].

Statistical analysis

SPSS version 19.00 (IBM Corporation, Armonk NY, USA) was used for data analysis. Continuous variables were expressed as mean standard ± deviation (S.D.), while discrete variables were assigned as numbers and percentages. The compliance of continuous variables with normal distribution was controlled with the Kolmogorov–Smirnov test. Whether Healthy Controls and Cluster Headache groups differed in terms of discrete variables was checked through Pearson's Chi Squared test ($\chi2$). Since continuous variables did not comply with a normal distribution, the Mann–Whitney U test was used for between group comparisons. Spearman's Rho correlation (ρ) was used to test between-variables relationships. We set statistical significance at $P \leq 0.05$.

Results

Patients characteristics and serum levels of kynurenine metabolites

Demographic and clinical features of patients affected by CH ($n = 21$) and age-matched healthy controls ($n = 35$) are shown in Table 1. The CH group, as expected, showed a prevalence of male gender (90.5 %), which was not significantly higher than in the group of selected HCs (77.1 %). Mean age was similar between the two groups (about 44 years) and mean frequency of headache attacks in CH patients was about 2 attacks/day. Six patients were affected by chronic CH, and the remaining 15 patients were affected by episodic CH. The latter patients were examined during the active phase of CH.

LC/MS-MS analysis of kynurenine metabolites showed significant reductions in serum levels of KYN (-36 %), KYNA (-34 %), 3-HK (-51 %), 3-HANA (-54 %), XA (-25 %), 5-HIAA (-39 %) and QUINA (-43 %) in the serum of the overall population of patients affected by CH, as compared to HCs (Table 1, Fig. 1). Serum levels of Trp and ANA were instead significantly increased in patients affected by CH (+18 % and +54 %, respectively).

Table 1 Demographic and clinical characteristics and serum kynurenine pathways metabolites levels in the study groups

	Healthy controls ($n = 35$)	Patients with CH ($n = 21$)	χ^2/U *p*
Gender (M, %)	27 (77.1)	19 (90.5)	1.59 0.19
Age (years; mean ± SD)	44.8 ± 7.64	44,4 ± 7.60	278 0.13
Chronic cluster headache (n, %)	-	6 (28.6 %)	-
Mean daily frequency of attacks (mean ± SD)	-	2.05 ± 0.86	-
Trp (μg/ml) (mean ± SD)	5.50 ± 1.71	6.50 ± 1.60	233 *0.01*
KYN (μg/ml) (mean ± SD)	0.36 ± 0.15	0.23 ± 0.11	165.5 *<0.01*
KYNA (ng/ml) (mean ± SD)	3.15 ± 1.39	2.09 ± 1.49	189 *0.03*
ANA (ng/ml) (mean ± SD)	1.85 ± 1.57	2.85 ± 1.37	199 *<0.01*
3-HK (ng/ml) (mean ± SD)	2.16 ± 1.58	1.05 ± 0.84	217 *0.01*
3-HANA (ng/ml) (mean ± SD)	9.76 ± 4.38	4.50 ± 1.52	67.5 *<0. 01*
QUINA (ng/ml) (mean ± SD)	16.3 ± 10.1	9.28 ± 2.28	115 *<0.01*
5-HIAA (ng/ml) (mean ± SD)	33.4 ± 13.7	20.5 ± 8.36	156.5 *<0.01*
XA (ng/ml) (mean ± SD)	1.77 ± 0.95	1.32 ± 1.53	148 *0.02*

Kynurenine metabolites levels in the serum of patients with chronic and episodic CH, and correlations with daily headache frequency

Analysis of serum levels of kynurenine metabolites in patients affected by episodic or chronic CH showed no differences between the two subgroups, with exception of KYN levels, which were significantly higher (+50 %) in patients affected by chronic CH (Table 2).

No significant correlations were found between any kynurenine metabolite and daily frequency of headache attacks (not shown).

Discussion

The profile of serum kynurenine metabolites in patients affected by CH was similar to that reported in the accompanying manuscript in patients with chronic migraine with two notable exceptions: (i) XA levels, which were decreased in patients with CH, but increased in patients with chronic migraine; and, (ii) ANA levels, which were increased to a much lower extent in patients

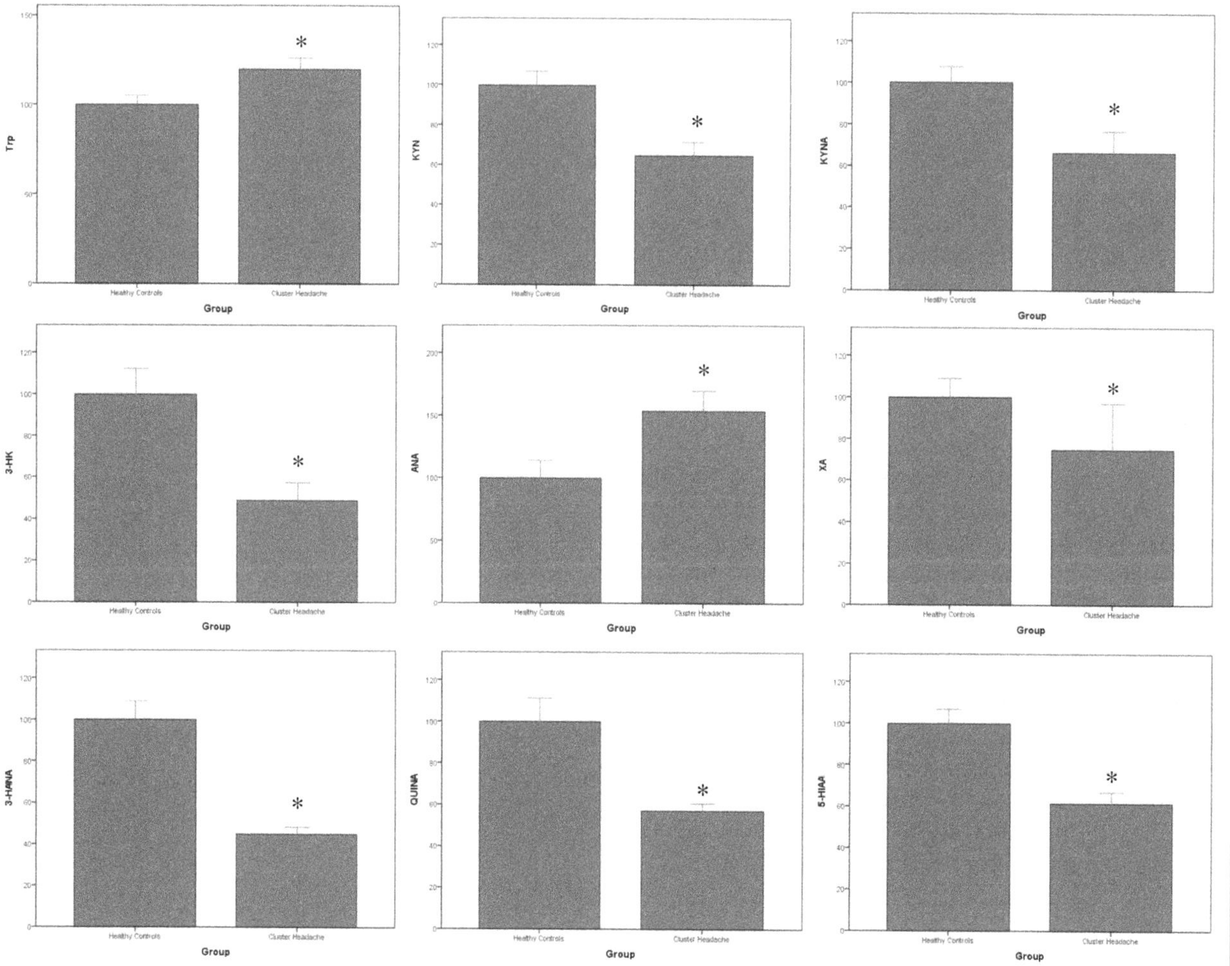

Fig. 1 Percent changes in serum kynurenine metabolites in patients affected by CH with respect to healthy controls. Data are presented as per cent of HC values for each metabolite. Values are means ± S.E.M. *$p < 0.05$ vs. healthy controls (HCs)

with CH than in patients with chronic migraine. As we have highlighted in the accompanying manuscript, serum levels of kynurenine metabolites may roughly mirror CNS levels because the constitutive action of the kynurenine pathway is low in the CNS, and at least KYN and 3-HK of peripheral source can cross the blood-brain barrier and fuel the pathway in the brain parenchyma [16]. The most relevant finding here is the reduction in KYNA levels, which, within the context of an enhanced release of glutamate might contribute to a hyperactivity of NMDA receptors resulting into nociceptive sensitization in CH. Thus, the reductions in KYNA levels found in patients affected by CH (present data) and in patients affected by chronic migraine (see accompanying manuscript) represent a nice clinical counterpart of the numerous experimental data that demonstrate the ability of KYNA to restrain the activation of the trigeminal system [18–22]. In fact, several preclinical studies demonstrated the mediatory and modulatory role of KYNA for glutamate and its receptors in central and peripheral pain processing [23]. Some of the identified roles are: the attenuation of the cutaneous nociceptors sensitization by the inactivation of peripheral glutamate receptors [24], the probable reduction of the first-order neurons activation and of the consecutive release of CGRP and nitric oxide from the nerve endings in the trigeminal nucleus caudalis [22] and the inhibition of the neural activity on brain stem structures such as the locus coeruleus, periaqueductal grey and nucleus raphe magnus [25–28].

The different behavior of XA in patients by CH and chronic migraine is interesting and deserves some comments. XA is a putative neurotransmitter [29] that activates mGlu2 and mGlu3 metabotropic glutamate receptors [17], and may also indirectly influence glutamatergic transmission by interacting with vesicular glutamate transporters [30]. Activation of mGlu2 receptors causes analgesia by negatively modulating glutamate release from primary afferent fibers [31], and preliminary data demonstrate the analgesic activity of XA in rodents (M. Bernabucci and F. Fazio, unpublished observation). Hence, the increase in

Table 2 Kynurenine pathway metabolites in Chronic and Episodic Cluster Headache groups

	Episodic CH ($n = 15$)	Chronic CH ($n = 6$)	U p
Trp (μg/ml) (mean ± SD)	6.60 ± 1.74	6.57 ± 1.32	43.5 0.91
KYN (μg/ml) (mean ± SD)	0.20 ± 0.07	0.31 ± 0.16	20.0 *0.05*
KYNA (ng/ml) (mean ± SD)	1.91 ± 1.43	2.52 ± 1.67	34.0 0.42
ANA (ng/ml) (mean ± SD)	2.67 ± 1.44	3.30 ± 1.18	30.0 0.27
3-HK (ng/ml) (mean ± SD)	1.21 ± 0.94	0.66 ± 0.29	30.5 0.27
3-HANA (ng/ml) (mean ± SD)	4.44 ± 1.69	4.22 ± 1.11	42.0 0.85
QUINA (ng/ml) (mean ± SD)	9.33 ± 2.36	8.54 ± 2.17	7.00 0.93
5-HIAA (ng/ml) (mean ± SD)	18.4 ± 6.32	25.8 ± 10.9	21.0 0.07
XA (ng/ml) (mean ± SD)	1.33 ± 1.59	1.18 ± 1.07	6.00 0.93

serum XA levels found in patients with chronic migraine has been interpreted as a defensive mechanism aimed at reducing the extent of headache in migraine. This potential defense was absent in patients with CH, where serum XA levels were reduced. We speculate on the possibility that a reduced production of XA contributes to the severity of pain attacks in CH, and that pharmacological strategies aimed at enhancing XA biosynthesis or reducing XA catabolism might cause analgesia in CH patients. This attractive hypothesis warrants further investigation. ANA levels were found to be increased in patients affected by both CH and chronic migraine, suggesting that, in both disorders, KYN is preferentially metabolized by kynureninase rather than by kynurenine monoxygenase or kynurenine aminotransferases (see also accompanying manuscript). Why ANA levels were much more elevated in chronic migraine than in CH is unknown. The only biochemical explanation is that ANA transformation into 3-HANA or other catabolites is dramatically reduced in chronic migraine, but not in CH. The incomplete knowledge of the metabolism of ANA makes this hypothesis difficult to prove. The marked difference in ANA levels between chronic migraine and CH suggests that this compound may serve as a peripheral biomarker that may facilitate the correct diagnosis of patients with chronic headache with mixed clinical features.

Alterations of serum kynurenine pathway metabolites have been found in other neuropsychiatric disorders [16], have been linked to chronic stress [32] and sleep deprivation [33]. Although we did not recruit patients affected by psychiatric comorbidities, we cannot exclude that the chronic stress associated to the active CH condition, often associated with sleep disturbances, might have affected tryptophan metabolism.

Conclusion

In conclusion, we have shown for the first time that CH is associated with abnormalities of the kynurenine pathway of tryptophan metabolism, as reflected by substantial alterations of all kynurenine metabolites in the peripheral blood. This manuscript and the accompanying manuscript reporting data obtained in patients with chronic migraine are in line with the increasing number of preclinical data that highlight the importance of the kynurenine pathway in the pathophysiology and treatment of chronic headache disorders.

Competing interests

AN received travel grants, honoraria consultancy and participated in Advisory Board from Allergan, ElectroCore, and Medtronic. PM received travel grants, honoraria consultancy and participated in Advisory Board from Allergan, Medtronic, and Mylan. MC, MC, FF, FP, FN, MS, LL, MAG: none. This research project received no specific grant from any funding agency in the public, commercial, or not-profit sectors.

Authors' contributions

MC, LL and PM designed the protocol. AN and PM recruited patients and collected the blood. MC, FF and LL performed the assessment of kynurenine serum levels. MC, FP and FN reviewed statistic content. MC, FP and LL drafted the manuscript. PM, MAG, MS and FN reviewed critically the final draft. All authors read and approved the final manuscript.

Disclosures

No author nor any immediate family member has financial relationships with commercial organizations that might appear to present a potential conflict of interest with the material presented.

Author details

[1]Department of Psychiatry, Harvard Medical School, Boston, MA, USA. [2]Department of Molecular Medicine, Sant'Andrea Medical Center, Sapienza University of Rome, Via di Grottarossa 1035-1039, Rome 00189, Italy. [3]Advanced Molecular Diagnostics, IDI-IRCCS, Rome, Italy. [4]Regional referral headache center, Sant'Andrea Hospital, Rome, Italy. [5]IRCCS Neuromed, Pozzilli, Italy. [6]Headache Center and Geriatrics Clinic, Department of Medicine and Science of Aging, "G. D'Annunzio" University, Chieti, Italy. [7]Department of Physiology and Pharmacology, Sapienza University of Rome, Rome, Italy.

References

1. Headache Classification Committee of the International Headache Society (IHS) (2013) The International Classification of Headache Disorders, 3rd edition (beta version). Cephalalgia 33:629–808
2. Edvardsson B (2014) Symptomatic cluster headache: a review of 63 cases. SpringerPlus 3:64
3. Nesbitt AD, Goadsby PJ (2012) Cluster headache. BMJ 344:e2407
4. Leroux E, Ducros A (2008) Cluster headache. Orphanet J Rare Dis 3:20
5. Ashkenazi A, Schwedt T (2011) Cluster headache–acute and prophylactic therapy. Headache 51:272–286

6. May A (2005) Cluster headache: pathogenesis, diagnosis, and management. Lancet 366:843–855
7. Waldenlind E, Gustafsson SA, Ekbom K, Wetterberg L (1987) Circadian secretion of cortisol and melatonin in cluster headache during active cluster periods and remission. J Neurol Neurosurg Psychiatry 50:207–213
8. Chazot G, Claustrat B, Brun J, Jordan D, Sassolas G, Schott B (1984) A chronobiological study of melatonin, cortisol growth hormone and prolactin secretion in cluster headache. Cephalalgia 4:213–220
9. Polleri A, Nappi G, Murialdo G, Bono G, Martignoni E, Savoldi F (1982) Changes in the 24-hour prolactin pattern in cluster headache. Cephalalgia 2:1–7
10. Sánchez del Rio M, Alvarez Linera J (2004) Functional neuroimaging of headaches. Lancet Neurol 3:645–651
11. Goadsby PJ (2005) New targets in the acute treatment of headache. Curr Opin Neurol 18:283–288
12. Gasparini CF, Griffiths LR (2013) The biology of the glutamatergic system and potential role in migraine. Int J Biomed Sci 9:1–8
13. Venturelli E, Rao R, Charles A (2010) Memantine for prevention of cluster headache: a possible new treatment? J Headache Pain 11(suppl 1):S63
14. Vécsei L, Szalárdy L, Fülöp F, Toldi J (2013) Kynurenines in the CNS:recent advances and new questions. Nat Rev Drug Discov 12:64–82
15. Curto M, Lionetto L, Fazio F, Mitsikostas DD, Martelletti P (2015) Fathoming the kynurenine pathway in migraine: why understanding the enzymatic cascades is still critically important. Intern Emerg Med 10:413–421
16. Schwarcz R, Bruno JP, Muchowski PJ, Wu HQ (2012) Kynurenines in the mammalian brain: when physiology meets pathology. Nat Rev Neurosci 13:465–477
17. Fazio F, Lionetto L, Curto M, Iacovelli L, Cavallari M, Zappulla C, Ulivieri M, Napoletano F, Capi M, Corigliano V, Scaccianoce S, Caruso A, Miele J, De Fusco A, Di Menna L, Comparelli A, De Carolis A, Gradini R, Nisticò R, de Blasi A, Girardi P, Bruno V, Battaglia G, Nicoletti F, Simmaco M (2015) Xanthurenic Acid Activates mGlu2/3 Metabotropic Glutamate Receptors and is a Potential Trait Marker for Schizophrenia. Sci Rep 5:17799
18. Knyihar-Csillik E, Toldi J, Mihály A, Krisztin-Péva B, Chadaide Z, Németh H, Fenyo R, Vécsei L (2007) Kynurenine in combination with probenecid mitigates the stimulation-induced increase of c-fos immunoreactivity of the rat caudal trigeminal nucleus in an experimental migraine model. J Neural Transm 114:417–421
19. Knyihar-Csillik E, Toldi J, Krisztin-Péva B, Chadaide Z, Németh H, Fenyo R, Vécsei L (2007) Prevention of electrical stimulation-induced increase of c-fos immunoreaction in the caudal trigeminal nucleus by kynurenine combined with probenecid. Neurosci Lett 418:122–126
20. Knyihar-Csillik E, Mihaly A, Krisztin-Peva B, Robotka H, Szatmari I, Fulop F, Toldi J, Csillik B, Vecsei L (2008) The kynurenate analog SZR-72 prevents the nitroglycerol-induced increase of c-fos immunoreactivity in the rat caudal trigeminal nucleus: comparative studies of the effects of SZR-72 and kynurenic acid. Neurosci Res 61:429–432
21. Vamos E, Párdutz A, Varga H, Bohár Z, Tajti J, Fülöp F, Toldi J, Vécsei L (2009) L-kynurenine combined with probenecid and the novel synthetic kynurenic acid derivative attenuate nitroglycerin-induced nNOS in the rat caudal trigeminal nucleus. Neuropharmacology 57:425–429
22. Vamos E, Fejes A, Koch J, Tajti J, Fülöp F, Toldi J, Párdutz A, Vécsei L (2010) Kynurenate derivative attenuates the nitroglycerin-induced CamKIIα and CGRP expression changes. Headache 50:834–843
23. Guo S, Vecsei L, Ashina M (2011) The L-kynurenine signalling pathway in trigeminal pain processing: a potential therapeutic target in migraine? Cephalalgia 31:1029–1038
24. Zhang YQ, Ji GC, Wu GC, Zhao ZV (2003) Kynurenic acid enhances electroacupuncture analgesia in normal and carrageenan-injected rats. Brain Res 966:300–307
25. Ennis M, Aston-Jones G, Shiekhattar R (1992) Activation of locus coeruleus neurons by nucleus paragigantocellularis or noxious sensory stimulation is mediated by intracoerulear excitatory amino acid neurotransmission. Brain Res 598:185–195
26. Jiang M, Behbehani MM (2001) Physiological characteristics of the projection pathway from the medial preoptic to the nucleus raphe magnus of the rat and its modulation by the periaqueductal gray. Pain 94:139–147
27. Murphy AZ, Behbehani MM (1993) Electrophysiological characterization of the projection from the nucleus raphe magnus to the lateral reticular nucleus: possible role of an excitatory amino acid in synaptic activation. Brain Res 606:68–78
28. Kristensen JD, Post C, Gordh T Jr et al (1993) Spinal cord morphology and antinociception after chronic intrathecal administration of excitatory amino acid antagonists in the rat. Pain 54:309–316
29. Copeland CS, Neale SA, Salt TE (2013) Actions of Xanthurenic acid, a putative endogenous Group II metabotropic glutamate receptor agonist, on sensory transmission in the thalamus. Neuropharmacology 66:133–142
30. Neale SA, Copeland CS, Uebele VN, Thomson FJ, Salt TE (2013) Modulation of hippocampal synaptic transmission by the kynurenine pathway member xanthurenic acid and other VGLUT inhibitors. Neuropsychopharmacol 38: 1060–1067
31. Chiechio S, Copani A, Zammataro M, Battaglia G, Gereau RW 4th, Nicoletti F (2010) Transcriptional regulation of type-2 metabotropic glutamate receptors: an epigenetic path to novel treatments for chronic pain. Trends Pharmacol Sci 31:153–160
32. O'Farrell K, Harkin A (2015) Stress-related regulation of the kynurenine pathway: Relevance to neuropsychiatric and degenerative disorders. Neuropharmacology. Dec 12. doi:10.1016/j.neuropharm.2015.12.004
33. Kuhn E, Rysánek K, Brodan V (1968) Alterations of tryptophan metabolism induced by sleep deprivation. Experientia 24:901–902

3

Headaches attributed to airplane travel: a Danish survey

Sebastian Bao Dinh Bui†, Torben Petersen†, Jeppe Nørgaard Poulsen and Parisa Gazerani*

Abstract

Background: Airplane headache (AH) is a headache that occurs during take-off and landing. The pain is described as severe, unilateral, and located in the fronto-orbital region. This study aimed at investigating the incidence of AH among Scandinavian air-travelers, and to elucidating potential risk factors.

Methods: An online, Danish-survey was developed. The questionnaire consisted of 14 questions and was distributed through the Facebook-pages of Scandinavian-airlines and interest organizations. Participants reached the questionnaire through a web-link.

Results: Out of 254 responses, 89 noted that they suffered from headaches associated to airplane travel. Of the 89, 21 cases the headache was severe and limited to 30 min duration, as described in the ICH's criteria of AH. The remaining 68 cases indicated that the headache lasted longer than 30 min. Our data demonstrated that High-Altitude Headache (HAH) is a risk factor for developing AH ($p < 0.05$). Triptans (19 %) and paracetamol (5 %) were reported effective to relieve AH.

Conclusion: This study indicates that up to 8.3 % of the studied population suffered from AH, with a higher incidence in those with a history of HAH. Self-medication by triptans and paracetamol were reported effective for relieving AH.

Keywords: Headache, Airplane headache, Flight, Triptans, High-altitude headache, Danish

Background

Airplane headache (AH) is an intense, short lasting headache - usually lasts around 30 min [1], and is exclusively related to airplane travels. AH has a sudden onset and may occur at any time during flight; although, with a high incidence during take-off and landing, with the highest frequency during the landing phase [1]. AH is thought to affect a small part of the population [2]. However, with occupancy of around 70 % and more than 3.3 billion commercially available airplane seats, the Bnai Zion Medical Center estimates more than 100 million cases of AH annually [3]. Population-based investigations on AH, and its underlying mechanisms, treatments, prevention strategies, and risk factors are limited. Hence, further investigation to provide a clear picture that will eventually lead to better diagnosis and treatment is warranted.

The pathogenesis of AH has not been clarified yet and considering a diverse group of patients, with a broad range of symptoms, it is complicated to define a clear underlying mechanism(s). It has been suggested that barotrauma to the sinuses may lead to vasodilation of the cerebral arteries, which in turn may play an essential role in development of AH [2, 4–7]. Hence, it is reasonable to consider that airplane headache may also be linked to dysregulation occurring in the cerebral arteries [8]. Previous studies have shown a high psychological impact, caused by fear of future attacks, and stress of flying [6]. No report is present that focus on a North-European population [2, 4–7, 9–11]. Hence, the present study was designed to provide an overview of AH in a Northern-European population. The outcome of this study might provide new evidence on the incidence and risk factors of AH.

* Correspondence: gazerani@hst.aau.dk
†Equal contributors
SMI®, Department of Health science and Technology, Faculty of Medicine, Aalborg University, Aalborg, Denmark

Methods

Study design and population

An online survey-based trial was designed to identify the incidence of AH among Scandinavian-air travelers, since no information was available regarding incidence or risk factors of AH in this population. The inclusion criteria admitted individuals with an age of ≥ 18 years, with a history of at least 3 flights (without restrictions on length of flight).

Participants were asked to rate their pain intensity on a scale of 1–10, where 1–3 was considered as mild headache, 4–7 reflected moderate headache, and 8–10 was considered as severe headache. Furthermore, the participants were asked to note their choice of medication as well as time of consumption.

Survey and recruitment

Participants were recruited through advertisements posted on the Facebook-pages of Scandinavian-airline companies, and other interest organizations, with a link directing them to a custom-designed Danish-questionnaire. The questionnaire was available in the period from the 15th October 2014 to the 1st of December 2014 (a total of 48 days). The questionnaire was composed of 14 questions with adequate space provided for a supplementary or descriptive text. The first 6 questions focused on the demographical information of the participants, including nationality, age, gender, migraine and HAH. Other questions focused on AH and more specifically on its symptoms and co-morbidities, while others focused on the flight composition. The questionnaire was designed and made available through Google Docs. All questions were designed in a way that they had to be answered before continuing to the next question, thus securing an answer to each question.

Statistical analysis

In the text and tables, data are presented as number of responses and percentages, except age, which is presented as mean +/− SD (standard deviation).

Statistical analysis was performed using SPSS (version 22.0, IBM, USA), and the level of significance was set at 0.05. A *t*-test was performed to determine if there was an age-difference between the headache group and the non-headache group. Fisher's Exact Test or chi-square was used to determine if gender distribution, migraine and HAH are significant risk factors of AH.

Results

A total number of 254 Scandinavian-air travelers participated in this survey. Among those, 89 (35 %) identified themselves to be a victim of headache attributed to airplane travel. However, based on the current version of the ICH's diagnostic criteria (version 3, beta) [1] for airplane headache, only 21 of them (8.3 %) met diagnostic criteria (i.e., headache lasts less than 30 min).

Therefore, two groups were defined for analysis of the collected data: AH group ($n = 21$) and the non-AH group ($n = 233$).

There was no statistical difference in the gender distribution between the AH and non-AH group. Overall, there was a tendency for more females responding to the questionnaire (≈62 %). The gender distribution is outlined in Table 1.

The average age for the AH group was 39 ± 14 years (range: 19–67, $p > 0.05$), there was no statistical age difference between the genders.

In total, 62 participants (24.4 %) indicated diagnosed with migraine. There was no statistical difference in the distribution of migraine between the two groups (7 in AH group (33 %) and 55 in non-AH group (24 %)), for gender distribution see Table 2). However, migraine appears to be more frequent in the AH group, although the population size does not allow a conclusive consideration. Fifty-five participants (22 %) indicated that they suffered from HAH. There was a statistical difference in the distribution of HAH between the two groups ($p < 0.001$, 13 in AH group (62 %) and 42 (18 %) in non-AH group, for gender distribution see Table 3).

The onset of headache was equally divided between take-off (first 30 min) and landing (last 30 min) with 8 participants in each category (38 %). Five participants (24 %) reported that the headache occurred sometime in between of take-off and landing (see Table 4).

The majority of AH participants (91 %) described their headache as unilateral, fronto-orbital or fronto-parietal. The headache was described mainly as "pressing" (43 %), but also pulsating (29 %) and stabbing (29 %). The intensity of headache was described as severe (57 %) or moderate (43 %).

When asked to provide a possible cause for their headache, changes in cabin pressure during take-off and landing was reported as the most possible cause of their AH (95 %).

The AH-group was divided into two subgroups: A medicated-group (24 %) and a non-medicated-group (76 %) (see Table 5). Among participants in the medicated-group, 1 (5 %) took paracetamol, and 4 (19 %) used triptans (Table 5). Among those who

Table 1 Gender distribution in AH-group and non-AH group

	AH-group	Non-AH-group	Total
Females	12 (5 %)	146 (57 %)	158 (62 %)
Males	9 (4 %)	87 (34 %)	96 (38 %)
Total	21 (9 %)	233 (91 %)	254 (100 %)

AH airplane headache. The numbers represent number of responses. Percentages are given in brackets

Table 2 Gender distribution and occurrence of migraine in AH group and non-AH group

	Migraine in AH-group	Migraine in Non-AH group	Total
Females	6 (50 %)	48 (33 %)	54 (34 %)
Males	1 (11 %)	7 (8 %)	8 (8 %)
Total	7 (33 %)	55 (24 %)	62 (24 %)

AH airplane headache. The numbers represent number of responses. Percentages are given in brackets

used triptans, 2 females and 1 male were diagnosed with migraine.

The participants were asked to note any chronic diseases, to rule out possible co-morbidities, as well as whether or not they had been suffering from recent bouts of influenza. One case of asthma and one case of epilepsy were noted in the AH group.

Discussion

The present study showed that up to 8.3 % ($n = 21$) of our study population suffered from AH. There might have been a skewed gender distribution due to the possibility of a mainly young audience using Facebook. Despite this, close to 40 participants were aged 60+, the average age was 38.2 years ± 15.8 (range 18–76). Although, larger population-based studies would be required to give a more precise estimate of the prevalence of AH in Northern Europe (i.e., Denmark). However, our findings are in line with findings from Southern Europe [2, 4, 6, 12]. Based on the current ICH's classification, AH is short-lived - usually around 30 min experienced when ascending or descending - with severe stabbing pain, usually on one side of the head, near the eye. Although, the clinical symptoms reported in our population is consistent with this classification; we also found 68 participants that claimed that they suffer from AH, however, we could not classify them based on the diagnostic criteria of AH, but noted that their headache occurred only while flying. Whether or not this group or some individuals in this group can still be identified as AH is not clear now, due to inadequate information.

However, the pain in AH-group ($n = 21$) was experienced as stabbing in only 29 % of the cases. The grading of severity was moderate and the onset of the attacks was equally divided between take-off and landing. Five participants experienced headache during the cruising, but the onset of the headaches could potentially have started after the take-off phase. Our findings in the AH group are not completely in accordance with the literature, where the headache is usually rated as severe, with a jabbing, stabbing or sometimes pulsating quality, and mostly occurs during the landing phase [2, 4, 6, 12].

Table 3 Gender distribution and occurrence of HAH in AH group and non-AH group

	HAH in AH group	HAH in Non-AH group	Total
Females	9 (75 %)	34 (23 %)	43 (27 %)
Males	4 (44 %)	8 (9 %)	12 (13 %)
Total	13 (62 %)	42 (18 %)	55 (22 %)

AH airplane headache, *HAH* high-altitude headache. The numbers represent number of responses. Percentages are given in brackets

Table 4 Onset of headache as reported by participants in the AH-group

	Take-off (first 30 min)	Landing (last 30 min)	During the flight	Total
Females	5 (63 %)	3 (37 %)	4 (80 %)	12 (57 %)
Males	3 (37 %)	5 (63 %)	1 (20 %)	9 (43 %)
Total	8 (38 %)	8 (38 %)	5 (24 %)	21 (100 %)

AH airplane headache. The numbers represent number of responses. Percentages are given in brackets

To identify potential risk factors of AH, we asked if the participants had experienced a cold or any other nasal congesting syndrome (that can be a cofounding factor). Two AH-participants noted cases of cold, however they indicated having AH is independent of cold.

The participants were also asked to note if they suffered from any chronic diseases to identify co-morbidities. Two chronic diseases, asthma and epilepsy, were listed by the participants in the AH group. Based on our data gender does not seems to be a risk factor for AH, although our data indicate a higher female AH-ratio, which is in contrast to previous studies suggesting a male dominance [4, 6, 13]. A skewed gender distribution is known from previous studies with a higher incidence in men than in women. A skewed gender distribution is also known from other types of headaches, such as tension type headache, where males have a higher risk than females [14]. However, the risk of migraines is three times higher in females than in males (18 % F, 7 % M) [15].

According to our findings AH primarily occurred during take-off, and landing. This is consistent with the previous findings [4, 6] and the ICH's criteria for AH [1]. Changes in cabin pressure when an airplane is ascending or descending could affect those passengers with a highly sensitive baroreflex [16]. One study has demonstrated that migraine patients may have a highly sensitive baroreflex compared with healthy controls [17]. If a

Table 5 Medication consumed by participants in the AH-group and its distribution (AH: airplane headache)

	No medication	Medication	Total
Females	9 (43 %)	3 (14 %)	12 (57 %)
Males	7 (33 %)	2 (10 %)	9 (43 %)
Total	16 (76 %)	5 (24 %)	21 (100 %)

The numbers represent number of responses. Percentages are given in brackets

similar sensitivity exists in AH, this might pose a possible pathway for the development of AH. Sensitive baroreceptors and the link with migraine remains to be properly proven [17]. Another mechanisms might be through trigeminal nerve stimulation of the mucosal tissue. Cabin pressure may also affect cranial arteries, causing vasodilatation and headache. The vasodilatation might be caused by an imbalance between internal and external air pressure [4, 18, 19]. Cabin pressure may also affect hypersensitive cranial arteries, possibly cerebral arteries, thereby causing vasodilation and headache [10, 11]. Based on our results, HAH is a risk factor for AH. HAH is short lasting condition, that may occur during changes in altitude (primarily; ascending over 2500 meters), and often seen in activities such as mountain climbing [1]. HAH is felt on both sides of the head with an intensity ranging from mild to moderate [1] different from AH, which is unilateral and severe in intensity [6]. A previous study has shown that the intensity of HAH increases at higher altitude [20]. Several studies have measured changes in cabin pressure during a flight [21], and a linear coherence has been shown between altitude and cabin pressure [21]. Cabin pressure would normally decrease with around 8 hPa for each 300 meters, until the plane reaches an altitude of 2500 m, at which, the cabin pressure stabilizes at an average of 846 hPa (≈0.85 bar) for the rest of the flight [21]. The decreased pressure might lead to different degrees of hypoxia and changing pressure in body tissues and cavities [22, 23]. As such, these changes might contribute to the development of HAH and AH in the ascending phase. A study has recently shown a possible relation between AH and "mountain descending headache", which is a condition with common symptoms comparable with AH [24]. We therefore speculate that both headaches are triggered by increasing atmospheric pressure during the descending phase, which will result in expanding the air in the cavities and thereby inducing the headache in the aforementioned phase. However, the mechanism(s) underlying HAH, mountain descending headache and AH remains to be identified [25].

Five participants of the AH group used medication (24 %) (prior to their flight) in an effort to prevent AH. One individual self-medicated with paracetamol and four took triptans. These medications were reported effective to prevent AH. Our results are in line with a former study that examined the effect of triptans by analyzing 5 flight travelers with AH who all used triptans during a flight, they all reported complete pain relief for the duration of the flight [5]. Triptans are reported to be the most effective when taken 30 min before a flight [5].

Conclusion

This study found that up to 8.3 % of our study group suffered from AH with an increased risk in those with a history of HAH. Triptans and paracetamol were used to alleviate AH. Population-based studies are called for identification of global AH incidence. In addition, further prospective studies are highly recommended to clarify the mechanisms underlying AH, its triggers and prevention strategies.

Competing interests

The authors declare that they have no competing interests.

Authors' contributions

SBDB and TP contributed equally in this study. SBDB and TP designed the study, analyzed data, and drafted the manuscript. JNP and PG made substantive intellectual contribution to this study, provided academic support, and revised the manuscript drafts. All authors have read and approved the final version of the manuscript prior to submission.

Acknowledgements

Research support to P. Gazerani provided by the Danish Research Council is greatly acknowledged. In addition, we would like to acknowledge Aalborg Airport, Sonderborg Airport, Alsie Express, Migrænikerforbundet and Migræne og Hovedpineforeningen for their valuable contributions to this report by posting our questionnaire on their Facebook-pages.

References

1. Headache Classification Committee of the International Headache Society (IHS) (2013) The International Classification of Headache Disorders, 3rd edition (beta version). Cephalalgia 33:629–808
2. Kararizou E, Anagnostou E, Paraskevas GP, Vassilopoulou SD, Naoumis D, Kararizos G, Spengos K (2011) Headache during airplane travel ("airplane headache"): first case in Greece. J Headache Pain 12:489–91
3. http://www.b-zion.org.il/default_e.aspx. Accessed Dec 2014
4. Berilgen MS, Mungen B (2011) A new type of headache, headache associated with airplane travel: preliminary diagnostic criteria and possible mechanisms of aetiopathogenesis. Cephalalgia 31:1266–73
5. Ipekdal HI, Karadas O, Oz O, Ulas UH (2011) Can triptans safely be used for airplane headache? Neurol Sci 32:1165–9
6. Mainardi F, Lisotto C, Maggioni F, Zanchin G (2012) Headache attributed to airplane travel ('airplane headache'): clinical profile based on a large case series. Cephalalgia 32:592–9
7. Mainardi F, Maggioni F, Lisotto C, Zanchin G (2013) Diagnosis and management of headache attributed to airplane travel. Curr Neurol Neurosci Rep 13:335. doi:10.1007/s11910-012-0335-y
8. Kim MW, Kim M (2011) Can migraine prophylaxis prevent acute mountain sickness at high altitude? Med Hypotheses 77:818–23
9. Atkinson V, Lee L (2004) An unusual case of an airplane headache. Headache 44:438–9
10. Berilgen MS, Mungen B (2006) Headache associated with airplane travel: report of six cases. Cephalalgia 26:707–11
11. Evans RW, Purdy RA, Goodman SH (2007) Airplane descent headaches. Headache 47:719–23
12. Mainardi F, Lisotto C, Palestini C, Sarchielli P, Maggioni F, Zanchin G (2007) Headache attributed to airplane travel ("airplane headache"): first Italian case. J Headache Pain 8:196–9
13. Potasman I, Rofe O, Weller B (2008) Flight-associated headaches-prevalence and characteristics. Cephalalgia 28:863–7.
14. McGeeney BE (2005) Cluster headache pharmacotherapy. Am J Ther 12:351–8
15. Peterlin BL, Calhoun AH, Balzac F (2012) Men, women, and migraine: the role of sex, hormones, obesity, and PTSD. J Fam Pract 61:S7–11
16. Pfund Z, Trauninger A, Szanyi I, Illes Z (2010) Long-lasting airplane headache in a patient with chronic rhinosinusitis. Cephalalgia 30:493–5

17. Nilsen KB, Tronvik E, Sand T, Gravdahl GB, Stovner LJ (2009) Increased baroreflex sensitivity and heart rate variability in migraine patients. Acta Neurol Scand 120:418–23
18. Mendonca JC, Bussoloti Filho I (2005) Craniofacial pain and anatomical abnormalities of the nasal cavities. Braz J Otorhinolaryngol 71:526–34
19. Wolf G, Saria A, Gamse R (1987) New aspects of the autonomic innervation of human nasal mucosa. Laryngol Rhinol Otol (Stuttg) 66:149–51
20. Serrano-Duenas M (2005) High altitude headache. A prospective study of its clinical characteristics. Cephalalgia 25:1110–6
21. Kelly PT, Seccombe LM, Rogers PG, Peters MJ (2007) Directly measured cabin pressure conditions during Boeing 747–400 commercial aircraft flights. Respirology 12:511–5
22. Matthys H (2011) Fit for high altitude: are hypoxic challenge tests useful? Multidiscip Respir Med 6:38–46
23. West JB (2006) Human responses to extreme altitudes. Integr Comp Biol 46:25–34
24. Mainardi F, Maggioni F, Lisotto C, Zanchin G (2013) Coexistence of "headache attributed to airplane travel" and "mountain descending headache". J Headache Pain 14:169. doi:10.1186/1129-2377-14-S1-P169
25. Brundrett G (2002) Sickness at high altitude: a literature review. J R Soc Promot Health 122:14–20

4

Comorbidities of psychiatric and headache disorders in Nepal: implications from a nationwide population-based study

Ajay Risal[1,2], Kedar Manandhar[1,2], Are Holen[1,3], Timothy J. Steiner[1,4] and Mattias Linde[1,5*]

Abstract

Background: Headache disorders, anxiety and depression – the major disorders of the brain – are highly comorbid in the western world. Whether this is so in South Asia has not been investigated, but the question is of public-health importance to countries in the region. We aimed to investigate associations, and their direction(s), between headache disorders (migraine, tension-type headache [TTH] and headache on ≥15 days/month) and psychiatric manifestations (anxiety, depression and neuroticism), and how these might affect quality of life (QoL).

Methods: In a nationwide, cross-sectional survey of the adult Nepalese population ($N = 2100$), trained interviewers applied: 1) a culturally-adapted version of the *Headache-Attributed Restriction, Disability, Social Handicap and Impaired Participation* (HARDSHIP) questionnaire to diagnose headache disorders; 2) a validated Nepali version of the *Hospital Anxiety and Depression Scale* (HADS) to detect anxiety (HADS-A), depression (HADS-D) and comorbid anxiety and depression (HADS-cAD); 3) a validated Nepali version of the *Eysenck Personality Questionnaire Revised Short Form-Neuroticism* (EPQRS-N); and 4) the *World Health Organization Quality of Life 8-question scale* (WHOQOL-8). Associations with headache types were analysed using logistic regression for psychiatric caseness and linear regression for neuroticism. Adjustments were made for age, gender, household consumption, habitat, altitude and use of alcohol and marijuana.

Results: HADS-A was associated with any headache ($p = 0.024$), most strongly headache on ≥15 days/month (AOR = 3.2) followed by migraine (AOR = 1.7). HADS-cAD was also associated with any headache ($p = 0.050$, more strongly among females than males [$p = 0.047$]) and again most strongly with headache on ≥15 days/month (AOR = 2.7), then migraine (AOR = 2.3). Likewise, neuroticism was associated with any headache ($p < 0.001$), most strongly with headache on ≥15 days/month (B = 1.6), followed by migraine (B = 1.3). No associations were found between HADS-D and any headache type, or between TTH and any psychiatric manifestation. Psychiatric caseness of any sort, when comorbid with migraine or TTH, aggravated the negative impact on QoL ($p < 0.001$).

Conclusion: Headache disorders are highly comorbid with anxiety and show associations with neuroticism in Nepal, with negative consequences for QoL. These findings call for reciprocal awareness, and a holistic coordinated approach to management and in the health service. Care for common headache and common psychiatric disorders should be integrated in primary care.

Keywords: Anxiety, Comorbidity, Depression, Headache disorders, Holistic care, Nepal, Neuroticism, Primary care, Questionnaire, South Asia, Global campaign against headache

* Correspondence: mattias.linde@ntnu.no
[1]Department of Neuroscience, Norwegian University of Science and Technology, Nevrosenteret Øst, St Olavs Hospital, 7006 Trondheim, Norway
[5]Norwegian Advisory Unit on Headache, St Olavs University Hospital, Trondheim, Norway
Full list of author information is available at the end of the article

Background

The term "comorbidity" refers to the coexistence of any additional ailment in a person with an index disease [1]. Headache disorders such as migraine and tension-type headache (TTH) and psychiatric disorders such as anxiety and depression are all very common among general populations worldwide. Accordingly, some level of comorbidity between them will arise by chance. However, epidemiological studies over 25 years have consistently indicated that headache disorders and anxiety and depression are excessively comorbid [2–20], with bidirectional [6] or syndromal [7] associations. Although most such studies have selectively considered migraine [8–11], some have looked at TTH [12], "chronic daily headache" (CDH) [13] or headache in general [14]. Furthermore there are studies showing associations between headache disorders and neuroticism [21, 22], a personality trait closely interlinked with psychological distress [23].

Headache disorders, anxiety and depression are collectively viewed as the major disorders of the brain (MDBs) [24], each occupying a place among the top ten causes of disability in the world [25, 26]. From a public-health perspective, worrying consequences for overall disease burden arise from these disorders being comorbid. Firstly, comorbidity increases morbidity, perhaps synergistically. For example, headache associated with psychopathology has exaggerated effects on quality of life (QoL) and disability [23, 27, 28]. Secondly, comorbid disorders may be mutually aggravating. Again for example, comorbid psychiatric illnesses are risk factors for headache becoming chronic [29]. Thirdly, comorbid headache and psychiatric disorders pose significant management challenges: treatment of each may be hindered by the other, with worse outcomes likely and increased health-care liabilities [30]. Fourthly, there is the possibility of causal relationships, in either or both directions.

Most data on this subject come from the western world. However, MDBs appear to be prevalent and burdensome everywhere. The Global Burden of Disease Study 2013 (GBD2013) extrapolations to South Asia indicated that years of life lost to disability (YLDs) in this Region from these conditions were in line with global rankings [25]. Our study from Nepal, the only nationwide study in this region so far, showed high prevalences of both headache and psychiatric disorders, including a much higher prevalence of migraine than the global mean [31] and prevalences of anxiety above and of depression at the upper limit of their respective global ranges [32]. Both anxiety and depression correlated positively with neuroticism and negatively with QoL [32]. The probability of comorbidity between these disorders in Nepal, and the implications arising therefrom, are consequently matters of considerable public-health importance and of interest to health policy.

Therefore, our aims were to examine the extent to which the common headache disorders (migraine, TTH and the group of headache disorders characterised by headache occurring on ≥15 days/month) and psychiatric disorders (anxiety and depression) are comorbid in Nepal, a country with unique geocultural diversity [33], and to look also for associations between these headache disorders and neuroticism. Our objective was to establish the public-health implications of any associations discovered. Our purpose was to guide national health policy.

Methods

Ethics

This study was part of a research project addressing MDBs in Nepal [33], approved by the Nepal Health Research Council, the Institutional Review Committee of Kathmandu University School of Medical Sciences, Dhulikhel Hospital, and the Regional Committee for Health and Research Ethics in Central Norway. Informed consent was collected from all participants.

Study design and sampling

This was a cross-sectional study in which unannounced household visits were made during May 2013 by trained interviewers using structured questionnaires. In order to obtain a representative sample of the adult general population of the country, we used a multistage random cluster sampling technique to select households in all three physiographic divisions of Nepal, and, within each division, all five development regions (Far-Western, Mid-Western, Western, Central and Eastern). From each household, we randomly selected one adult aged 18–65 years. The details of the sampling and data collection procedures, including the steps taken to ensure a very high participation rate, have been published elsewhere [34].

Survey instrument

We used the Headache-Attributed Restriction, Disability, Social Handicap and Impaired Participation (HARDSHIP) questionnaire [35], translated and culturally adapted for Nepal. It included demographic enquiry followed by modules assessing headache, psychiatric comorbidities, neuroticism and QoL.

All parts of the instrument, including these modules, were interviewer-administered.

Headache enquiry

The screening question asked "Did you have headache in the last 12 months?" Those who answered "no" were classified as headache-free and served as the reference group. Those responding "yes" were asked a series of diagnostic questions based on the International Classification of Headache Disorders (ICHD-3 beta) [36]. Participants reporting more than one headache type were requested to focus only on the most bothersome type in response to these questions. Diagnoses were made algorithmically. Participants with headache on ≥15 days/month were first separated; those who were also overusing acute or symptomatic medication for headache were diagnosed as probable MOH (pMOH), and the remainder as "other headache on ≥15 days/month". To all other participants, the algorithm applied ICHD-3 beta criteria, with modifications, in the order: definite migraine, definite TTH, probable migraine, probable TTH. Any remaining cases were unclassifiable. In the subsequent analyses, definite and probable migraine were considered together as migraine, and definite and probable TTH as TTH. This procedure, and the necessary adaptations made to certain of the ICHD-3 beta criteria, have been described in detail earlier [31].

Assessment of psychiatric comorbidities

Imported as a module into the HARDSHIP questionnaire was a validated Nepali version of the Hospital Anxiety and Depression Scale (HADS) [37]. This scale consists of 14 items in two subscales, HADS-Anxiety and HADS-Depression, each with seven items [38]. Each item expresses the subjective experience of the respondent in the preceding week, and is rated 0–3 (3 indicating maximum symptom severity) so that the sum of each subscale has a potential range of 0–21. In accordance with the original description of HADS [38] and our validation of the Nepali version [37], a threshold of 11 on the respective subscale was taken to indicate caseness for anxiety or depression. Participants scoring above the threshold on only one subscale were regarded as cases of anxiety (HADS-A) only or depression (HADS-D) only; those scoring above 11 on both were regarded as cases of comorbid anxiety and depression (HADS-cAD).

Assessment of neuroticism

Also imported as a module into the HARDSHIP questionnaire was a similarly validated version of the Eysenck Personality Questionnaire Revised Short Form-Neuroticism (EPQRS-N) [39]. It has 12 questions, each with the response options "no" (scored 0) and "yes" (scored 1) to assess the degree of neuroticism in a respondent [40]: the sum of responses has a potential range of 0–12, with higher values indicating more neuroticism.

Assessment of quality of life

Finally imported into the HARDSHIP questionnaire was a culturally-adapted version of the World Health Organization Quality-of-Life 8-question scale WHOQOL-8 [41]. This consists of eight questions addressing perceived aspects of the respondent's QoL in four principal domains: psychological, physical, social and environmental. Each question has five response options on a Likert scale, scored from 1 (worst) to 5 (best); the summed score has the potential range of 8–40, with higher scores indicating better QoL.

Statistical analysis

Analyses were carried out using IBM SPSS Statistics 21.

We used logistic regression analysis to examine associations between headache (all, and its different types: migraine, TTH or headache on ≥15 days/month) and psychiatric caseness (HADS-A, HADS-D or HADS-cAD). Both bivariate and multivariate analyses were undertaken with headache (or its types) as the independent variable; multivariate analyses were repeated with each of HADS-A, HADS-D and HADS-cAD as the independent variable. Odds ratios (ORs) with 95 % confidence intervals (CIs) are presented as the measure of association.

We used a general linear regression model (GLM) to identify associations between total neuroticism score and all headache or its types. The regression coefficient (B) represents the difference in neuroticism scores between participants with headache (or a headache type) and those with no headache (the reference category in both analyses).

In the logistic regression analyses as well as the GLM model, we adjusted for age (categorized 18–25, 26–35, 36–45, 46–55, 56–65 years), gender, annual household consumption (categorized ≤950, 950–1200, >1200 USD/year), habitat (urban *versus* rural), altitude (<2000 *versus* ≥2000 m) and the use of alcohol or marijuana (no *versus* yes). Potential interactions of headache types with demographic (age, gender) or environmental (habitat, altitude) factors in the associations with psychiatric caseness or total neuroticism score were tested by creating an interaction term (the product of the two independent variables: *eg*, age category*headache type) which was added to the regression model. If the interaction term reached statistical significance ($p < 0.05$), subgroup-specific results were derived.

We compared WHOQOL-8 scores among participants with each type of headache with or without psychiatric comorbidity, and among psychiatric cases with or without comorbid headache. We used Student's t-test to compare differences in mean scores. We set $p < 0.05$ as the level of significance in all analyses.

Results

There were 2100 participants, with a participation rate of 99.6 % (males: 861 [41.0 %]; females: 1239 [59.0 %]; mean age 36.4 ± 12.8 years). The majority (1328; 63.2 %) were rural inhabitants, and over one fifth (470; 22.4 %) lived at an altitude of ≥2000 m. Well over one third (822; 39.1 %) were in the lowest category of annual household consumption. A detailed description of the sample characteristics has been reported previously [34].

Having any headache was significantly associated with HADS-A caseness (17.2 %) compared with having no headache (10.5 %; AOR 1.6; 95 % CI: 1.1–2.3; $p = 0.024$) (Table 1). In relation to headache types, the strongest association with HADS-A was observed for headache on ≥15 days/month (AOR 3.2) followed by migraine (AOR 1.7); there was no significant association between TTH and HADS-A (Table 1). No interaction effects were seen with any of the factors analysed.

There were no significant associations between having headache and HADS-D caseness (Table 2).

Having any headache was significantly associated with HADS-cAD caseness (7.0 %) compared with having no headache (3.6 %; AOR 1.9; 95 % CI: 1.0–3.6; $p = 0.050$) (Table 3). Again the strongest association with HADS-cAD was seen for headache on ≥15 days/month (AOR 2.7) followed by migraine (AOR 2.3), and there was no significant association between TTH and HADS-cAD.

In tests for interaction, we found only a weakly significant effect of gender ($p = 0.047$) with any headache. A subgroup analysis, however, suggested that the association of any headache with HADS-cAD was specific to females (AOR 4.3 [95 % CI: 1.3–13.8] *versus* AOR 1.0 [95 % CI: 0.4–2.2] in males). Numbers were low in the reference group in these analyses. No significant interactions were seen with any of the headache types.

Linear regression analysis showed a significant association between all headache and neuroticism score (B = 0.9; 95 % CI: 0.5–1.2; $p < 0.001$). Among headache types, headache on ≥15 days/month showed the strongest association (B = 1.6; 95 % CI: 0.9–2.2; $p < 0.001$), followed by migraine (B = 1.3; 95 % CI: 0.8–1.7; $p < 0.001$); the association between TTH and neuroticism was weak, although significant (B = 0.4; 95 % CI: 0.02–0.8; $p = 0.040$). All these analyses were adjusted for age, gender, household consumption, habitation, altitude and use of alcohol and marijuana. Tests for interaction revealed no significant effects with regard to any headache. However, in relation to migraine, the association with neuroticism demonstrated some gender-specificity, being stronger among males (B = 1.9; 95 % CI: 1.3–2.5) than females (B = 0.8; 95 % CI: 0.1–1.4).

Tables 4 and 5 summarise the data from Tables 1, 2 and 3, presenting them from a clinical management perspective: what was the probability (expressed as a percentage and AOR) that a patient with either headache (of a specific type) or psychiatric disorder (as HADS caseness) had the other as a comorbid condition? HADS-A was the most prevalent HADS caseness comorbid with each of the headache types: a patient with headache on ≥15 days/month had almost 30 % probability (AOR 3.2) of also having HADS-A. Migraine was the most prevalent headache comorbid with each of HADS-A, HADS-D and HADS-cAD: a patient with HADS-cAD had 46.7 % probability (AOR 2.5) of also having migraine.

Tables 6 and 7 show how the effects of comorbid headache and HADS caseness interacted on QoL, being additive (reducing WHOQOL score) in almost all cases. The only exceptions were that the presence or absence of TTH made little difference to QoL in those with HADS-A or HADS-cAD. In general, the additive effects of comorbid HADS caseness were highly significant; those of HADS-cAD were strongest and those of HADS-A least strong. None of the effects of the headache types were significant although, apart from those of TTH, they were consistent; headache on ≥15 days/month had, numerically, the strongest effect (Table 7).

Discussion

This is the first nationwide, population-based survey in any country of South Asia to explore the comorbidity of headache and psychiatric disorders, which are both highly prevalent in Nepal [31, 32]. Comorbidity occurred more than was expected by chance, at least with regard to migraine and headache on ≥15 days/month on the one hand, and HADS-A and HADS-cAD on the other, the associations thereby indicated (with AORs in the range 1.7–3.2) likely to be bidirectional. There were also significant associations between headache, especially headache occurring on ≥15 days/month, and neuroticism.

Table 1 Logistic regression analysis showing association of headache disorders with anxiety (HADS-A)

Headache type	HADS-A caseness			p
	n (%)[a]	OR [95 % CI]	AOR [95 % CI]	
No headache (N = 306)	32 (10.5)	Reference		
Any headache (N = 1794)	308 (17.2)	1.8 [1.2–2.6]	1.6 [1.1–2.3]	0.024
Migraine (N = 728)	134 (18.4)	1.9 [1.3–2.9]	1.7 [1.1–2.6]	0.013
Tension-type headache (N = 863)	121 (14.0)	1.4 [0.9–2.1]	1.3 [0.8–1.9]	0.29
Headache on ≥15 d/m (N = 161)	48 (29.8)	3.6 [2.2–5.9]	3.2 [1.9–5.4]	<0.001

[a]Number (n) of cases with anxiety (HADS-A) and their proportion (%) among those (N) with the headache type; OR: odds ratio, AOR: adjusted odds ratio (adjusted for age, gender, annual household consumption, habitation, altitude and use of alcohol and marijuana), d/m: days/month

Table 2 Logistic regression analysis showing association of headache disorders with depression (HADS-D)

Headache type	HADS-D caseness			*p*
	n (%)[a]	OR [95 % CI]	AOR [95 % CI]	
No headache (*N* = 306)	15 (4.9)	Reference		
Any headache (*N* = 1794)	94 (5.2)	1.1 [0.6–1.9]	1.2 [0.6–2.0]	0.66
Migraine (*N* = 728)	44 (6.0)	1.3 [0.7–2.3]	1.3 [0.7–2.3]	0.49
Tension-type headache (*N* = 863)	36 (4.2)	0.8 [0.5–1.6]	0.9 [0.5–1.8]	0.91
Headache on ≥15 d/m (*N* = 161)	11 (6.8)	1.4 [0.6–3.2]	1.5 [0.6–3.4]	0.38

[a]Number (n) of cases with depression (HADS-D) and their proportion (%) among those (N) with the headache type; OR: odds ratio, AOR: adjusted odds ratio (adjusted for age, gender, annual household consumption, habitation, altitude and use of alcohol and marijuana), d/m: days/month

There were no associations between any headache and HADS-D, and none between TTH and any HADS caseness. Additive and possibly synergistic effects of comorbid headache and HADS caseness were evident on QoL, highly significantly so when migraine or TTH was the index disorder and HADS caseness the comorbid disorder.

Before considering the implications of these findings, we would compare them with others as a test of veracity; but as we have noted, there are none from this Region. Outside South Asia, most studies exploring psychiatric associations with headache disorders have focused on migraine [3–11]. A Zürich cohort study first demonstrated strong relationships between migraine and both anxiety and depression [3], which were subsequently reported in the United States (US) [4, 9] and Canada [42]. Other US studies found that people with migraine had high levels of neuroticism [43, 44]. In Nepal, we found strong associations between migraine and HADS-A, HADS-cAD and neuroticism, but not HADS-D.

There is relatively little evidence regarding psychiatric associations with episodic TTH [45]. A large Swiss epidemiological study found no associations with depressive or anxiety disorders [7], and neither did we. Episodic TTH is usually a less painful disorder than migraine, and less troublesome since it lacks the range of associated symptoms that contribute to the burden of migraine [35]. Hence people with episodic TTH may not express the same extent of subjective emotional experiences as those with migraine [46].

People with chronic TTH, on the other hand, demonstrate strong psychiatric associations [47]: in the US, almost half had either a depressive or an anxiety disorder [48] while those in a Norwegian study had high levels of neuroticism [22]. We did not analyse chronic TTH specifically because it could not reliably be diagnosed by lay interviewers using a questionnaire [35], but among our participants with other headache on ≥15 days/month would have been some with this disorder. The category of headaches occurring on ≥15 days/month corresponds with what is elsewhere referred to as "CDH" [49], which has been associated with high frequencies of both depressive and anxiety symptoms [13, 50]. We found, in the Nepalese population, that headache on ≥15 days/month was associated with HADS-A, HADS-cAD and neuroticism, but not HADS-D.

Our findings, therefore, are not entirely in accord with others regarding depression. The explanation may be methodological. We found no association between HADS-D and any headache type, in line with French [27] and Norwegian studies [51] that also used HADS to establish psychiatric caseness. The studies from Switzerland [3], the US [4] and Canada [42], which found strong associations between depression and headache, instead used structured interviews based on Diagnostic and Statistical Manual (DSM) criteria [52]. A

Table 3 Logistic regression analysis showing association of headache disorders with comorbid anxiety and depression (HADS-cAD)

Headache type	HADS-cAD caseness			*p*
	n (%)[a]	OR [95 % CI]	AOR [95 % CI]	
No headache (*N* = 306)	11 (3.6)	Reference		
Any headache (*N* = 1794)	126 (7.0)	2.0 [1.1–3.8]	1.9 [1.0–3.6]	0.050
Migraine (*N* = 728)	64 (8.8)	2.6 [1.3–4.9]	2.3 [1.2–4.4]	0.016
Tension-type headache (*N* = 863)	42 (4.9)	1.4 [0.7–2.7]	1.4 [0.7–2.8]	0.34
Headache on ≥15 d/m (*N* = 161)	17 (10.6)	3.2 [1.4–6.9]	2.7 [1.2–6.1]	0.014

[a]Number (n) of cases with comorbid anxiety and depression (HADS-cAD) and their proportion (%) among those (N) with the headache type; OR: odds ratio, AOR: adjusted odds ratio (adjusted for age, gender, annual household consumption, habitation, altitude and use of alcohol and marijuana), d/m: days/month

Table 4 Prevalence of psychiatric disorder among participants with headache, by headache type

Headache type	HADS-A caseness (*N* = 340)		HADS-D caseness (*N* = 109)		HADS-cAD caseness (*N* = 137)	
	n (%)	AOR [95 % CI]	*n* (%)	AOR [95 % CI]	n (%)	AOR [95 % CI]
Migraine (*N* = 728)	134 (18.4)	1.7 [1.1–2.6]	44 (6.0)	1.3 [0.7–2.3]	64 (8.8)	2.3 [1.2–4.4]
Tension-type headache (*N* = 863)	121 (14.0)	1.3 [0.8–1.9]	36 (4.2)	0.9 [0.5–1.8]	42 (4.9)	1.4 [0.7–2.8]
Headache on ≥15 d/m (*N* = 161)	48 (29.8)	3.2 [1.9–5.4]	11 (6.8)	1.5 [0.6–3.4]	17 (10.6)	2.7 [1.2–6.1]

AOR: adjusted odds ratio (multivariate logistic regression analysis, using participants with no headache as reference and adjusted for age, gender, household consumption, habitation, altitude and use of alcohol and marijuana), d/m: days/month

recent study from South Korea [53] obtained similar findings using the self-administered Patient Health Questionnnaire-9 (PHQ-9) [54], as did another US study [48] using the Beck Depression Inventory (BDI) [55]. Cultural factors determining how moods are expressed [56] may contribute: in many Asian countries, depression is often manifested somatically [57, 58], while HADS does not capture the somatic domains of depression so well [38]. HADS may therefore underestimate any association of depression *alone* with headache.

However, as was pointed out in a recent review [20] and revealed in the French study [27], depression in migraine rarely occurs alone but is almost always comorbid with anxiety. A stronger association of migraine with combined anxiety-depression than with either independently was seen in the early Zürich study [3], and similar findings in relation to the other headache types came later in Norway [51]. In our study, HADS-cAD occurred twice as often among all headache sufferers and those with migraine, and almost three times in those with headache on ≥15 days/month. Hence the association of headache with depression in our population, though not apparent in HADS-D, may have manifested in HADS-cAD. There was, however, a gender influence in this association: for any headache, the association with HADS-cAD appeared specific to females (AOR 4.3 *versus* 1.0 in males).

Summarising these arguments, we believe use of HADS – a screening rather than diagnostic instrument for depression – is valid among people with headache although it may underestimate caseness prevalence. We could not establish any association between headache disorders and HADS-D in Nepal, but this limitation should be taken into account.

We also note other limitations. It is a general limitation of cross-sectional studies that, while associations can be demonstrated, causality cannot. However, public-health purposes are served in the first instance by uncovering these relationships, which have important policy implications; subsequent research can investigate causation. It is a limitation of HADS that it cannot go beyond detecting caseness of anxiety or depression, which encompass heterogeneous mental disorders. This renders it difficult to identify and make provision in health-service planning for issues that might be related to particular types of these disorders. By a similar token, our headache diagnostic questionnaire captured episodic migraine and TTH, while all chronic cases were subsumed under headache on ≥15 days/month [35]. Comorbidities associated with these subtypes were likely to be different in view of their high-frequency, long-duration, intractable symptoms coupled with problems in management, but the prevalence of each would have been about 1 % or less. Categorically assessing these multiple types and subtypes would have been a cumbersome exercise requiring much greater investment. We believe that our approach, with simple validated interviewer-administered culturally-validated instruments, was a more practical option in a population with high illiteracy, and it best served our public-health purpose. Furthermore, our study had notable strengths: tried and tested methodology [33–35, 59], large sample size, high participation rate and good representativeness of the diverse population of Nepal [33, 34].

Table 5 Prevalence of headache among participants with psychiatric disorder, by HADS caseness

HADS caseness	Migraine (*N* = 728)		Tension-type headache (*N* = 863)		Headache on ≥15 d/m (*N* = 161)	
	n (%)	AOR [95 % CI]	*n* (%)	AOR [95 % CI]	*n* (%)	AOR [95 % CI]
HADS-A (*N* = 340)	134 (39.4)	1.8 [1.2–2.7]	121 (35.6)	1.2 [0.8–1.8]	48 (14.1)	3.2 [1.9–5.5]
HADS-D (*N* = 109)	44 (40.4)	1.3 [0.7–2.4]	36 (33.0)	0.9 [0.5–1.9]	11 (10.1)	1.1 [0.5–2.8]
HADS-cAD (*N* = 137)	64 (46.7)	2.5 [1.2–4.8]	42 (30.7)	1.4 [0.7–2.9]	17 (12.4)	2.8 [1.2–6.5]

AOR: adjusted odds ratio (multivariate logistic regression analysis, using participants with no psychiatric disorder as reference and adjusted for age, gender, household consumption, habitation, altitude and use of alcohol and marijuana), d/m: days/month

Conclusion

Headache disorders, highly prevalent in Nepal, are excessively comorbid with anxiety and associated with neuroticism, and these relationships aggravate their negative impact on QoL. These findings call for reciprocal awareness, and a holistic coordinated approach to management and in the health service. Care for common headache and common psychiatric disorders should be integrated in primary care.

Abbreviations

AOR: adjusted odds ratio; BDI: Beck Depression Inventory; cAD: comorbid anxiety and depression; CI: confidence interval; CMD: common mental disorder; CDH: chronic daily headache; DSM: Diagnostic and Statistical manual of Mental disorders; EPQRS-N: Eysenck Personality Questionnaire Revised Short Form-Neuroticism; GBD: Global Burden of Disease; HADS: Hospital Anxiety and Depression Scale; HARDSHIP: Headache-Attributed Restriction Disability, Social Handicap and Impaired Participation; ICD: International Classification of Diseases; ICHD: International Classification of Headache Disorders; LAMI: low-and-middle-income; MDB: major disorders of the brain; NTNU: Norwegian University of Science and Technology; OR: odds ratio; PHQ: Patient Health Questionnaire; pMOH: probable medication-overuse headache; QoL: quality of life; SPSS: Statistical Package for Social Science; TTH: tension-type headache; US: United States; WHOQOL-8: World Health Organization Quality-of-Life 8-question scale; YLD: year of life lost to disability.

Competing interests

TJS is a Director and Trustee of *Lifting The Burden*.

Authors' contributions

All authors were involved in conception and design of the study. AR and KM, with support from ML and TJS, were responsible for data acquisition. All authors engaged in data analysis and interpretation. AR drafted the manuscript. All authors revised it critically for intellectual content, and approved the version submitted.

Acknowledgements

This project was funded by grants from Samarbeidsorganet, the Liaison Committee between the Central Norway Regional Health Authority and the Norwegian University of Science and Technology (NTNU). The study was a research collaboration between NTNU Department of Neuroscience, Kathmandu University School of Medical Sciences (KUSMS), and *Lifting The Burden*, a UK-registered non-governmental organization directing the Global Campaign against Headache in official relations with the World Health Organization. We thank Dhulikhel Hospital, Kathmandu University Hospital, for assistance and logistic support during the planning phase. We are grateful to Professor Grethe Albrektsen, Professor in Medical Statistics, Faculty of Medicine Department of Public Health and General Practice, NTNU, for advice in statistical analysis.

Author details

[1]Department of Neuroscience, Norwegian University of Science and Technology, Nevrosenteret Øst, St Olavs Hospital, 7006 Trondheim, Norway. [2]Dhulikhel Hospital, Kathmandu University Hospital, Dhulikhel, Kavre, Nepal. [3]Pain Unit, St Olavs University Hospital, Trondheim, Norway. [4]Division of Brain Sciences, Imperial College London, London, UK. [5]Norwegian Advisory Unit on Headache, St Olavs University Hospital, Trondheim, Norway.

References

1. Feinstein AR (1970) The pre-therapeutic classification of co-morbidity in chronic disease. J Chronic Dis 23(7):455–468
2. Pompili M, Serafini G, Di Cosimo D, Dominici G, Innamorati M, Lester D, Forte A, Girardi N, De Filippis S, Tatarelli R, Martelletti P (2010) Psychiatric comorbidity and suicide risk in patients with chronic migraine. Neuropsychiatr Dis Treat 6:81–91
3. Merikangas KR, Angst J, Isler H (1990) Migraine and psychopathology. Results of the Zürich cohort study of young adults. Arch Gen Psychiatry 47(9):849–853
4. Breslau N, Davis GC (1993) Migraine, physical health and psychiatric disorder: a prospective epidemiologic study in young adults. J Psychiatr Res 27(2):211–221
5. Lake AE 3rd, Rains JC, Penzien DB, Lipchik GL (2005) Headache and psychiatric comorbidity: historical context, clinical implications, and research relevance. Headache 45(5):493–506. doi:10.1111/j.1526-4610.2005.05101.x
6. Baskin SM, Smitherman TA (2009) Migraine and psychiatric disorders: comorbidities, mechanisms, and clinical applications. Neurol Sci 30(Suppl 1):S61–S65. doi:10.1007/s10072-009-0071-5
7. Merikangas KR, Merikangas JR, Angst J (1993) Headache syndromes and psychiatric disorders: association and familial transmission. J Psychiatr Res 27(2):197–210
8. Merikangas KR, Stevens DE (1997) Comorbidity of migraine and psychiatric disorders. Neurol Clin 15(1):115–123
9. Breslau N, Lipton RB, Stewart WF, Schultz LR, Welch KM (2003) Comorbidity of migraine and depression: investigating potential etiology and prognosis. Neurology 60(8):1308–1312
10. Wang SJ, Chen PK, Fuh JL (2010) Comorbidities of migraine. Front Neurol 1:16. doi:10.3389/fneur.2010.00016
11. Buse DC, Silberstein SD, Manack AN, Papapetropoulos S, Lipton RB (2013) Psychiatric comorbidities of episodic and chronic migraine. J Neurol 260(8):1960–1969. doi:10.1007/s00415-012-6725-x
12. Puca F, Genco S, Prudenzano MP, Savarese M, Bussone G, D'Amico D, Cerbo R, Gala C, Coppola MT, Gallai V, Firenze C, Sarchielli P, Guazzelli M, Guidetti V, Manzoni G, Granella F, Muratorio A, Bonuccelli U, Nuti A, Nappi G, Sandrini G, Verri AP, Sicuteri F, Marabini S (1999) Psychiatric comorbidity and psychosocial stress in patients with tension-type headache from headache centers in Italy. The Italian Collaborative Group for the Study of Psychopathological Factors in Primary Headaches. Cephalalgia 19(3):159–164
13. Verri AP, Proietti Cecchini A, Galli C, Granella F, Sandrini G, Nappi G (1998) Psychiatric comorbidity in chronic daily headache. Cephalalgia 18(Suppl 21):45–49
14. Samaan Z, Farmer A, Craddock N, Jones L, Korszun A, Owen M, McGuffin P (2009) Migraine in recurrent depression: case-control study. Br J Psychiatry 194(4):350–354. doi:10.1192/bjp.bp.108.054049
15. Breslau N, Davis GC, Schultz LR, Peterson EL (1994) Migraine and major depression: a longitudinal study. Headache 34(7):387–393
16. Holm JE, Penzien DB, Holroyd KA, Brown TA (1994) Headache and depression: confounding effects of transdiagnostic symptoms. Headache 34(7):418–423
17. Mitsikostas DD, Thomas AM (1999) Comorbidity of headache and depressive disorders. Cephalalgia 19(4):211–217
18. Lipton RB, Hamelsky SW, Kolodner KB, Steiner TJ, Stewart WF (2000) Migraine, quality of life, and depression: a population-based case-control study. Neurology 55(5):629–635
19. Smitherman TA, Penzien DB, Maizels M (2008) Anxiety disorders and migraine intractability and progression. Curr Pain Headache Rep 12(3):224–229
20. Smitherman TA, Kolivas ED, Bailey JR (2013) Panic disorder and migraine: comorbidity, mechanisms, and clinical implications. Headache 53(1):23–45. doi:10.1111/head.12004
21. Rasmussen BK (1992) Migraine and tension-type headache in a general population: psychosocial factors. Int J Epidemiol 21(6):1138–1143
22. Aaseth K, Grande RB, Leiknes KA, Benth JS, Lundqvist C, Russell MB (2011) Personality traits and psychological distress in persons with chronic tension-type headache. The Akershus study of chronic headache. Acta Neurol Scand 124(6):375–382. doi:10.1111/j.1600-0404.2011.01490.x
23. Boye B, Lundin KE, Leganger S, Mokleby K, Jantschek G, Jantschek I, Kunzendorf S, Benninghoven D, Sharpe M, Wilhelmsen I, Blomhoff S, Malt UF, Jahnsen J (2008) The INSPIRE study: do personality traits predict general quality of life (Short form-36) in distressed patients with ulcerative colitis and Crohn's disease? Scand J Gastroenterol 43(12):1505–1513. doi:10.1080/00365520802321196
24. Gustavsson A, Svensson M, Jacobi F, Allgulander C, Alonso J, Beghi E, Dodel R, Ekman M, Faravelli C, Fratiglioni L, Gannon B, Jones DH, Jennum P, Jordanova A, Jonsson L, Karampampa K, Knapp M, Kobelt G, Kurth T, Lieb R, Linde M, Ljungcrantz C, Maercker A, Melin B, Moscarelli M, Musayev A, Norwood F, Preisig M, Pugliatti M, Rehm J, Salvador-Carulla L, Schlehofer B,

Simon R, Steinhausen HC, Stovner LJ, Vallat JM, Van den Bergh P, van Os J, Vos P, Xu W, Wittchen HU, Jonsson B, Olesen J (2011) Cost of disorders of the brain in Europe 2010. Eur Neuropsychopharmacol 21(10):718–779
25. Vos T, Barber RM, Bell B, Bertozzi-Villa A, Biryukov S, Bolliger I, Charlson F, Davis A, Degenhardt L, Dicker D, Duan L, Erskine H, Feigin VL, Ferrari AJ, Fitzmaurice C, Fleming T, Graetz N, Guinovart C, Haagsma J, Hansen GM, Hanson SW, Heuton KR, Higashi H, Kassebaum N, Kyu H, Laurie E, Liang X, Lofgren K, Lozano R, et al. (2015) Global, regional, and national incidence, prevalence, and years lived with disability for 301 acute and chronic diseases and injuries in 188 countries, 1990–2013: a systematic analysis for the Global Burden of Disease Study 2013. Lancet 386(9995):743–800. doi:10.1016/s0140-6736(15)60692-4
26. Steiner TJ, Birbeck GL, Jensen RH, Katsarava Z, Stovner LJ, Martelletti P (2015) Headache disorders are third cause of disability worldwide. J Headache Pain 16:58. doi:10.1186/s10194-015-0544-2
27. Lanteri-Minet M, Radat F, Chautard MH, Lucas C (2005) Anxiety and depression associated with migraine: influence on migraine subjects' disability and quality of life, and acute migraine management. Pain 118(3):319–326. doi:10.1016/j.pain.2005.09.010
28. Beghi E, Allais G, Cortelli P, D'Amico D, De Simone R, d'Onofrio F, Genco S, Manzoni GC, Moschiano F, Tonini MC, Torelli P, Quartaroli M, Roncolato M, Salvi S, Bussone G (2007) Headache and anxiety-depressive disorder comorbidity: the HADAS study. Neurol Sci 28(Suppl 2):S217–S219. doi:10.1007/s10072-007-0780-6
29. Gambini O, Islam L, Demartini B, Scarone S (2010) Psychiatric issues in patients with headaches. Neurol Sci 31(Suppl 1):S111–S113. doi:10.1007/s10072-010-0300-y
30. Pesa J, Lage MJ (2004) The medical costs of migraine and comorbid anxiety and depression. Headache 44(6):562–570. doi:10.1111/j.1526-4610.2004.446004.x
31. Manandhar K, Risal A, Steiner TJ, Holen A, Linde M (2015) The prevalence of primary headache disorders in Nepal: a nationwide population-based study. J Headache Pain 16(1):95. doi:10.1186/s10194-015-0580-y
32. Risal A, Manandhar K, Linde M, Steiner TJ, Holen A (2016) Anxiety and depression in Nepal: Prevalence, comorbidity and associations. BMC Psychiatry 16(1):1–9. doi: 10.1186/s12888-016-0810-0.
33. Risal A, Manandhar K, Steiner TJ, Holen A, Koju R, Linde M (2014) Estimating prevalence and burden of major disorders of the brain in Nepal: cultural, geographic, logistic and philosophical issues of methodology. J Headache Pain 15(1):51. doi:10.1186/1129-2377-15-51
34. Manandhar K, Risal A, Steiner TJ, Holen A, Koju R, Linde M (2014) Estimating the prevalence and burden of major disorders of the brain in Nepal: methodology of a nationwide population-based study. J Headache Pain 15(1):52. doi:10.1186/1129-2377-15-52
35. Steiner TJ, Gururaj G, Andree C, Katsarava Z, Ayzenberg I, Yu S-Y, Jumah MA, Tekle-Haimanot R, Birbeck GL, Herekar A, Linde M, Mbewe E, Manandhar K, Risal A, Jensen R, Queiroz LP, Scher AI, Wang S-J, Stovner LJ (2014) Diagnosis, prevalence estimation and burden measurement in population surveys of headache: presenting the HARDSHIP questionnaire. J Headache Pain 15:3
36. Headache Classification Committee of the International Headache Society (2013) The international classification of headache disorders, 3rd edition (beta version). Cephalalgia 33(9):629–808. doi:10.1177/0333102413485658
37. Risal A, Manandhar K, Linde M, Koju R, Steiner TJ, Holen A (2015) Reliability and Validity of a Nepali-language Version of the Hospital Anxiety and Depression Scale (HADS). Kathmandu Univ Med J 50(2):115–124
38. Zigmond AS, Snaith RP (1983) The hospital anxiety and depression scale. Acta Psychiatr Scand 67(6):361–370
39. Manandhar K, Risal A, Linde M, Koju R, Steiner TJ, Holen A (2015) Measuring neuroticism in Nepali: Reliability and validity of the Neuroticism Subscale of the Eysenck Personality Questionnaire Kathmandu. Univ Med J 50(2):156–161
40. Eysenck SBG, Eysenck HJ, Barrett P (1985) A revised version of the psychoticism scale. Person Individ Difl 6(1):21–29
41. The WHOQOL Group (1998) The World Health Organization Quality of Life assessment (WHOQOL): Development and general psychometric properties. Soc Sci Med 46:1569–1585
42. Jette N, Patten S, Williams J, Becker W, Wiebe S (2008) Comorbidity of migraine and psychiatric disorders–a national population-based study. Headache 48(4):501–516. doi:10.1111/j.1526-4610.2007.00993.x
43. Breslau N, Andreski P (1995) Migraine, personality, and psychiatric comorbidity. Headache 35(7):382–386
44. Breslau N, Chilcoat HD, Andreski P (1996) Further evidence on the link between migraine and neuroticism. Neurology 47(3):663–667
45. Semenov IA (2015) Tension-type headaches. Dis Mon 61(6):233–235. doi:10.1016/j.disamonth.2015.03.006
46. Nicholson RA (2010) Chronic headache: the role of the psychologist. Curr Pain Headache Rep 14(1):47–54. doi:10.1007/s11916-009-0087-9
47. Heckman BD, Holroyd KA (2006) Tension-type headache and psychiatric comorbidity. Curr Pain Headache Rep 10(6):439–447
48. Holroyd KA, Stensland M, Lipchik GL, Hill KR, O'Donnell FS, Cordingley G (2000) Psychosocial correlates and impact of chronic tension-type headaches. Headache 40(1):3–16
49. Murinova N, Krashin D (2015) Chronic daily headache. Phys Med Rehabil Clin N Am 26(2):375–389. doi:10.1016/j.pmr.2015.01.001
50. Juang KD, Wang SJ, Fuh JL, Lu SR, Su TP (2000) Comorbidity of depressive and anxiety disorders in chronic daily headache and its subtypes. Headache 40(10):818–823
51. Zwart JA, Dyb G, Hagen K, Odegard KJ, Dahl AA, Bovim G, Stovner LJ (2003) Depression and anxiety disorders associated with headache frequency. The Nord-Trondelag Health Study. Eur J Neurol 10(2):147–152
52. American Psychiatric Association (2000) Diagnostic and statistical manual of mental disorders (4th ed., text rev.). doi:10.1176/appi.books.9780890423349.
53. Oh K, Cho SJ, Chung YK, Kim JM, Chu MK (2014) Combination of anxiety and depression is associated with an increased headache frequency in migraineurs: a population-based study. BMC Neurol 14:238. doi:10.1186/s12883-014-0238-4
54. Kroenke K, Spitzer RL, Williams JB (2001) The PHQ-9: validity of a brief depression severity measure. J Gen Intern Med 16(9):606–613
55. Beck AT, Steer RA, Brown GK (1996) Manual for the Beck Depression Inventory-II. Psychological Corporation, San Antonio, TX
56. Steel Z, Marnane C, Iranpour C, Chey T, Jackson JW, Patel V, Silove D (2014) The global prevalence of common mental disorders: a systematic review and meta-analysis 1980–2013. Int J Epidemiol 43(2):476–493. doi:10.1093/ije/dyu038
57. Yong N, Hu H, Fan X, Li X, Ran L, Qu Y, Wang Y, Tan G, Chen L, Zhou J (2012) Prevalence and risk factors for depression and anxiety among outpatient migraineurs in mainland China. J Headache Pain 13(4):303–310. doi:10.1007/s10194-012-0442-9
58. Shen YC, Zhang MY, Huang YQ, He YL, Liu ZR, Cheng H, Tsang A, Lee S, Kessler RC (2006) Twelve-month prevalence, severity, and unmet need for treatment of mental disorders in metropolitan China. Psychol Med 36(2):257–267. doi:10.1017/s0033291705006367
59. Stovner LJ, Al Jumah M, Birbeck GL, Gururaj G, Jensen R, Katsarava Z, Queiroz LP, Scher AI, Tekle-Haimanot R, Wang SJ, Steiner TJ (2014) The methodology of population surveys of headache prevalence, burden and cost: Principles and recommendations from the Global Campaign against Headache. J Headache Pain 15(1):5. doi:10.1186/1129-2377-15-5
60. World Health Organization and *Lifting The Burden* (2011) Atlas of Headache Disorders and Resources in the World 2011. WHO, Geneva
61. Kessler RC, Aguilar-Gaxiola S, Alonso J, Chatterji S, Lee S, Ormel J, Ustun TB, Wang PS (2009) The global burden of mental disorders: an update from the WHO World Mental Health (WMH) surveys. Epidemiol Psichiatr Soc 18(1):23–33
62. Risal A (2011) Common mental disorders. Kathmandu Univ Med J (KUMJ) 9(35):213–217

5

Headache: an important factor associated with muscle soreness/pain at the two-year follow-up point among patients with major depressive disorder

Ching-I Hung[1,2], Chia-Yih Liu[1,2], Ching-Hui Yang[3] and Shuu-Jiun Wang[4,5*]

Abstract

Background: No study has compared the associations of headache, anxiety, and depression at baseline with muscle soreness or pain (MS/P) at baseline and at the two-year follow-up point among outpatients with major depressive disorder (MDD). This study aimed to investigate the above issue.

Methods: This study enrolled 155 outpatients with MDD at baseline, and 131 attended a two-year follow-up appointment. At baseline, migraine was diagnosed based on the *International Classification of Headache Disorders*, 2nd edition. MDD and anxiety disorders were diagnosed using the Structured Clinical Interview for DSM-IV-TR. The visual analog scale was used to evaluate the intensities of headache and MS/P in the neck, shoulder, back, upper limbs, and lower limbs. Depression and anxiety were evaluated using the Hospital Anxiety and Depression Scale. Multiple linear regressions were used to compare the associations of these factors with MS/P.

Results: Compared with anxiety disorders, migraine was more strongly associated with MS/P in all areas at baseline and in the upper and lower limbs at follow-up. Headache intensity at baseline was the factor most strongly associated with MS/P in all areas at baseline and follow-up after controlling for depression and anxiety. Headache intensity at baseline predicted MS/P at baseline and follow-up.

Conclusions: Migraine and headache intensity are important factors related to MS/P at baseline and follow-up among patients with MDD. Integrating depression and headache treatment might be indicated to improve MS/P.

Keywords: Depression, Anxiety, Migraine, Pain, Muscle soreness

Background

Depression and muscle soreness or pain (MS/P) are closely related and interact [1–3]. Chronic muscle pain is frequently accompanied by symptoms of depression [2]. Major depressive disorder (MDD) is common among chronic pain patients with myofascial pain syndrome [4]. Co-occurrence of musculoskeletal pain and depressive symptoms is strongly related to poor self-rated physical work ability [3]. Among patients with depression, muscle soreness is one of the factors that independently predict a slower remission after controlling for the baseline severity of depression [5].

Headache, depression, and anxiety are closely related and interact [6–8]. A strong bidirectional association between migraine and psychiatric disorders has been documented [8]. Migraine is common among patients with MDD and bipolar disorders [9–11]. Migraine is related to poorer recovery of health-related quality of life after acute pharmacotherapy among patients with MDD [12]. MDD patients with migraine are associated with greater severities of depression, anxiety, and somatic and pain symptoms [9, 10, 13, 14]. Migraine is also associated with an increased frequency of suicidal ideation and suicide attempts in patients with MDD [8]. Migraine and

* Correspondence: sjwang@vghtpe.gov.tw
[4]Faculty of Medicine, National Yang-Ming University School of Medicine and Neurological Institute, Taipei Veterans General Hospital, Taipei, Taiwan
[5]Department of Neurology, Taipei Veterans General Hospital, No. 201 Shi-Pai Road, Section 2, Taipei 112, Taiwan

other headaches in a general population are associated with increased musculoskeletal symptoms [15].

Anxiety is associated with musculoskeletal symptoms [1, 16]. Increased muscle tension is one criterion for generalized anxiety disorder (GAD) [17]. Fifty percent of workers with persistent musculoskeletal pain undergoing work rehabilitation initially exhibited GAD symptoms [18]. Anxiety and/or depression are factors related to poor outcomes and disability related to musculoskeletal pain [19, 20]. Anxiety, depression, and migraine were associated with pain in the back, neck, orofacial area, abdomen, joints, and chest, but the associations of migraine with the six pains weakened substantially after correction for the severity of anxiety and depression [21]. Therefore, a considerable part of the comorbidity of migraine and the six pains might be explained by depression and anxiety [21].

As mentioned above, MS/P, migraine, depression, and anxiety are closely related and interact. Investigation of factors related to MS/P among patients with MDD is important, because MS/P is related to a poor treatment prognosis of depression and associated with occupational disability [3, 5, 20]. Although previous studies have reported associations of migraine or other headaches with MS/P among patients with headaches or in a general population [15, 22, 23], the associations of migraine or headaches with MS/P among patients with MDD have been neglected. No study has compared the associations of migraine and anxiety disorders with MS/P in addition to comparing the associations of headache indices, depression, and anxiety with MS/P at baseline and during long-term follow-up among patients with MDD.

The aims of this study were to compare the associations of headaches, anxiety, and depression evaluated at baseline with MS/P at baseline and at the two-year follow-up point among patients with MDD.

We hypothesized that the association of headaches with MS/P is not inferior to the associations of anxiety and depression with MS/P after controlling for demographic and other variables.

Methods

Subjects

The study was approved by the Institutional Review Board of Chang Gung Memorial Hospital, a medical center in northern Taiwan. This project was conducted in the psychiatric outpatient clinics of the same hospital from September 2005 to August 2009. Written informed consent, based on the guidelines regulated in the Declaration of Helsinki, was obtained from all subjects prior to their entrance into the study.

Study participants, aged 18–65 years, were recruited from consecutive outpatients who met the DSM-IV- text revision (TR) criteria for MDD [17] and were experiencing a current major depressive episode (MDE) and had not taken antidepressants or other psychotropic drugs within the previous four weeks. Three exclusion criteria were established in order to prevent depression and pain symptoms from being confounded by psychotic symptoms, substance abuse, or other medical conditions: 1) psychotic symptoms, severe psychomotor retardation, mental retardation, or catatonic features; 2) a history of substance dependence or abuse without full remission in the previous month; and 3) chronic medical diseases such as diabetes mellitus, hypertension, severe neurological disorders, and other medical diseases, except for headaches. The Structured Clinical Interview for DSM-IV-TR Axis I Disorders was used to diagnose MDD and anxiety disorders [24].

Assessment of headaches

A structured headache intake form was designed to meet the operational criteria of the *International Classification of Headache Disorders*, 2nd edition (ICHD-2) [25]. Questions regarding headache pattern, intensity, frequency, location, duration, aggravation by physical activities, aura, nausea, vomiting, phonophobia, photophobia, precipitating factors and medication usage for headache were included. At baseline, subjects completed the structured headache intake form. An experienced headache specialist, who was masked to the results of psychiatric evaluations, interviewed all patients after they had completed the headache intake form and made diagnoses. Patients who fulfilled the criteria of migraine without aura and/or migraine with aura were categorized as the "migraine" group, while the other subjects were categorized as the "non-migraine" group.

The average headache intensity in the past week was evaluated using a visual analog scale (VAS), with 0 representing "no pain" and 10 representing "pain as severe as I can imagine". The number of headache days in the past week was recorded as the headache frequency. The intensity and frequency were evaluated at baseline and at two-year follow-up.

Assessment of anxiety disorders

One board-certified psychiatrist, who was masked to the diagnoses of headaches and the psychometric results, used the Structured Clinical Interview to diagnose the following anxiety disorders: panic disorder, agoraphobia, specific phobia, social phobia, obsessive–compulsive disorder, post-traumatic stress disorder, and GAD [24]. Patients with any one of the anxiety disorders in a current episode or partial remission were categorized as the "anxiety disorders" group, while the others were classified as the "non-anxiety disorders" group.

Assessment of muscle soreness or pain, depression, and anxiety

The average MS/P in the past week was evaluated by using a VAS, with 0 representing "no pain" and 10 representing "pain as severe as I can imagine". MS/P in five areas was evaluated, including the neck, shoulder, back, upper limbs, and lower limbs.

The severities of depression and anxiety were evaluated by the Hospital Anxiety and Depression Scale (HADS). The HADS includes 7 items for the anxiety subscale (HADS-A) and 7 for the depression subscale (HADS-D), with the scores for each subscale ranging from 0 to 21 [26, 27]. The HADS was used because it does not include any somatic or pain symptoms, which might be related to MS/P. The HADS and MS/P were measured at baseline and follow-up.

Procedures

After enrollment, subjects were treated for four weeks with venlafaxine extended-release, one 75 mg capsule per day, and zolpidem. After the four-week treatment, these patients were treated as general psychiatric outpatients without controlling their pharmacotherapy. In the following two years, some patients continued pharmacotherapy and others dropped out. Two years later, the subjects were followed-up. Subjects with pharmacotherapy in the index follow-up month were categorized into the treated group and those without were categorized into the not treated group.

Statistical methods

All statistical analyses were performed using SPSS for Windows 12.0 (SPSS Inc., Chicago, IL, USA). The independent *t* test, the Mann-Whitney *U* test, the paired *t* test, Pearson's correlation, Spearman's correlation and the Chi-square test were used as appropriate.

Two models of multiple linear regressions with forward selection were used to compare the associations of these independent variables with MS/P in the five areas at baseline and two-year follow-up after controlling for other factors. The first regression model compared the associations of two categorical variables (migraine and anxiety disorders) diagnosed at baseline with MS/P in the five areas at baseline and at the two-year follow-up point. The second model compared the associations of four continuous variables (headache intensity, headache frequency, HADS-D score and HADS-A score) evaluated at baseline with MS/P in the five areas at baseline and at the two-year follow-up point. In the first and second models, the dependent variables were MS/P (VAS scores) in the five areas at baseline and follow-up. In the first model, the independent variables included five demographic variables (gender, age, marital status, educational years, and employment status), with pharmacotherapy or not at follow-up, with migraine or not at baseline, and with anxiety disorders or not at baseline. In the second model, the independent variables included five demographic variables, the four continuous variables (headache intensity, headache frequency, HADS-D score and HADS-A score) at baseline, and whether or not pharmacotherapy is being used at follow-up.

A two-tailed P value <0.05 was considered statistically significant. In the comparison of MS/P in the five areas between groups, Bonferroni correction was used and a two-tailed P value <0.01 was considered to indicate a significant difference.

Results

Subjects

At baseline, 155 patients were enrolled (Table 1). At the two-year follow-up, 131 patients agreed to participate in the follow-up, 11 patients refused to participate, and 13 patients were unable to be contacted by phone and mail. There were no significant differences in the five demographic variables, the percentages of migraine and anxiety comorbidities, the HADS scores, or the headache indices between the patients who were followed-up and those who were not followed-up.

At the two-year follow-up, of 30 patients in the treated group, 18 (60.0 %) and 12 were treated with venlafaxine (mean dosage of 102.1 ± 49.5 mg per day) and other antidepressants, respectively. Benzodiazepine or other hypnotics were used in 19 (63.3 %) subjects.

Table 1 Demographic variables and comorbidities among patients with major depressive disorder

	Baseline	Two years
Case number	155	131
Age (years)	30.3 ± 8.0	32.5 ± 8.3
Educational years	13.4 ± 2.5	13.5 ± 2.5
Female (%)	68.4	66.4
In employment (%)	59.4	58.8
Married (%)	38.7	40.5
With pharmacotherapy (%)	–	22.9
With migraine (%)	47.1	46.6
With anxiety disorders (%)	45.2	45.8
HADS-D scores[a]	14.4 ± 3.4	7.1 ± 5.3
HADS-A scores[a]	14.8 ± 3.4	8.7 ± 4.6
Headache intensity[b]	4.2 ± 3.1	2.1 ± 2.6
Headache frequency[c]	3.4 ± 2.6	2.2 ± 2.5

HADS-D the depression subscale of the Hospital Anxiety and Depression Scale (HADS), HADS-A the anxiety subscale of the HADS

[a]50.3 and 56.1 % of the subjects had severe depression and anxiety at baseline, respectively, with HADS-D and HADS-A scores ranging from 15 to 21

[b]The average headache intensity, measured using a visual analog scale, in the past week

[c]The headache days in the past week

Headache and psychiatric diagnoses

Among the 155 subjects at baseline, 73 (47.1 %) had migraine, including 16 subjects with chronic migraine, 2 with chronic migraine and medication overuse headache, 49 with episodic migraine without aura, and 6 with episodic migraine both with and without aura. The other 82 participants included 27 with probable migraine without aura, 1 with chronic tension-type headache (TTH), 30 with episodic TTH, 6 with probable episodic TTH, 9 with headache unspecified, and 9 without any headaches.

At baseline, 70 (45.2 %) patients had at least one anxiety disorder, including 15 (9.7 %) with panic disorder and/or agoraphobia, 38 (24.5 %) with social phobia, 28 (18.1 %) with specific phobia, 18 (11.6 %) with post-traumatic stress disorder, 10 (6.5 %) with obsessive-compulsive disorder, and 11 (7.1 %) with GAD.

MDD subjects with migraine had a higher risk of comorbidity with any one of the anxiety disorders (63.4 % vs. 28.0 %, odds ratio = 4.64, P <0.001) as compared with MDD subjects without migraine.

Differences in the severities of MS/P between groups

Table 2 shows the severities of MS/P at baseline and follow-up. For the full sample at baseline and follow-up, there was a trend that MS/P in the shoulder was of the greatest severity, followed by the neck, back, and limbs. At baseline, the patients with migraine had significantly (post-Bonferroni correction; P <0.01) greater severities of MS/P in the five areas as compared with the patients without migraine. Compared with patients without anxiety disorders, patients with anxiety disorders also had significantly (P <0.01) higher pain intensities in the five areas, except for neck soreness or pain.

At the two-year follow-up point, differences in MS/P in all areas post-correction were not significant between patients with and without migraine or between patients with and without anxiety disorders, both in the treated and not treated groups.

At the two-year follow-up point, the severities of MS/P in the five areas, HADS-A, HADS-D, and headache indices had significantly (P <0.05) decreased both in the treated and not treated groups compared with these variables at baseline, except for the severities of MS/P in the upper and lower limbs and two headache indices in the treated group.

The correlations of MS/P with headache indices, depression, and anxiety

Table 3 shows the correlations of MS/P at baseline and follow-up with headache indices, depression, and anxiety at baseline. At baseline, the correlations of MS/P in all areas with headache intensity, headache frequency, and HADS-A scores were significant. However, the correlations of MS/P with the HADS-D scores were not significant, except for MS/P in the shoulder.

At the two-year follow-up point, the headache intensity at baseline was significantly correlated with MS/P in all areas in the treated and not-treated group, except for MS/P in the neck in the not-treated group and in the

Table 2 The intensities of muscle soreness/pain between groups among patients with major depressive disorder at baseline and follow-up[a]

Time points	Treatment	Comorbidities at baseline[b]		Number	Neck	Shoulder	Back	Upper limbs	Lower limbs
Baseline		Full sample		155	5.0 ± 3.5	5.1 ± 3.6	3.8 ± 3.6	2.6 ± 3.2	2.3 ± 3.0
	No Tx	Migraine	Yes	73	6.4 ± 3.2**	6.8 ± 3.2**	5.1 ± 3.7**	3.5 ± 3.4**	3.3 ± 3.2**
	No Tx	Migraine	No	82	3.7 ± 3.3	3.7 ± 3.3	2.6 ± 3.1	1.7 ± 2.8	1.4 ± 2.4
	No Tx	Anxiety	Yes	70	5.7 ± 3.5*	6.1 ± 3.5**	4.6 ± 3.9**	3.4 ± 3.4**	3.1 ± 3.3**
	No Tx	Anxiety	No	85	4.4 ± 3.5	4.3 ± 3.5	3.1 ± 3.2	1.9 ± 2.9	1.7 ± 2.6
Two years	–	Full sample		131	3.0 ± 3.2	3.3 ± 3.1	2.0 ± 2.8	1.3 ± 2.3	1.5 ± 2.3
	No Tx	Migraine	Yes	43	3.2 ± 3.6	3.9 ± 3.5	2.6 ± 3.3	1.9 ± 3.0*	2.0 ± 2.8*
	No Tx	Migraine	No	58	2.8 ± 3.0	2.8 ± 2.8	1.8 ± 2.6	0.8 ± 1.4	1.1 ± 1.6
	No Tx	Anxiety	Yes	45	3.4 ± 3.5	4.0 ± 3.4*	2.7 ± 3.3	1.9 ± 3.0*	2.0 ± 2.8*
	No Tx	Anxiety	No	56	2.7 ± 3.0	2.7 ± 2.8	1.7 ± 2.5	0.7 ± 1.4	1.0 ± 1.6
	Tx	Migraine	Yes	17	3.7 ± 2.8*	4.3 ± 2.9	2.2 ± 2.4	1.7 ± 2.6	2.1 ± 2.9
	Tx	Migraine	No	13	1.5 ± 3.0	2.0 ± 3.1	1.2 ± 2.5	1.1 ± 1.8	1.2 ± 2.3
	Tx	Anxiety	Yes	16	3.7 ± 3.2	4.0 ± 3.3	1.9 ± 2.7	1.3 ± 2.0	1.9 ± 2.7
	Tx	Anxiety	No	14	1.7 ± 2.6	2.5 ± 3.0	1.7 ± 2.2	1.5 ± 2.7	1.5 ± 2.6

Tx accepted pharmacotherapy in the index follow-up month

[a]The independent t test and the Mann-Whitney U test were used where appropriate

[b]Anxiety comorbidities represented patients with at least one of following anxiety disorders: panic disorder, agoraphobia, social phobia, specific phobia, post-traumatic stress disorder, obsessive–compulsive disorder, and generalized anxiety disorder

$^*P < 0.05$; $^{**}P < 0.01$

Table 3 The correlations of muscle soreness/pain at baseline and two-year follow-up with headache indices, depression, and anxiety at baseline

Time points	Treatment	Number		Neck	Shoulder	Back	Upper limbs	Lower limbs
Baseline	No Tx	155	HI	0.46**	0.45**	0.36**	0.29**	0.37**
	No Tx	155	HF	0.36**	0.36**	0.20*	0.16*	0.16*
	No Tx	155	HADS-D	0.12	0.17*	0.12	0.01	0.08
	No Tx	155	HASD-A	0.26**	0.32**	0.33**	0.17*	0.19*
Two years	No Tx	101	HI	0.13	0.31**	0.21*	0.26**	0.27**
	No Tx	101	HF	0.02	0.21*	0.12	0.15	0.14
	No Tx	101	HADS-D	−0.02	−0.03	−0.04	−0.02	−0.05
	No Tx	101	HASD-A	0.01	0.07	0.06	0.11	0.21*
	Tx	30	HI	0.56**	0.41*	0.45*	0.32	0.39*
	Tx	30	HF	0.42*	0.33	0.31	0.34	0.44*
	Tx	30	HADS-D	0.08	0.03	−0.15	0.03	0.20
	Tx	30	HASD-A	0.22	0.08	−0.02	−0.24	−0.07

HADS-D the depression subscale of the Hospital Anxiety and Depression Scale (HADS), HADS-A the anxiety subscale of the HADS, HI average headache intensity in the past week, HF headache frequency measured by the headache days in the past week, Tx accepted pharmacotherapy in the index follow-up month
*$P < 0.05$; **$P < 0.01$

upper limbs in the treated group. Headache frequency at baseline was significantly correlated with MS/P in the shoulder in the not-treated group and MS/P in the neck and lower limbs in the treated group. The correlations of HADS-D and HADS-A scores with MS/P in all areas were not significant in both groups, except for the correlation of HADS-A with MS/P in the lower limbs in the not-treated group.

Comorbidities independently associated with MS/P

In the first regression model (Table 4), migraine at baseline was an independent factor related to MS/P in the all areas at baseline after controlling for demographic variables. At the two-year follow-up point, migraine at baseline was also an independent factor related to MS/P in the upper and lower limbs. A trend was noted that the association of migraine with MS/P had decreased at the two-year follow-up point. Anxiety disorder at baseline was an independent factor related to MS/P in the shoulder at the two-year follow-up.

Table 4 Independent comorbidities associated with muscle soreness/pain among patients with major depressive disorder[a,b]

Areas	Independent variable	Beta	R^2 change	t	P
$Neck_{(B)}$	$Migraine_{(B)}$	0.40	0.16	5.3	<0.01
$Neck_{(2Y)}$	No	–	–	–	–
$Shoulder_{(B)}$	$Migraine_{(B)}$	0.43	0.19	6.0	<0.01
$Shoulder_{(2Y)}$	Anxiety $disorders_{(B)}$	0.21	0.05	2.5	0.01
$Back_{(B)}$	$Migraine_{(B)}$	0.35	0.12	4.6	<0.01
$Back_{(2Y)}$	No	–	–	–	–
Upper $limbs_{(B)}$	$Migraine_{(B)}$	0.27	0.07	3.5	<0.01
Upper $limbs_{(2Y)}$	$Migraine_{(B)}$	0.22	0.05	2.6	0.01
Lower $limbs_{(B)}$	$Migraine_{(B)}$	0.32	0.10	4.2	<0.01
Lower $limbs_{(2Y)}$	$Migraine_{(B)}$	0.21	0.04	2.4	0.02

[a]The case numbers were 155 and 131 at baseline and two-year follow-up, respectively
[b]"(B)" and "(2Y)" were used to represent the variable evaluated at baseline and two-year follow-up, respectively

Headache, depression, and anxiety independently associated with MS/P

In the second regression model (Table 5), headache intensity was the most important factor (with the greatest R square change) related to MS/P in all areas at baseline and follow-up after controlling for other factors. Headache frequency did not enter these regressions.

Anxiety (HADS-A score) was a factor independently associated with MS/P in three areas at baseline. However, anxiety was not a significant factor related to MS/P in all areas at follow-up. Depression (HADS-D score) was not a significant factor related to MS/P in all areas at baseline and follow-up.

Discussion

Migraine at baseline was an independent factor related to MS/P after controlling for other factors. The association of migraine with MS/P was not limited to baseline measurements, but persisted to the two-year follow-up point in the upper and lower limbs. Previous studies have reported that migraine is associated with increased musculoskeletal symptoms and increased self-reported muscle tension [15, 23, 28]. This might result from the fact that migraine is related to increased intracranial and extracranial mechanical sensitivities and associated with somatosensory amplification [29, 30]. Repeated migraine attacks might cause central sensitization, which is related to allodynia, hyperalgesia and spontaneous pain

Table 5 Independent factors associated with muscle soreness/pain among patients with major depressive disorder[a,b]

Areas	Independent variable	Beta	R^2 change	t	P
$Neck_{(B)}$	$HI_{(B)}$	0.42	0.21	5.8	<0.01
	$HADS\text{-}A_{(B)}$	0.16	0.02	2.2	0.03
$Neck_{(2Y)}$	$HI_{(B)}$	0.22	0.05	2.6	0.01
$Shoulder_{(B)}$	$HI_{(B)}$	0.38	0.20	5.3	<0.01
	$HADS\text{-}A_{(B)}$	0.24	0.05	3.3	<0.01
	$gender_{(B)}$	−0.17	0.03	−2.4	0.02
$Shoulder_{(2Y)}$	$HI_{(B)}$	0.33	0.11	4.0	<0.01
$Back_{(B)}$	$HI_{(B)}$	0.29	0.13	3.9	<0.01
	$HADS\text{-}A_{(B)}$	0.27	0.06	3.6	<0.01
	$gender_{(B)}$	−0.15	0.02	−2.1	0.04
$Back_{(2Y)}$	$HI_{(B)}$	0.25	0.06	3.0	<0.01
Upper $limbs_{(B)}$	$HI_{(B)}$	0.29	0.09	3.8	<0.01
Upper $limbs_{(2Y)}$	$HI_{(B)}$	0.27	0.08	3.2	<0.01
Lower $limbs_{(B)}$	$HI_{(B)}$	0.37	0.14	4.9	<0.01
Lower $limbs_{(2Y)}$	$HI_{(B)}$	0.30	0.09	3.5	<0.01

HADS-A the anxiety subscale of the Hospital Anxiety and Depression Scale, HI = average headache intensity in the past week

[a]The case numbers were 155 and 131 at baseline and two-year follow-up, respectively

[b]"(B)" and "(2Y)" were used to represent the variable evaluated at baseline and two-year follow-up, respectively

[29, 31]. Therefore, MDD patients with migraine might become more sensitive to other pains. One previous study reported that the impact of migraine on physical and pain symptoms might be greater than that of a MDE among psychiatric outpatients [10]. The upper and lower limbs were the areas continuously associated with migraine at the two-year follow-up point. Previous studies have reported that limb pain is associated with migraine and has been considered part of migrainous syndrome [32–34]. In this study, migraine was more associated with MS/P in most areas than anxiety disorders. Therefore, clinicians should not ignore migraine when treating MS/P in patients with MDD.

Headache intensity at baseline was the factor most strongly associated with MS/P at baseline and at the two-year follow-up point. This demonstrated that the association of headache intensity with MS/P was greater than the associations of the severities of depression and anxiety with MS/P. Previous studies have reported that headache is related to musculoskeletal symptoms [15, 23]. Therefore, headache might be an important factor related to central sensitization among patients with MDD. Our results implied that headache intensity at baseline might be an important marker related to MS/P among patients with MDD. MDD patients with a greater intensity of headache during a MDE might have greater severities of MS/P at long-term follow-up. However, further evidence may be needed in order to prove these hypotheses.

Three points were worthy of note. 1) One longitudinal population-based cohort study found a bidirectional relationship between headache and chronic musculoskeletal complaints [22]. Therefore, the pathophysiology of headache and chronic musculoskeletal complaints might overlap or be closely related. The study concluded that chronic musculoskeletal complaints should be treated not only to relieve them but also to prevent the development of chronic daily headache, and vice versa [22]. This conclusion hinted that treatment of migraine and headache might be helpful to improve MS/P among patients with MDD. 2) Depression, migraine, and fibromyalgia are often comorbid with each other and interact [9, 10, 35–37]. Our study showed that migraine and headache intensity were factors related to MS/P, an important characteristic of fibromyalgia [38], among patients with MDD. Our study provided further evidence of correlations between depression, migraine, headache, and fibromyalgia. 3) Our study demonstrated that headache intensity was associated with MS/P to a greater extent than headache frequency. One previous study reported that frequency of headache had a higher impact than headache diagnosis on the association between headache and musculoskeletal symptoms [15]. The impact ranking of headache intensity, headache frequency, and headache diagnoses associated with musculoskeletal symptoms should be further investigated.

Several limitations or methodological issues should be addressed. 1) In the clinical neutral study, subjects in the treated and not treated groups were not divided by randomization, but by patients' decisions. This might cause bias. Moreover, the division caused small sample sizes, which hindered assessment of the statistical significance. 2) Although pharmacotherapy was listed as an independent factor in the regression model, the content of pharmacotherapy was not controlled at follow-up. Analysis of the impacts of different medications on MS/P would be hindered by the small sample sizes. 3) The headache intensity and frequency in the past week were recalled by subjects. A more reliable method would be to record headache parameters in a prospective headache diary. 4) Our sample was collected from a medical center. Expansion of the results of this study to the general population should be performed cautiously. 5) This study only focused on the association of migraine with MS/P. Some patients with migraine might have comorbidity with TTH, which is also related to muscle tension. The association of TTH with MS/P should be investigated in future studies.

Conclusion

Compared with anxiety disorders, migraine was more strongly associated with MS/P in all areas at baseline and in the upper and lower limbs at the two-year follow-up point among patients with MDD. Headache intensity was the factor most strongly associated with MS/P in all areas at baseline and follow-up after controlling for depression, anxiety, and other factors. Headache intensity evaluated at baseline had impacts on MS/P in all areas not only at baseline, but also at the two-year follow-up point. Migraine and headache intensity should not be neglected in the treatment of MS/P in patients with MDD. Simultaneously, treatment of depression and headache might improve MS/P.

Abbreviations
GAD, generalized anxiety disorder; HADS, Hospital Anxiety and Depression Scale; HADS-A, anxiety subscale of the HADS; HADS-D, depression subscale of the HADS; ICHD-2, International Classification of Headache Disorders 2nd edition; MDD, major depressive disorder; MDE, major depressive episode; MS/P, muscle soreness or pain; TTH, tension-type headache, VAS visual analog scale

Acknowledgement
This study was supported in part by grants from the National Science Council of Taiwan (NSC 95-2314-B-182A-188-MY2) and Chang Gung Memorial Hospital Research Programs (CLRPG 3D0041and CMRPG3E0991). The funding sources had no further role in study design; in the collection, analysis and interpretation of data; in the writing of the report; and in the decision to submit the paper for publication.

Authors' contributions
SJW and CIH participated in the design of the study and wrote the protocol. CIH, CHY, and CYL collected the data. CIH performed the statistical analysis. CIH, CHY, and CYL interpreted the results. CIH wrote the first draft of the manuscript. All authors contributed to and have approved the final version.

Competing interests
All authors declare that they have no conflicts of interest.

Author details
[1]Department of Psychiatry, Chang Gung Memorial Hospital, Linkou, Taiwan. [2]Chang Gung University College of Medicine, Tao-Yuan, Taiwan. [3]Department of Nursing, Chang Gung University of Science and Technology, Tao-Yuan, Taiwan. [4]Faculty of Medicine, National Yang-Ming University School of Medicine and Neurological Institute, Taipei Veterans General Hospital, Taipei, Taiwan. [5]Department of Neurology, Taipei Veterans General Hospital, No. 201 Shi-Pai Road, Section 2, Taipei 112, Taiwan.

References
1. Means-Christensen AJ, Roy-Byrne PP, Sherbourne CD, Craske MG, Stein MB (2008) Relationships among pain, anxiety, and depression in primary care. Depress Anxiety 25:593–600
2. Björnsdóttir SV, Jónsson SH, Valdimarsdóttir UA (2014) Mental health indicators and quality of life among individuals with musculoskeletal chronic pain: a nationwide study in Iceland. Scand J Rheumatol 43:419–423
3. Shiri R, Kaila-Kangas L, Ahola K, Kivekäs T, Viikari-Juntura E, Heliövaara M, Miranda H, Leino-Arjas P (2013) The relation of co-occurring musculoskeletal pain and depressive symptoms with work ability. J Occup Environ Med 55:1281–1285
4. Altindag O, Gur A, Altindag A (2008) The relationship between clinical parameters and depression level in patients with myofascial pain syndrome. Pain Med 9:161–165
5. Karp JF, Scott J, Houck P, Reynolds CF 3rd, Kupfer DJ, Frank E (2005) Pain predicts longer time to remission during treatment of recurrent depression. J Clin Psychiatry 66:591–597
6. Zebenholzer K, Lechner A, Broessner G, Lampl C, Luthringshausen G, Wuschitz A, Obmann SM, Berek K, Wöber C (2016) Impact of depression and anxiety on burden and management of episodic and chronic headaches – a cross-sectional multicentre study in eight Austrian headache centres. J Headache Pain 17:15
7. Innamorati M, Pompili M, Erbuto D, Ricci F, Migliorati M, Lamis DA, Amore M, Girardi P, Martelletti P (2015) Psychometric properties of the stagnation scale in medication overuse headache patients. J Headache Pain 16:2
8. Pompili M, Serafini G, Di Cosimo D, Dominici G, Innamorati M, Lester D, Forte A, Girardi N, De Filippis S, Tatarelli R, Martelletti P (2010) Psychiatric comorbidity and suicide risk in patients with chronic migraine. Neuropsychiatr Dis Treat 6:81–91
9. Oedegaard KJ, Fasmer OB (2005) Is migraine in unipolar depressed patients a bipolar spectrum trait? J Affect Disord 84:233–242
10. Hung CI, Liu CY, Wang SJ (2013) Migraine predicts physical and pain symptoms among psychiatric outpatients. J Headache Pain 14:19
11. Fornaro M, De Berardis D, De Pasquale C, Indelicato L, Pollice R, Valchera A, Perna G, Iasevoli F, Tomasetti C, Martinotti G, Koshy AS, Fasmer OB, Oedegaard KJ (2015) Prevalence and clinical features associated to bipolar disorder-migraine comorbidity: a systematic review. Compr Psychiatry 56:1–16
12. Hung CI, Liu CY, Yang CH, Wang SJ (2012) The negative impact of migraine on quality of life after four weeks of treatment in patients with major depressive disorder. Psychiatry Clin Neurosci 66:8–16
13. Hung CI, Liu CY, Cheng TY, Wang SJ (2009) Migraine: a missing link between somatic symptoms and major depressive disorder. J Affect Disord 117:108–115
14. Hung CI, Liu CY, Chen CY, Yang CH, Wang SJ (2014) The impacts of migraine and anxiety disorders on painful physical symptoms among patients with major depressive disorder. J Headache Pain 15:73
15. Hagen K, Einarsen C, Zwart JA, Svebak S, Bovim G (2002) The co-occurrence of headache and musculoskeletal symptoms amongst 51 050 adults in Norway. Eur J Neurol 9:527–533
16. Poleshuck EL, Bair MJ, Kroenke K, Damush TM, Tu W, Wu J, Krebs EE, Giles DE (2009) Psychosocial stress and anxiety in musculoskeletal pain patients with and without depression. Gen Hosp Psychiatry 31:116–122
17. American Psychiatric Association (2000) Diagnostic and Statistical Manual of Mental Disorders, Fourth Edition Text Revision (DSM-IV-TR). American Psychiatric Association, Washington, DC
18. Coutu MF, Durand MJ, Marchand A, Labrecque ME, Berbiche D, Cadieux G (2013) Factors associated with generalized anxiety in workers undergoing work rehabilitation for persistent musculoskeletal pain. Disabil Rehabil 35:1599–1607
19. Mallen CD, Peat G, Thomas E, Dunn KM, Croft PR (2007) Prognostic factors for musculoskeletal pain in primary care: a systematic review. Br J Gen Pract 57:655–661
20. Vranceanu AM, Barsky A, Ring D (2009) Psychosocial aspects of disabling musculoskeletal pain. J Bone Joint Surg Am 91:2014–2018
21. Ligthart L, Gerrits MM, Boomsma DI, Penninx BW (2013) Anxiety and depression are associated with migraine and pain in general: an investigation of the interrelationships. J Pain 14:363–370
22. Hagen K, Linde M, Steiner TJ, Zwart JA, Stovner LJ (2012) The bidirectional relationship between headache and chronic musculoskeletal complaints: an 11-year follow-up in the Nord-Trondelag Health Study (HUNT). Eur J Neurol 19:1447–1454
23. Blaschek A, Milde-Busch A, Straube A, Schankin C, Langhagen T, Jahn K, Schröder SA, Reiter K, von Kries R, Heinen F (2012) Self-reported muscle pain in adolescents with migraine and tension-type headache. Cephalalgia 32:241–249
24. First MB, Spitzer RL, Gibbon M, Williams JBW (2002) Structured Clinical Interview for DSM-IV-TR Axis I Disorders, Research Version, Patient Edition (SCID-I/P). Biometrics Research, New York State Psychiatric Institute, New York
25. Headache Classification Subcommittee of the International Headache Society (2004) The International Classification of Headache Disorders, 2nd ed. Cephalalgia 24:1–160
26. Hung CI, Liu CY, Wang SJ, Yao YC, Yang CH (2012) The cut-off points of the Depression and Somatic Symptoms Scale and the Hospital Anxiety and Depression Scale in detecting non-full remission and a current major depressive episode. Int J Psychiatry Clin Pract 16:33–40
27. Zigmond AS, Snaith RP (1983) The hospital anxiety and depression scale. Acta Psychiatr Scand 67:361–370
28. Hung CI, Liu CY, Chen JJ, Wang SJ (2008) Migraine predicts self-reported muscle tension in patients with major depressive disorder. Psychosomatics 49:502–510

29. Aguggia M, Saracco MG, Cavallini M, Bussone G, Cortelli P (2013) Sensitization and pain. Neurol Sci 34:S37–S40
30. Yavuz BG, Aydinlar EI, Dikmen PY, Incesu C (2013) Association between somatic amplification, anxiety, depression, stress and migraine. J Headache Pain 14:53
31. Tietjen GE, Brandes JL, Peterlin BL, Eloff A, Dafer RM, Stein MR, Drexler E, Martin VT, Hutchinson S, Aurora SK, Recober A, Herial NA, Utley C, White L, Khuder SA (2009) Allodynia in migraine: association with comorbid pain conditions. Headache 49:1333–1344
32. Tarantino S, Capuano A, Torriero R, Citti M, Vollono C, Gentile S, Vigevano F, Valeriani M (2014) Migraine equivalents as part of migraine syndrome in childhood. Pediatr Neurol 51:645–649
33. Prakash S, Shah ND, Dholakia SY (2009) Recurrent limb pain and migraine: case reports and a clinical review. Cephalalgia 29:898–905
34. Saito Y, Fusayasu E, Iitsuka T, Takeshima T, Ohno K (2006) Familial limb pain in childhood: unusual manifestation of migraine? Brain Dev 28:660–662
35. Giamberardino MA, Affaitati G, Martelletti P, Tana C, Negro A, Lapenna D, Curto M, Schiavone C, Stellin L, Cipollone F, Costantini R (2015) Impact of migraine on fibromyalgia symptoms. J Headache Pain 17(1):28
36. Pae CU, Luyten P, Marks DM, Han C, Park SH, Patkar AA, Masand PS, Van Houdenhove B (2008) The relationship between fibromyalgia and major depressive disorder: a comprehensive review. Curr Med Res Opin 24:2359–2371
37. Küçükşen S, Genç E, Yilmaz H, Sallı A, Gezer İA, Karahan AY, Salbaş E, Cingöz HT, Nas Ö, Uğurlu H (2013) The prevalence of fibromyalgia and its relation with headache characteristics in episodic migraine. Clin Rheumatol 32:983–990
38. Jones GT, Atzeni F, Beasley M, Flüß E, Sarzi-Puttini P, Macfarlane GJ (2015) The prevalence of fibromyalgia in the general population: a comparison of the American college of rheumatology 1990, 2010, and modified 2010 classification criteria. Arthritis Rheumatol 67:568–575

Table 6 Quality of life (WHOQOL scores) among participants with headache, by headache type, with and without comorbid psychiatric disorder

Headache type	WHOQOL score (mean ± SD)								
	HADS-A caseness (*N* = 340)			HADS-D caseness (*N* = 109)			HADS-cAD caseness (*N* = 137)		
	Present	Absent	*p**	Present	Absent	*p**	Present	Absent	*p**
Migraine (*N* = 728)	25.7 ± 4.1	26.9 ± 3.9	<0.001	24.6 ± 2.9	26.9 ± 3.9	<0.001	22.7 ± 3.6	27.1 ± 3.7	<0.001
Tension-type headache (*N* = 863)	27.2 ± 3.8	28.4 ± 3.7	<0.001	24.9 ± 3.2	28.4 ± 3.7	<0.001	24.4 ± 3.2	28.4 ± 3.6	<0.001
Headache on ≥15 d/m (*N* = 161)	25.1 ± 4.2	26.2 ± 3.9	0.10	24.0 ± 3.2	25.9 ± 4.1	0.11	21.6 ± 3.4	26.4 ± 3.8	<0.001

*Student's t-test, d/m: days/month

Implications for Nepal

From the public-health perspective, there is reason for alarm in the high prevalences of these MDBs in Nepal. We found a clear negative impact on QoL in people with headache and comorbid psychiatric disorder. GBD2013 provides disability weights for these disorders [25], which, multiplied by prevalence, yield estimates of disability burden. Migraine, MOH, depression and anxiety are all in the top 20 causes of YLDs globally [25], while all seem to be more prevalent in Nepal than their respective global means [31, 32]. These facts, together with evidence of excessive comorbidity between headache disorders and anxiety, and indications of aggravated burden when they are comorbid, signal an urgent need for action backed by health policy. The global context is not good, either for headache, which is undertreated everywhere [60] (a failure that should not discourage attempts at remediation [26]), or for psychiatric disorders, for which only a minority of affected people receive adequate treatment in most countries around the world [61]. In Nepal, an underdeveloped country with multiple adversities [33], the challenges brought forward by these comorbid conditions are considerable; this resource-deficient country is not prepared to cope with them.

From the clinical perspective, patients with headache disorders can be expected to have an excess of psychiatric manifestations, and *vice versa*. Physicians in Nepal treating headache patients should be looking out among them for anxiety and depression as potentially aggravating comorbid factors likely to hinder management. Moreover, psychiatrists and others treating depression and anxiety can expect to encounter migraine and headache on ≥15 days/month at high levels. We summarise this as a need for reciprocal awareness.

We propose that a coordinated effort offers a solution from both perspectives – public-health and clinical. It requires training of health-care providers encountering headache patients to think beyond the somatic dimension: screening for both anxiety and depression, and collaborating with mental-health personnel in patient education on lifestyle, psychological treatment and behavioural strategies, may be appropriate options in addition to offering usual pharmacological interventions. This already happens to an extent in some cities where headache patients may be referred directly to psychiatrists, but these are a small minority. In the rural areas and in the high hills, such referrals are generally not possible. In these areas, and in the cities also, most headache care is and should be provided in primary care, for reasons related both to logistics and cost [60], as well as because it is feasible. In primary care is also where most depression and anxiety are encountered [62]. Bringing the management of common headache and common psychiatric disorders together under one primary-care roof, supported by educational initiatives and referral channels to specialist services, appears to be good health policy. We recommended its trial implementation in a circumscribed area as a first step, and enter a plea for urgency in this action.

Table 7 Quality of life (WHOQOL scores) among participants with HADS caseness, with and without comorbid headache

HADS caseness	WHOQOL score (mean ± SD)								
	Migraine (*N* = 728)			Tension-type headache (*N* = 863)			Headache on ≥15 d/m (*N* = 161)		
	Present	Absent	*p**	Present	Absent	*p**	Present	Absent	*p**
HADS-A (*N* = 340)	25.7 ± 4.1	26.5 ± 2.8	0.30	27.2 ± 3.8	26.5 ± 2.8	0.36	25.1 ± 4.2	26.5 ± 2.8	0.096
HADS-D (*N* = 109)	24.6 ± 2.9	26.5 ± 3.9	0.055	24.9 ± 3.2	26.5 ± 3.9	0.15	24.0 ± 3.2	26.5 ± 3.9	0.094
HADS-cAD (*N* = 137)	22.7 ± 3.6	24.2 ± 3.2	0.21	24.4 ± 3.2	24.2 ± 3.2	0.86	21.6 ± 3.4	24.2 ± 3.2	0.060

*Student's t-test, d/m: days/month

6

Post procedure headache in patients treated for neurovascular arteriovenous malformations and aneurysms using endovascular therapy

Sabrina Khan[1*], Faisal Mohammad Amin[1], John Hauerberg[2], Markus Holtmannspötter[3], Julie Falkenberg Petersen[1], Zainab Fakhril-Din[1], David Gaist[4,5] and Messoud Ashina[1]

Abstract

Background: Though endovascular therapy (EVT) is increasingly applied in the treatment of intracranial vascular lesions, little is known about the effect of EVT on post-procedure headache. We aimed to investigate the prevalence of headache in patients who have undergone EVT for cerebral arteriovenous malformations (AVMs) and aneurysms.

Methods: A total of 324 patients underwent EVT treatment for aneurysms and AVMs at the Danish National Hospital from January 2012 to December 2014. We applied strict exclusion criteria in order to minimize the effect of other factors on headache occurrence, e.g., craniotomy. Eligible subjects were phone-interviewed using a purpose-developed semi-structured questionnaire. Headaches were classified according to ICHD-III beta criteria.

Results: The 59 patients underwent treatment of aneurysms ($n = 43$), cranial dural fistulas ($n = 11$), and AVMs ($n = 5$). There was a significant increase in overall headache ($p = 0.017$) and tension-type headache (TTH) ($p = 0.012$) within the first 3 months after EVT compared to 1 month before EVT. However, at interview time (median 2.5 years post-EVT), the increase in overall headache, migraine, and tension-type headache was not statistically significant. A minority of patients experienced headaches for the first time within 3 months of their EVT (migraine 4, TTH 10). At interview time, 50 % of these new headaches still persisted.

Conclusion: Our results suggest a temporary increase in headache in the first 3 months after EVT, which normalizes over time. Clinicians may use this knowledge to better inform their patients of functional outcomes after their EVT procedure.

Keywords: Endovascular therapy, Arteriovenous malformation, Aneurysm, Headache, Post procedure, Risk

Background

Endovascular treatment (EVT) of intracranial vascular lesions as aneurysms or arteriovenous malformations (AVMs) has been increasingly applied in the last decades. Evidence suggests a reduction of post-treatment mortality and morbidity with the transition from open surgery to EVT [1]; however, functional outcomes such as headache after EVT have received only little attention. These vascular lesions may predispose to headache in their own right [2, 3], and several studies describe headache as a presenting symptom of both conditions [4, 5]. What is less known, is how this headache is affected by endovascular treatment procedures, and the expected time frame of headache resolution. Current studies in this field are contradictory, some showing headache improvement after EVT, others worsening of preexisting headaches [6–9]. Furthermore, it is unknown whether

* Correspondence: sabrina.khan@regionh.dk
[1]Danish Headache Center, Department of Neurology, Rigshospitalet Glostrup, Faculty of Health and Medical Sciences, University of Copenhagen, Nordre Ringvej 57, Glostrup 2600, Denmark

the treatment itself may induce headache in a patient without previous headache.

From a clinical perspective, uncovering any risk of post treatment headache and the temporal evolution of such a headache is important for optimal counseling of patients with treatment demanding vascular lesions.

The aim of the present study was to investigate the prevalence of headache in patients with intracranial aneurysms and AVMs after EVT, and to uncover whether EVT treatment predisposes to onset of new headache. For this purpose we retrospectively assessed headache characteristics in a cohort of patients with AVMs and aneurysms who had undergone EVT at a single institution.

Methods

Patients and data collection

Using a computerized registry maintained by the Department of Radiology, we identified all patients who underwent EVT for cerebral AVMs and aneurysms at a tertiary referral center at Rigshospitalet (the Danish National Hospital), Copenhagen, Denmark between January 2012 and December 2014. The first author assessed the medical records of all identified cases and based on this information, excluded those fulfilling one or more of the following exclusion criteria: 1) EVT undergone for conditions other than AVM and aneurysms, 2) non-EVT treatment of vessel malformation, e.g., open surgery, 3) multiple EVT treatments, 4) multiple records for the same patient, 5) other intracranial illnesses, 6) head trauma resulting in unconsciousness and hospitalization, 7) aphasia, or no command of Danish or English, 8) aged below 18 years at time of EVT, and 9) unreachable after 5 efforts.

The remaining eligible patients were interviewed via telephone using a purpose-developed semi-structured questionnaire aimed at eliciting any history of headache as well as possible headache after EVT. Headache status was established for the following time periods: (i) 1 year before EVT; (ii) 1 month before EVT; (iii) 3 months after EVT; and (iv) at time of interview. The semi-structured interview allowed for diagnosis of headaches according to the International Classification of Headache Disorders 3 beta version. Headaches where classified as migraine (with and without aura), tension-type headache, and "overall headache". Overall headache included migraine, tension-type headache, probable migraine, probable tension-type headache, cluster headache, and headaches that could not be classified due to lack of information. The first author and two medical students trained by the first author conducted all interviews in the period of August 2014 to February 2016.

The Committee on Health Research Ethics, Capital Region approved the study. All patients provided written informed consent.

Statistical analysis

Frequencies and percentages were calculated for categorical variables and medians and range were calculated for continuous variables. For comparisons of categorical data we used McNemars test. All p-values were two-sided and we considered p-values below 0.05 to be statistically significant. All analyses were performed using IBM® SPSS® Statistics version 23.

Results

A total of 830 patients were identified in the register. Of these patients, 324 had undergone EVT for aneurysms ($n = 239$) or AVMs ($n = 85$) (Fig. 1). The AVM group comprised patients that had undergone embolization for various malformations including arteriovenous fistulas, spinal dural arteriovenous fistulas, and dural arteriovenous fistulas (DAVFs). After application of exclusion criteria, a total of 59 eligible subjects were included in the study (43 treated for aneurysms, 16 treated for AVMs). Median age at time of EVT was 57 years (range: 30–87 years). Median time from EVT procedure to interview was 2.5 years (range: 1.2–3.8 years). Clinical and demographic characteristics of study participants are outlined in Table 1.

Patients treated for aneurysms underwent coiling, stenting, coiling and stenting combined, and placement of web-devices (table 1). Fifteen of the aneurysms had ruptured, 28 were unruptured. Patients treated with aneurysm coiling ($n = 26$) received standard antithrombotic care after EVT, which in Denmark consists of aspirin treatment for 2 months. Patients where aneurysms were treated with stent placement ($n = 11$), were prescribed aspirin for 6 months along with an additional antiplatelet medication for the first 3 months.

AVMs were treated with embolization solely (2 partial occlusions, 3 complete occlusions), while DAVFs were treated with embolization or embolization and coiling combined (2 partial occlusions, 9 complete occlusions). The most common localizations of vascular malformations, fistulas, and aneurysms were the internal carotid arteries and the basilar artery (Fig. 2).

Headache status before and after EVT

A similar number of patients experienced overall headaches 3 months after EVT compared with 1 year before the procedure (31 versus 32 patients; 23 treated for aneurysms, 8 treated for AVMs) (Fig. 3, Table 2). All but one patient with migraine continued to experience migraine attacks post-EVT (9 versus 8 subjects). Slightly more subjects experienced TTH 3 months after EVT compared with the year before the procedure (20 versus 24 subjects, $p = 0.5$). However, none of the above comparisons were statistically significant. Extending the post-EVT window of comparison from 3 months to "time of interview" (on average 2.5 years after EVT) had

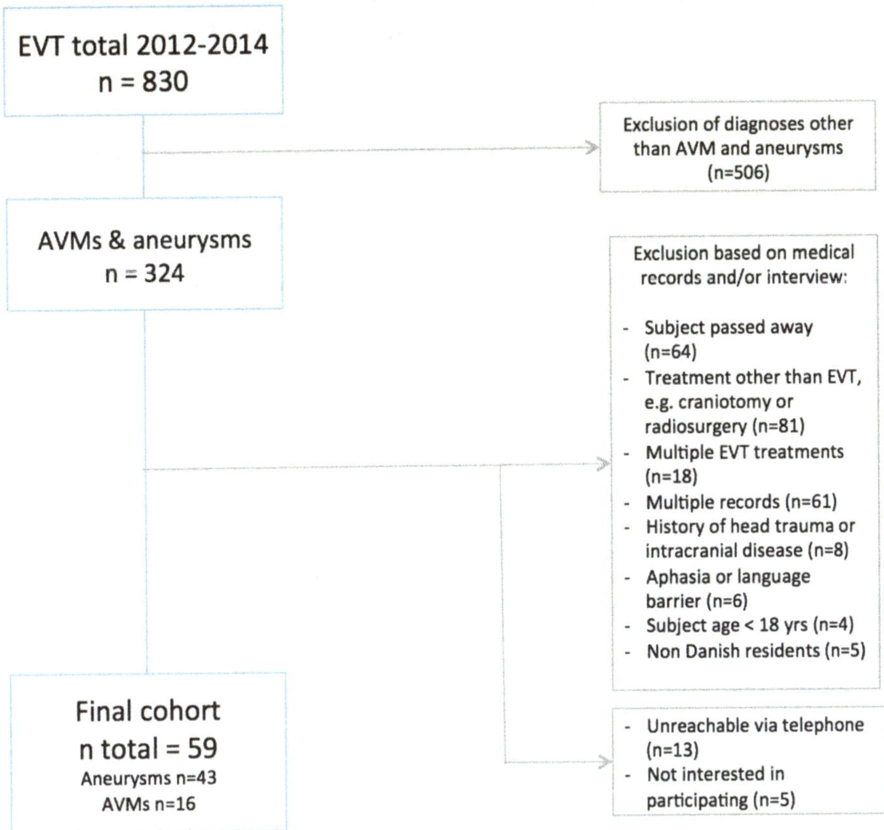

Fig. 1 Study enrolment

little impact on TTH (20 versus 19 subjects), while for migraine headaches; a larger albeit not statistically significant reduction was observed (9 versus 6 subjects, $p = 0.5$).

We also compared patients' headache status 1 month before EVT with 3 months after EVT, as an expression of peri-procedural headache status. Here we found an increase in overall headache (19 versus 31 subjects, $p = 0.017$), tension-type headache (12 versus 24 subjects, $p = 0.012$), and migraine (4 versus 8 subjects, $p = 0.3$) within the first 3 months after EVT. At interview time, there was still an increase in overall headache (19 versus 27 subjects, $p = 0.1$; 19 treated for aneurysms, 8 treated for AVMs), migraine (4 versus 6 subjects, $p = 0.7$) and tension-type headache (12 versus 19 subjects, $p = 0.1$), though none of these results reached statistical significance.

We also asked patients about headaches experienced at any time prior to EVT, as a measure of pre-intervention lifetime headache prevalence in this patient group. Compared to headache experienced at interview time, there was a significant decrease in overall headache (45 versus 27 subjects, $p < 0.001$) and migraine (15 versus 6 subjects, $p = 0.022$).

In patients treated for aneurysms and who reported headache after EVT, coiling was the most prevalent procedure followed by stenting, both at 3 months after EVT (23 subjects with overall headache; coiling = 13, stent = 7) and at time of interview (19 subjects with overall headache; coiling = 11, stent = 5, coiling + stent = 12).

Headache frequency before and after EVT

Comparing migraine frequency before and after EVT, there was an increase in headache days during the first 3 months post-procedure (31–45 headache days per 3 months) compared to both 1 year, and 1 month before EVT (6–12 headache days per month) (Table 3). However, at interview time, the frequency had regressed towards 1–5 headache days per month.

Headache frequency of TTH showed a similar pattern over time, although far less pronounced, with an increase in headache days the first 3 months after EVT (6–12 headache days per 3 months) and a regression to pre-EVT frequency at time of interview (1–5 headache days per month).

De novo headaches after EVT

In all, 10 of 24 subjects with TTH post-procedure experienced this headache type for the first time in their lives during the first 3 months after EVT (Fig. 4). By the time

Table 1 Clinical and demographic characteristics of endovascularly treated patients

Characteristics	
Median age and range	57,4 (30–87)
Males	21
Right-handed	50
Median height and range (cm)	169 (154 – 203)
Median weight and range (kg)	74 (48 – 106)
Median BMI and range (kg/m^2)	25 (17–39)
Vascular disorder	
- Aneurysms	43
- AVMs	5
- DAVFs	11
Aneurysm procedures	
- Coiling	26
- Stenting	11
- Coiling + stenting	4
- Web device	2
AVM procedures	
- Embolization	5
DAVF procedures	
- Embolization	9
- Embolization + coiling	2

AVM arteriovenous malformation, DAVF dural arteriovenous fistula

of interview, only 5 patients still experienced these headaches.

First time ever attacks of migraine were experienced by 4 subjects in the 3 month period after EVT, and two of these patients still experienced migraine attacks at time of interview (2.1 and 2.6 years after EVT, respectively), with a median frequency of 25–45 headache days per 3 months.

There was no correlation between side of procedure and headache laterality (data not shown).

Discussion

Existing studies on post-EVT headache in patients with aneurysms and AVMs show diverging results, generally favoring improvement of headache after treatment [8, 9]. Where an exacerbation was found, it was typically reported to be temporary and to resolve within days or months [6–8, 10]. Nevertheless, however short-lived these headaches may be, the majority still defy the strict time frame defined by the International Headache Classification, stating that headaches attributed to intracranial endovascular procedures develop within seconds and resolve within 24 h of the procedure [2]. For this reason, it has been suggested that ICHD-III beta criteria may not properly reflect clinical reality in terms of the temporal aspect of a possible headache after EVT [11]. Our data support this notion, as we found an increase in headache prevalence within the first three months after EVT compared to one month before EVT. At time of interview, this increase had regressed towards prevalence estimates similar to those reported in studies of the general Danish population for subjects with migraine. For tension-type headache, the prevalence also decreased over time, but was generally lower than corresponding numbers from Danish population-studies.

Possible reasons for these temporary headaches after EVT include local inflammation due to placement of foreign objects such as stents, coils or glue, and mechanical stimulation of the arterial wall [6, 8, 10]. Other explanations include changes in flow dynamics after EVT causing the release or stress of a venous overload [5, 11], possibly leading to post-procedural headache. This mechanism may be particularly true of AVMs.

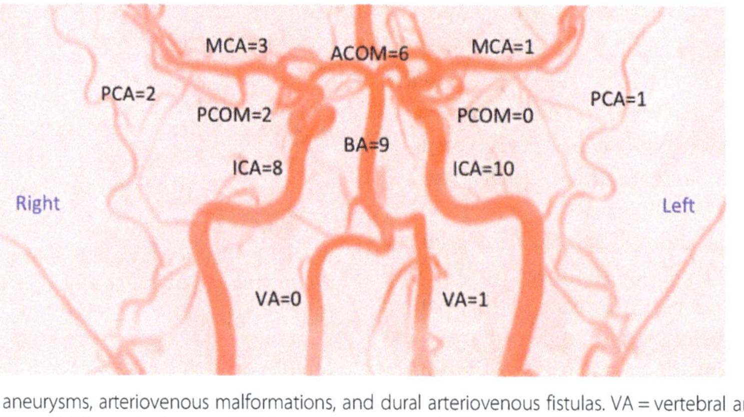

Fig. 2 Localization of treated aneurysms, arteriovenous malformations, and dural arteriovenous fistulas. VA = vertebral artery, BA = basilar artery, ICA = internal carotid artery, MCA = middle cerebral artery, ACOM = anterior communicating artery, PCOM = posterior communicating artery, PCA = posterior cerebral artery. Another 16 localizations were distributed as follows: Left MCA + ICA = 1; bilateral ICA = 1; ophthalmic artery = 1; cavernous sinus = 1; left sigmoid sinus = 1, and unspecified locations (n = 11)

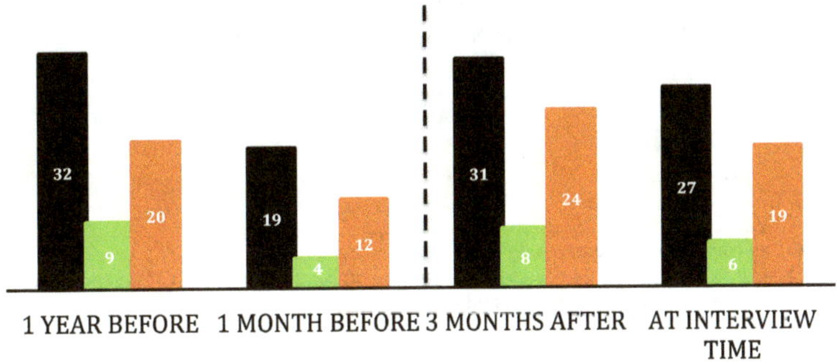

Fig. 3 Headache status before and after endovascular treatment. Numbers represent patients. Overall headache includes migraine with aura, migraine without aura, tension-type headache, probable migraine, probable tension-type headache, cluster headache, and unclassified headache. Red dotted line represents the endovascular procedure

A sub-group analysis of our cohort suggests that post-EVT headache may be more prevalent after coiling of aneurysms, followed by stent-placements. This is in line with previous studies, suggesting that use of a stent device is associated with increase of headache [6, 8]. It also seems that post-procedure headache is more prevalent in patients treated for aneurysms compared to AVMs. However, aneurysms are overrepresented in our cohort, and for this reason, along with generally small numbers in this subgroup analysis, we acknowledge that no firm conclusions can be made based on our tentative findings.

A potential correlation between aneurysms, AVMs and headache is no new concept, and studies have suggested that for patients harboring these vascular anomalies, headache may be more prevalent than in the general population [3, 4, 12]. Based on epidemiological studies of the general Danish population, the lifetime cumulated prevalence for both sexes is 16–18 % for migraine and 78 % for tension-type headache [13, 14]. With this study, we report a lifetime prevalence of 25 % for migraine, and 46 % for tension-type headache, suggesting that patients with aneurysms and AVMs are predisposed specifically to migraine. The pathophysiological mechanism responsible for this increase in migraine prevalence may be related to the very angioarchitecture of these vascular conditions, which, per definition, is abnormal. Lebedeva et al. suggested that increased sensory input from sensory nerve endings around the aneurysms may sensitize the central nervous system decreasing the threshold for developing spontaneous migraine attacks [4]. Other possible mechanisms predisposing to headache include local thrombosis, meningeal inflammation, expansion and inflammation of the aneurysm, and bleeding within the vessel wall; ultimately activating nociceptive C-fibers of the trigeminal nerve [4, 15]. For AVMs, Galletti et al. showed the location of AVMs to be significantly associated with migraine-like headache presentation, leading the authors to suggest that hemodynamic and structural

Table 2 Comparison of 59 patients' headache status before and after endovascular treatment

	Anytime before (n)	Interview time (n)[a]		*P*-value
Overall headache	45	27		0.0003*
Migraine	15	6		0.022*
Tension-type headache	27	19		0.077
	1 year before (n)	Interview time (n)	Change (%)	*P*-value
Overall headache	32	27	−16	0.302
Migraine	9	6	−33	0.453
Tension-type headache	20	19	−5	1.000
	1 month before (n)	3 months after (n)	Change (%)	*P*-value
Overall headache	19	31	+63	0.017*
Migraine	4	8	+100	0.289
Tension-type headache	12	24	+100	0.012*

[a]Median time from EVT procedure to interview: 2.5 years
**P*-values under 0.05

Table 3 Headache frequency before and after endovascular treatment

	Headache day score in relation to endovascular procedure			
	1 year before	1 month before	3 months after	At interview time
Migraine	2 (1 – 7) $n = 9$	2.5 (2 – 3) $n = 4$	5 (1 – 7) $n = 8$	1 (1 – 4) $n = 6$
Tension-type headache	3 (1 – 7) $n = 20$	1 (1 – 3) $n = 12$	2 (0 – 7) $n = 24$	1 (0 – 4) $n = 19$

Frequency represented as a headache score corresponding to following intervals: 0 = no headache days, 1 = 1–5 headache days, 2 = 6–12 headache days, 3 = 13–24 headache days, 4 = 25–30 headache days, 5 = 31–45 headache days, 6 = 46–60 headache days, and 7 = more than 60 headache days. Headache scores listed as median and range

changes caused by AVMs in the occipital lobe may trigger spreading depression and thus migraine [5].

For 1-year prevalence of headache, our data support the general knowledge of migraine prevalence, with 15 % reporting migraine in our cohort (9 out of 59 subjects within the last year prior to EVT) versus 10 % in the general Danish population [14]. The 1-year prevalence of tension-type headache is smaller in our cohort, with a prevalence of 34 % versus 74 % in the general Danish population [14]. In contrast to our results, Lebedeva et al. found a significant increase in the 1-year prevalence of migraine without aura in subjects with aneurysms (42.2 %) compared to controls (8.8 %), but no significant change in tension-type headache (19.6 % versus 23.1 %) [4]. However, important methodological differences exist between the studies, which impede direct comparisons. Subjects in the study by Lebedeva et al. were interviewed at time of admission to hospital upon rupture of their aneurysm. As thunderclap headache is the common presentation of aneurysms, the painful condition of the subjects at time of interview may have biased their recall of headaches. Conversely, in our study we interviewed patients after EVT, and it can be argued that the overall success of the procedure as seen from a patient perspective, may have influenced the subjects' recollection of their headaches, e.g., with a successful procedure leading to less focus on or recall of concomitant headache. It can be argued that the inclusion of 15 patients with ruptured aneurysms at the time of EVT could influence our results in so far that patients with this condition can experience headaches up to 1 month after the event [2]. However, in a post hoc analysis we excluded these 15 patients, and found similar results (1 month before vs. 3 months after, migraine: 3 subjects vs 6 subjects; TTH: 7 subjects vs 19 subjects).

In our cohort, a fraction of patients experienced onset of new headache after EVT. Three months post EVT, 10 subjects experienced tension-type headache, and 4 subjects experienced migraine; these numbers declined to 5 and 2 subjects, respectively, at time of interview. Albeit small in numbers, these de novo headaches may still be indicative of a causal relationship between EVT and headache, especially when considering the cohort median age of 57 years. Migraine onset in this age group is highly unusual [16]. We also note that some patients experience only temporary headache after EVT while others progress to persistent headache. Schwedt and colleagues suggest that central sensitization may contribute to the persistence of any such new headache following EVT [8].

In terms of classification of these post-procedural headaches, any de novo headache occurring for the first time after EVT is a secondary headache and would optimally be classified as a "headache attributed to

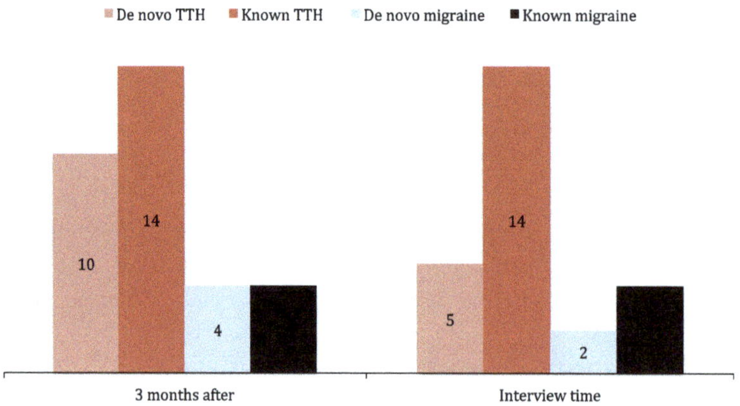

Fig. 4 Distribution of de novo headaches and known headache after endovascular treatment. Numbers represent patients. TTH = tension-type headache

intracranial endovascular procedure" [2]. However, as per the current definition, this headache resolves within 24 h after EVT, thus not fitting the temporal pattern of headache observed in our cohort. By comparison, the classification for "acute headache attributed to craniotomy" allows for headache duration of up to 3 months after surgical intervention. We believe this time frame to be more appropriate for our results, which suggested an increased prevalence of headache for the first 3 months after EVT that thereafter regresses over time. Faced with these classification complexities, we chose to classify all post-procedural headaches as primary headaches, although we fully acknowledge that de novo headaches with a causal and temporal relation to EVT can be conceived as secondary headaches.

Strengths of this study include a subject group comprised of two vascular conditions both treated with the introduction of foreign bodies including coils, glue, and stenting. Subjects were consecutively included at a single tertiary referral center. All interviews were conducted by medical specialists trained in diagnosing headaches according to the ICHD-III beta, using purpose-developed questionnaires and through direct, telephone contact. Also, to describe the evolution of headaches over time, we specifically collected information on subjects' headaches at multiple time-points before and after EVT. Finally, we pooled subjects with aneurysms and AVMs, as these conditions both comprise vascular anomalies and may predispose to headache by way of similar angioarchitectural mechanisms.

Because of its retrospective nature, recall bias is an inherent limitation of our study. Remembering characteristics of headaches occurring several years prior to EVT may pose a considerable challenge to some patients, which can result in some degree of headache diagnosis inaccuracy. Also, we recognize the limitation of our sample size. However, the relatively small sample size was partly due to a conscious choice on our behalf, i.e., our adherence to strict exclusion criteria so as to minimize bias introduced by inclusion of other conditions or treatments than the ones under study. Nonetheless, we cannot rule out the impact of clinical diversity on our results due to inter- and intra-group heterogeneities (e.g., aneurysms versus AVMs and a large aneurysm versus a small aneurysm, ruptured versus unruptured aneurysms, etc.), which we could only address in a limited fashion, i.e., in analyses stratified by type of vascular malformation (aneurysm vs. AVM).

For headache after EVT, we lack information on the time period between 3 months after EVT and up to the time of the interview, which took place 2.5 years after EVT on average. This would have provided us with a more detailed understanding of the evolution of a post--procedural headache.

Finally, one could argue that headache in the wake of such serious and potentially debilitating conditions is only a minor concern. Nevertheless, we do find it important to investigate functional outcomes after EVT in this patient group, particularly for those patients who are successfully treated for their primary condition, but where EVT results in other negative consequences such as persistent headache, which indeed may be highly disabling for the affected individual.

Conclusion

In conclusion, our results indicate that EVT performed in subjects with intracranial aneurysms and AVMs leads to a temporary increase in headache for the first three months after EVT. Over time, this increase in headache status regresses towards prevalence estimates resembling those of the general Danish population. Also, new onset of headache in a smaller fraction of subjects experienced in the first three months after EVT resolves over time in half of the cases. This knowledge of a potentially short-lived headache after EVT holds significant clinical value, as it may lead to better counseling of subjects about to undergo EVT and optimization of treatment efforts in cases where post-procedural headache does occur. Finally, we tentatively suggest that the current ICHD-3 beta definition of headache attributed to intracranial vascular procedures may be sub-optimal, as our results show that any such headache may well last more than the allowed 24 h. Prospective studies are warranted to closely follow headache patterns within shorter time intervals after EVT. This will allow us to further uncover even small exacerbations in headache, which inadvertently may affect the quality of life for the individual patient, however temporary these changes may prove to be.

Funding

We thank the Lundbeck Foundation (R155-2014-171), the Novo Nordisk Foundation (NNF11OC1014333), and the European Union's Seventh Framework programme (FP7-EUROHEADPAIN-no.602633).

Authors' contributions

SK designed and performed the study, with the help of FMA, DG and MA. SK performed interviews, and drafted the manuscript. SK and FMA performed the statistical analyses. JH and MH contributed with access to the patient data registry and valuable input to the manuscript, along with DG and MA. JFP and ZFD participated in interviewing of subjects. All authors read and approved the final manuscript.

Competing interests

The authors declare that they have no competing interests.

Author details

[1]Danish Headache Center, Department of Neurology, Rigshospitalet Glostrup, Faculty of Health and Medical Sciences, University of Copenhagen, Nordre Ringvej 57, Glostrup 2600, Denmark. [2]Department of Neurosurgery, Rigshospitalet, Faculty of Health and Medical Sciences, University of Copenhagen, Copenhagen, Denmark. [3]Department of Radiology, Rigshospitalet, Faculty of Health and Medical Sciences, University of Copenhagen, Copenhagen, Denmark. [4]Department of Neurology, Odense University Hospital, Odense, Denmark. [5]Department of Clinical Research,

Faculty of Health Sciences, University of Southern Denmark, Odense, Denmark.

References

1. Alshekhlee A, Mehta S, Edgell RC, Vora N, Feen E, Mohammadi A et al (2010) Hospital mortality and complications of electively clipped or coiled unruptured intracranial aneurysm. Stroke 41(7):1471–1476
2. Headache Classification Committee of the International Headache Society (IHS). Cephalalgia : an international journal of headache. 2013;33(9):629–808.
3. Esmanhotto BB, Piovesan EJ, Lange MC (2016) Brazilian experience of the influence of endovascular treatment on headache in patients with ruptured intracranial aneurysms. Acta Neurol Scand 5:10–14
4. Lebedeva ER, Gurary NM, Sakovich VP, Olesen J (2013) Migraine before rupture of intracranial aneurysms. J Headache Pain 14(1):15
5. Galletti F, Sarchielli P, Hamam M, Costa C, Cupini LM, Cardaioli G et al (2011) Occipital arteriovenous malformations and migraine. Cephalalgia 31(12):1320–1324
6. Choi K-S, Lee J-H, Yi H-J, Chun H-J, Lee Y-J, Kim D-W (2014) Incidence and risk factors of postoperative headache after endovascular coil embolization of unruptured intracranial aneurysms. Acta Neurochir (Wien) 156(7):1281–1287
7. Hwang G, Jeong E-A, Sohn JH, Park H, Bang JS, Jin S-C et al (2012) The characteristics and risk factors of headache development after the coil embolization of an unruptured aneurysm. AJNR Am J Neuroradiol 33(9): 1676–1678
8. Schwedt TJ, Gereau RW, Frey K, Kharasch ED (2011) Headache outcomes following treatment of unruptured intracranial aneurysms: a prospective analysis. Cephalalgia 31(10):1082–1089
9. Qureshi AI, Suri MFK, Kim SH, Olson K, Siddiqui AM, Yahia AM et al (2003) Effect of endovascular treatment on headaches in patients with unruptured intracranial aneurysms. Headache 43(10):1090–1096
10. Martins IP, Baeta E, Paiva T, Campos J, Gomes L (1993) Headaches during intracranial endovascular procedures: a possible model of vascular headache. Headache 33(5):227–233
11. Baron EP, Moskowitz SI, Tepper SJ, Gupta R, Novak E, Hussain MS et al (2012) Headache following intracranial neuroendovascular procedures. Headache 52(5):739–748
12. Waltimo O, Hokkanen E, Pirskanen R (2007) Intracranial arteriovenous malformations and headache. Book 23(1):12–14
13. Russell MB, Rasmussen BK, Thorvaldsen P, Olesen J (1995) Prevalence and sex-ratio of the subtypes of migraine. Int J Epidemiol 24(3):612–618
14. Rasmussen BK, Jensen R, Schroll M, Olesen J (1991) Epidemiology of headache in a general population–a prevalence study. J Clin Epidemiol 44(11):1147–1157
15. Raps EC, Rogers JD, Galetta SL, Solomon RA, Lennihan L, Klebanoff LM et al (1993) The clinical spectrum of unruptured intracranial aneurysms. Arch Neurol 50(3):265–268
16. Olesen J, Goadsby PJ, Ramadan NM, Tfelt-Hansen P, Welch KMA. The Headaches. 3rd ed. Philadelphia: Lippincott Williams & Wilkins; 2006.

7

Headache yesterday in Karnataka state, India: prevalence, impact and cost

Timothy J. Steiner[1,2*], Girish N. Rao[3], Girish B. Kulkarni[4], Gopalkrishna Gururaj[3] and Lars J. Stovner[1,5]

Abstract

Background: The Global Campaign against Headache has pioneered evaluation of the prevalence and impact of headache on the preceding day ("headache yesterday") as a new approach to the estimation of headache-attributed burden, avoiding recall error. We report its application in Karnataka State, southern India.

Methods: In a door-to-door survey, biologically unrelated adults (aged 18–65 years) were randomly sampled from urban and rural areas in and around Bengaluru and interviewed by trained researchers using a validated, structured questionnaire. Enquiry into headache applied ICHD-II diagnostic criteria and included questions about headache on the day preceding the interview (headache yesterday [HY]).

Results: There were 2329 participants (participation proportion 92.6 %; males 1141 [49.0 %], females 1188 [51.0 %]; mean age 38.0 [±12.7] years; 1103 [47.4 %] from rural areas, 1226 [52.6 %] urban). HY was reported by 138 participants (males 33 [2.9 %], females 105 [8.8 %]): the 1-day prevalence of headache was 5.9 %. Mean duration of HY was 7.0 ± 8.5 h, so that 1.7 % of the population (5.9 % * 7.0/24), on average, had headache at any moment in time yesterday. Mean intensity on a scale of 1–3 was 2.0 [±0.8]. Lost productivity due to HY was reported by 83.3 % of participants with HY: 37.7 % able to do less than half of what they had planned and 13.0 % able to do nothing. Productivity loss at population level (being the productivity loss within the entire adult population, every single day, attributable to headache) was 3.0 %.

Conclusions: This method of enquiry, free from recall error, confirmed a very high level of headache-attributed burden in Karnataka: previous estimates based on 3-month recall may even have been too low. Until another study is done in the country, these are the best data for all India. They demonstrate need for action nationwide to mitigate this burden, and correct action will ultimately almost certainly be cost-saving.

Keywords: Headache yesterday, Migraine, Tension-type headache, Medication-overuse headache, Burden, Cost, Health policy, India, Global Campaign against Headache

Background

The very heavy disability burden attributable to headache disorders is becoming increasingly clear [1, 2]. The Global Burden of Disease Study 2010 (GBD2010) ranked tension-type headache (TTH) and migraine as the second and third most common diseases worldwide [3], but many of the data included in this world survey derived from heterogeneous studies performed with varying methods over a period of nearly 30 years. In all regions except the Far East, more recent studies–of migraine in particular–have generally yielded higher prevalence estimates than the global mean estimates of GBD2010 [3] or GBD2013 [1]. This has been particularly apparent in low- and lower-middle-income countries: Georgia [4], India [5], Nepal [6], Zambia [7], Ethiopia (unpublished) and Pakistan (unpublished). In part this is explained by the careful methodology of recent studies [8, 9]. To a greater extent it may be because many earlier published studies excluded probable migraine: many reports are silent on how ICHD diagnostic criteria were applied with respect to definite and probable migraine; some explicitly excluded the latter, but a larger number may have done so without making this clear.

* Correspondence: t.steiner@imperial.ac.uk
[1]Department of Neuroscience, Norwegian University of Science and Technology (NTNU), Edvard Griegs Gate, Trondheim NO-7491, Norway
[2]Division of Brain Sciences, Imperial College London, London, UK

The expectation, as the Global Campaign against Headache [10, 11] continues its drive to conduct population-based studies in those parts of the world where data are currently lacking–mostly in low- and lower-middle-income countries, is that global mean prevalence estimates will continue to rise. With them, estimates of burden will rise also, as they have done through the iterative GBD studies since 2000 [2]. These estimates are the basis of needs assessments informing health policy and allocation of health-care resources.

When disease burdens are large and the call upon resources is substantial, estimates need to be as accurate as possible. The methodology for measuring headache-attributed burden is a relatively new and still developing science [8, 9]: in the last 30 years, many population-based studies of headache have assessed prevalence only. It is a field of innovation to which *Lifting The Burden* (LTB) [12, 13] has actively contributed in leading the Global Campaign against Headache. The components of headache-attributed burden are wide-ranging, and some are challenging to measure [9]. Symptom burden can be measured in terms of frequency, intensity and duration. The GBD studies use frequency and duration to estimate the proportion of time spent with symptoms, and apply a disability weight to this proportion of time to calculate the associated health loss [3]. For socioeconomic impact, the Headache-Attributed Lost Time (HALT) Index [14] enquires into effect of headache on productivity. In its original form (HALT-90), it relied upon a respondent's recall over the 3 months prior to the interview, that period of enquiry being intended to gather a representative view of each participant's lost productive time. This approach has its uses, but is subject to the limitations, errors and possible biases of recall over such a long period.

LTB has pioneered an alternative approach to avoid the problems associated with recall error, which is enquiry into headache occurring on the day before the interview ("headache yesterday"; HY) [8]. Recollection of HY, its symptoms and whatever impact they may have had, is likely to be highly reliable. While what happened yesterday is not representative, or therefore indicative, of an individual's headache-attributed burden over longer periods of time, at population level it is. This approach does, however, require a large number of participants, since far fewer people have headache in 1 day than in 3 months.

A question subset concerning HY [9] has been included in several recent large epidemiological studies supported by LTB within the Global Campaign against Headache: in China [15], Russia [16], countries of the Eurolight project [17] and several others not yet published. Here we report the analysis of HY in Karnataka State, southern India, and make comparisons with estimates based on 3 months' recall [18]. We apply the analysis in making an estimate of socioeconomic burden attributable to headache disorders in Karnataka State, and consider extrapolating this to all India.

Methods

The methods of the study have been published in detail previously [19] and are described only briefly here.

Study design and sampling

This was a cross-sectional survey, conducted during May to November 2009. It sampled urban and rural areas in and around Bengaluru: Kempegowdanagara, an urban administrative ward in the city of Bengaluru, and Uyamballi and Doddaaladahalli, two large villages located 75–80 Km from Bengaluru. Trained interviewers selected households randomly through multistage cluster sampling. They called at each household unannounced, listed all adult members (aged 18–65 years), randomly selected one and interviewed that person.

Enquiry and diagnosis

The survey instrument was a cultural adaptation of LTB's structured HARDSHIP questionnaire [9], translated into the local language (Kannada) in accordance with LTB's translation protocol for hybrid documents [20], and validated [19]. It began with demographic enquiry. The headache screening question ("Have you had headache during the last year?") and diagnostic questions based on ICHD-II [21] were followed, for those reporting headache, by multiple question sets enquiring into various aspects of burden, including the HALT questionnaire [14]. Participants reporting more than one headache type were asked to focus only on the one that was subjectively the most bothersome for purposes of diagnosis and burden attribution.

Diagnoses were made algorithmically. Participants with headache on ≥15 days/month were first identified; among these, any with medication overuse were diagnosed as probable MOH (pMOH), the remainder as "other headache on ≥15 days/month". The algorithm then applied ICHD-II criteria to all other cases in hierarchical sequence: first for definite migraine, then for definite TTH, then for probable migraine and finally for probable TTH. Remaining cases were considered unclassifiable. In the analysis, definite migraine and probable migraine were grouped as migraine, and definite TTH and probable TTH as TTH.

Questions on HY (in response to "Did you have headache yesterday?") included duration of HY (in hours up to 24), intensity of HY (reported by participants on a three-point categorical score ["not bad", "quite bad" and "very bad"]) and usage of acute medications. Lost productivity because of HY was reported as what had been done yesterday considered with regard to what had been planned or expected to be done: "everything", "more than half ", "less than half" or "nothing". The analysis of HALT offsets those who had done less than half against those who had done more than half, counting the former as doing nothing and the latter as doing everything [9, 14].

Statistics and analyses

Data were entered into a secure database and statistical analyses were performed using EPI INFO [22] and SPSS version 15.

We used proportions (%) to report prevalences, with 95 % confidence intervals (CIs) when appropriate. We used means, with standard deviations (SDs) and/or standard errors (SEs), and medians to summarise the distributions of continuous variables. Headache intensity responses "not bad", "quite bad" and "very bad" were equated to "mild", "moderate" and "severe" and converted to a numerical rating scale 1–3, which we treated as continuous data. We used Fisher's exact test for significance of differences. We set the level of significance at $p < 0.05$.

We calculated the predicted 1-day prevalence of any headache and of headache types from the 1-year prevalence and estimated mean frequency (F) in days/year (extrapolated from the last 3 months) using the formula:

$$\text{1-day prevalence} = \text{1-year prevalence} * F/365$$

We calculated total lost productivity as a proportion (%), the numerator being the sum of those reporting nothing or less than half done and the denominator the number (N) who reported HY.

Results

There were 2329 participants (1141 [49.0 %] male, 1188 [51.0 %] female; mean age 38.0 [±12.7] years; 1103 [47.4 %] from rural areas, 1226 [52.6 %] urban). The participation proportion was 92.6 % (eligible population n = 2514). The distributions of gender, age and habitation in the participating sample have been described in detail previously and were comparable to those of the population of Karnataka [19]. As reported previously, the 1-year prevalence of any headache was 63.9 %; the age-standardised 1-year prevalence of migraine was 25.2 % and of TTH was 35.1 %; the age-standardised prevalence of all causes of headache on ≥15 days/month was 3.0 % and of pMOH was 1.2 % [5].

Headache yesterday

HY was reported by 138 participants, representing a 1-day prevalence of headache of 5.9 %. The predicted 1-day prevalence of any headache calculated from its 1-year prevalence of 63.9 % and estimated mean frequency of 32.0 days/year [5] was 5.6 %, a very close match.

HY was reported by over three times as many females (8.8 %) as males (2.9 %) (Table 1). Reporting of HY varied with age, but with wide and overlapping confidence intervals. Almost three quarters of HY (73.9 %) was reported by rural participants, despite that they made up less than half (47.4 %) of the participating sample. These data are also shown in Table 1.

HY was reported to be typical of their usual most bothersome (diagnosed) headache by only 95 (68.8 %) of those with HY. This limited the inferences we could draw about HY diagnostically. Among these 95 only, we could make reasonable assumptions as to diagnosis; on these, we based calculations of predicted 1-day prevalences by headache type (Table 2). There was an exact match for migraine and a close match for pMOH; TTH and other headache on ≥15 days/month were underreported yesterday, and may have been preferentially among the cases of HY not considered typical of the usual most bothersome headache. For all HY, as noted above, there was a good match.

Mean duration of HY was 7.0 ± 8.5 h. From this we calculated that 1.7 % of the population (5.9 % * 7.0/24), on average, had headache at any moment in time yesterday. The median was 3 h; therefore HY was quite short-lasting in more than half of cases. If this reflected usage of acute medications, these were taken by 46.3 % of participants with HY–that is, 2.5 % of the total survey sample. By implication this meant that, on any day, 2.5 % of the adult population were using acute medication for headache. A further 36.9 % used local applications of various sorts, including 4.3 % who used both medication and local applications. Headache intensity was severe in 29.7 %, moderate in 46.4 % and mild in 23.9 %. Mean intensity on a scale of 1–3 was therefore 2.0 [±0.8] (SE: 0.07).

Lost productivity due to HY was reported to some degree by 83.3 % of participants with HY: 37.7 % had been able to do less than half of what they had planned and 13.0 % could do nothing. Applying the concept behind the analysis of HALT (see Methods [14]), we found that HY cost those affected by HY half (50.7 %) of their productivity yesterday. We looked at this by diagnosis in those for whom we had diagnostic information (Table 3). This analysis indicated that migraine cost much more lost productivity than TTH ($p = 0.048$ [Fisher's exact, 2-tailed]), while pMOH eclipsed even migraine (but with small numbers, $p = 0.75$). To calculate the productivity loss due to HY at population level we multiplied 50.7 % by the overall prevalence of HY of 5.9 %; this gave an estimate of 3.0 % as the productivity loss within the entire adult population, every single day, attributable to headache.

Table 1 Characteristics of participants reporting headache yesterday (HY) and population prevalence of HY by group ($N = 2329$)

Characteristic	Reported cases of HY in defined group n (%)	N in defined group	Population prevalence of HY in defined group (%) [95 % CI]
All cases of HY	138 (100.0)	2329	5.9 [5.0–7.0]
Gender			
Male	33 (24.0)	1141	2.9 [2.1–4.0]
Female	105 (76.0)	1188	8.8 [7.4–10.6]
Age (years)			
<25	18 (13.0)	353	5.1 [3.3–7.9]
25 to 34	35 (25.4)	627	5.6 [4.0–7.7]
35 to 44	41 (29.7)	603	6.8 [5.1–9.1]
45 to 54	23 (16.7)	409	5.6 [3.8–8.3]
55 to 65	21 (15.2)	337	6.2 [4.1–9.3]
Habitat			
Rural	102 (73.9)	1103	9.3 [7.7–11.1]
Urban	36 (26.1)	1226	2.9 [2.1–4.0]

Discussion

The principal finding was a 1-day prevalence of headache of 5.9 %, with the implication that this proportion of the adult population (one in 17) had headache on each and every day. Mean duration of HY was 7.0 ± 8.5 h, so that 1.7 % of the population (5.9 % * 7.0/24), on average, had headache at any moment in time yesterday (and, again by implication, at any moment on any day). Mean intensity on a scale of 1–3 was 2.0. Lost productivity was reported by most (83.3 %) participants with HY, of whom 37.7 % could do less than half of what they had planned and 13.0 % could do nothing. Productivity loss due to HY at population level (being the productivity loss within the entire adult population, every single day, attributable to headache) was 3.0 %.

The large difference in prevalence of HY between rural (9.3 %) and urban populations (2.9) was in part explained by the higher rural 1-year prevalence of headache (71.2 % versus 57.3 %), thought to be due to adverse rural socioeconomic conditions (diet, stress and relative poverty) [5]. In addition, the poor rural availability and utilization of health-care facilities were likely to contribute to more frequent headache and therefore more HY. Probable MOH was more prevalent in rural (1.5 %) than in urban areas (0.9 %) [5]; because of its high frequency, this disorder is a major contributor to HY despite its low prevalence.

It is a limitation of enquiry into HY that diagnosis cannot reliably be based on a single headache episode; unless a respondent is able to assert that HY was typical of a recurrent headache that has been diagnosed, its nature will not be known. In this survey, only two thirds could do this, with the result that our inferences on headache types, as opposed to all headache, are unavoidably constrained. From a public-health perspective this may not be of great importance; the key messages here emphasise the ubiquity of headache, its frequency, its symptom

Table 2 Prevalence of headache yesterday according to diagnosis (when recognized as most bothersome headache), and comparison with predicted 1-day prevalence based on reported frequency and 1-year prevalence

Headache type	Headache yesterday: with diagnosis ($N = 95$) or all cases ($N = 138$)		Predicted 1-day prevalence		
	n (%)	Observed 1-day prevalence (%) ($N = 2329$)	1-year prevalence [a] (%)	Mean headache days/year	Calculated 1-day prevalence (%)
Migraine	44/95 (46.3 %)	1.9	25.2	28 [b]	1.9
Tension-type headache	23/95 (24.2 %)	1.0	35.1	17 [b]	1.6
Probable medication-overuse headache	13/95 (13.7 %)	0.6	1.2	226 [b]	0.7
Other headache on ≥15 days/month	15/95 (15.8 %)	0.6	1.8	259 [b]	1.3
Unknown headache yesterday	43/138	1.8	-	-	-
All headache yesterday	138	5.9	63.9	32.0 [a]	5.6 [a]

[a]From reference [5]
[b]From reference [18]

Table 3 Lost productivity because of headache yesterday according to diagnosis (when recognized as most bothersome headache)

Amount of lost productivity	Headache yesterday with diagnosis ($N = 95$)				Any headache yesterday ($N = 138$)
	Migraine	Tension-type headache	Probable MOH	Other headache on ≥15 days/month	
N reporting headache yesterday (X)	44	23	13	15	138
Could do nothing at all (n) (Y)	6	1	2	2	18
Could do less than half (n) (Z)	20	6	7	3	52
Estimated lost productivity yesterday ([Y + Z]/X) (%)	60.5	30.4	69.2	33.3	50.7

MOH medication-overuse headache

burden, which can be assessed regardless of headache type, and its impact at population level (3.0 % loss of productivity).

This is the fourth published analysis of HY, following those in China [15], eight countries of Europe [17] and Russia [16]. Comparison with Russia is of most interest because headache prevalences in China are much lower [23] and the data from the Eurolight study were not entirely population-based [24]. In Russia, 14.5 % of participants, also aged 18–65 years, reported HY [16]. This much higher proportion (14.5 % versus 5.9 %) reflected a lower prevalence of migraine in Russia than in Karnataka (20.3 % versus 25.2 %) and lower prevalence of TTH (30.9 % versus 35.1 %), but a much higher prevalence of headache on ≥15 days/month (10.5 % versus 3.0 %) [5, 25]. As noted above, high-frequency headache has a dominant influence on HY.

The mean duration of HY of 7 h in Karnataka compared with 6 h in Russia, where there was a higher rate of medication use [16]. While we calculated that 1.7 % of the adult population in Karnataka had headache at any moment in time, in Russia, the proportion was much higher (3.6 % [16])–more than double. However, China reported a very similar 1.8 % [15]. In terms of pain intensity, the mean of 2.0 on a scale of 1–3 was much the same as the 2.1 reported in Russia [16], and expected to be disabling. The consequences were seen in the per-person lost productivity of 50.7 % and population-level lost productivity of 3.0 %. Per-person lost productivity was lower in Russia, at 39.8 %, but, with the higher prevalence, population-level lost productivity attributed to HY was quite a lot higher than in Karnataka, at 5.8 % [16]. Notwithstanding this, the 3.0 % losses in Karnataka represent a major socioeconomic drain.

While 5.9 % of participants reported HY in Karnataka, this number was closely corroborated by the predicted 1-day prevalence of headache of 5.6 %. In all three earlier published studies of HY, similar internal consistency has been seen between reported HY and prediction of 1-day headache prevalence based on estimated 1-year prevalence and recalled frequency during the preceding 3 months [15–17]. What was underestimated in recall over 3 months was the productivity loss, which was calculated at population level in Karnataka at only 1.8 % [18])–seemingly a major error. Similar underestimates in recall were reported in Russia [16].

The crucial question, which has been raised before [5, 18], is whether and to what extent these findings are representative of this culturally and environmentally very diverse country and can, therefore, be extrapolated to all India. The truth is that we do not know: we have drawn attention to the need for at least one further similar study in the country, perhaps in the north, seeking corroboration [18]. In the meantime, we reiterate that these are the best data available for the country. If it is the case that 1.7 % of the Indian adult population (approximately 14 million people), or anything in the region of this number, have disabling headache at every moment, this signals a pressing need to do something about it: cost-effective treatments are available [26]. At the least, the further study we have called for should be commissioned urgently. The do-nothing option is not cost-free: it incurs the estimated 3.0 % lost productivity, which is likely to be reflected in a correspondingly diminished gross domestic product. It should be noted that this survey was conducted among the population aged 18–65 years: ie, those of working age, among whom productivity losses have most impact on the population economy. The cost is therefore huge.

The strengths of our study were several. Enquiry into headache yesterday is a powerful approach to population-based burden-of-headache studies, virtually eliminating recall error and any bias that may follow from this [9]. Our sample was large and representative, and the non-participation proportion was low (7.4 %) [5, 19]. Through cold-calling and face-to-face interviews, we avoided the previously described bias of "headache today" [17]: participants with headache on the day they receive a questionnaire by post may defer responding until the first day of headache-freedom, and then spuriously report HY.

Conclusions

Using HY as a method of enquiry free from recall error, we have confirmed a very high level of headache-attributed burden in Karnataka. Previous estimates based on 3-month recall [18] may even have been too low. Until another study is done in the country, these are the best data for all India. We repeat our call for action, reiterating that correct action will ultimately almost certainly be cost-saving [27].

Acknowledgements
This work was financially supported by *Lifting The Burden*, a UK-registered non-governmental organization conducting the Global Campaign against Headache in official relations with the World Health Organization. We are grateful to Mr Remees Raj, Data Manager, Centre for Public Health, NIMHANS, for support in data analysis.

Authors' contributions
TJS and LJS conceived the study and drafted the protocol and study questionnaire, which were subsequently refined in discussion with GG. GG oversaw the study in Karnataka and took responsibility for quality control. GBK and GNR took charge of conduct of the study in the field, with GG acting as principal investigator. GNR took responsibility for the statistical analysis. TJS drafted the manuscript. All authors reviewed and approved the final version.

Competing interests
TJS and LJS are directors and trustees of *Lifting The Burden*.

Author details
[1]Department of Neuroscience, Norwegian University of Science and Technology (NTNU), Edvard Griegs Gate, Trondheim NO-7491, Norway. [2]Division of Brain Sciences, Imperial College London, London, UK. [3]Department of Epidemiology, National Institute of Mental Health and Neuro Sciences (NIMHANS), Bengaluru, India. [4]Department of Neurology, National Institute of Mental Health and Neuro Sciences (NIMHANS), Bengaluru, India. [5]Norwegian Advisory Unit on Headache, Nevrosenteret Øst, St Olavs University Hospital, Trondheim, Norway.

References
1. Vos T, Barber RM, Bell B, Bertozzi-Villa A, Biryukov S, Bolliger I, Charlson F, Davis A, Degenhardt L, Dicker D, Duan L, Erskine H, Feigin VL, Ferrari AJ, Fitzmaurice C, Fleming T, Graetz N, Guinovart C, Haagsma J, Hansen GM, Hanson SW, Heuton KR, Higashi H, Kassebaum N, Kyu H, Laurie E, Liang X, Lofgren K, Lozano R, MacIntyre MF, Moradi-Lakeh M, Naghavi M, Nguyen G, Odell S, Ortblad K et al (2015) Global, regional, and national incidence, prevalence, and years lived with disability for 301 acute and chronic diseases and injuries in 188 countries, 1990–2013: a systematic analysis for the Global Burden of Disease Study 2013. Lancet 386:743–800
2. Steiner TJ, Birbeck GL, Jensen RH, Katsarava Z, Stovner LJ, Martelletti P (2015) Headache disorders are third cause of disability worldwide. J Headache Pain 16:58
3. Vos T, Flaxman AD, Naghavi M, Lozano R, Michaud C, Ezzati M, Shibuya K, Salomon JA, Abdalla S, Aboyans V, Abraham J, Ackerman I, Aggarwal R, Ahn SY, Ali MK, Alvarado M, Anderson HR, Anderson LM, Andrews KG, Atkinson C, Baddour LM, Bahalim AN, Barker-Collo S, Barrero LH, Bartels DH, Basáñez MG, Baxter A, Bell ML, Benjamin EJ, Bennett D, Bernabé E, Bhalla K, Bhandari B, Bikbov B, Bin Abdulhak A et al (2012) Years lived with disability (YLDs) for 1160 sequelae of 289 diseases and injuries 1990–2010: a systematic analysis for the Global Burden of Disease Study 2010. Lancet 380:2163–2196
4. Katsarava Z, Dzagnidze A, Kukava M, Mirvelashvili E, Djibuti M, Janelidze M, Jensen R, Stovner LJ, Steiner TJ (2009) Primary headache disorders in the Republic of Georgia: prevalence and risk factors. Neurology 73:1796–1803
5. Kulkarni GB, Rao GN, Gururaj G, Stovner LJ, Steiner TJ (2015) Headache disorders and public ill-health in India: prevalence estimates in Karnataka State. J Headache Pain 16:67
6. Manandhar K, Risal A, Steiner TJ, Holen A, Linde M (2015) The prevalence of primary headache disorders in Nepal: a nationwide population-based study. J Headache Pain 16:95
7. Mbewe E, Zairemthiama P, Yeh HH, Paul R, Birbeck GL, Steiner TJ (2015) The epidemiology of primary headache disorders in Zambia: a population-based door-to-door survey. J Headache Pain 16:30
8. Stovner LJ, Al Jumah M, Birbeck GL, Gururaj G, Jensen R, Katsarava Z, Queiroz LP, Scher AI, Tekle-Haimanot R, Wang SJ, Steiner TJ (2014) The methodology of population surveys of headache prevalence, burden and cost: Principles and recommendations from the Global Campaign against Headache. J Headache Pain 15:5
9. Steiner TJ, Gururaj G, Andrée C, Katsarava Z, Ayzenberg I, Yu S-Y, Al Jumah M, Tekle-Haimanot R, Birbeck GL, Herekar A, Linde M, Mbewe E, Manandhar K, Risal A, Jensen R, Queiroz LP, Scher AI, Wang SJ, Stovner LJ (2014) Diagnosis, prevalence estimation and burden measurement in population surveys of headache: presenting the HARDSHIP questionnaire. J Headache Pain 15:3
10. Steiner TJ (2004) Lifting the burden: the global campaign against headache. Lancet Neurol 3:204–205
11. Steiner TJ (2005) *Lifting The Burden*: The global campaign to reduce the burden of headache worldwide. J Headache Pain 6:373–377
12. Steiner TJ, Birbeck GL, Jensen R, Katsarava Z, Martelletti P, Stovner LJ (2010) *Lifting The Burden*: the first 7 years. J Headache Pain 11:451–455
13. Steiner TJ, Stovner LJ, Dua T, Birbeck GL, Jensen R, Katsarava Z, Martelletti P, Saxena S (2011) Time to act on headache disorders. J Headache Pain 12:501–503
14. Steiner TJ (2007) The HALT and HART indices. J Headache Pain 8(Suppl 1):S22–S25
15. Yu S, He M, Liu R, Feng J, Qiao X, Yang X, Cao X, Zhao G, Fang Y, Steiner TJ (2013) Headache yesterday in China: a new approach to estimating the burden of headache, applied in a general-population survey in China. Cephalalgia 33:1211–1217
16. Ayzenberg I, Katsarava Z, Sborowski A, Obermann M, Chernysh M, Osipova V, Tabeeva G, Steiner TJ (2015) Headache yesterday in Russia: its prevalence and impact, and their application in estimating the national burden attributable to headache disorders. J Headache Pain 16:7
17. Andrée C, Steiner TJ, Barré J, Katsarava Z, Lainez JM, Lampl C, Lantéri-Minet M, Rastenyte D, Ruiz de la Torre E, Tassorelli C, Stovner LJ (2014) Headache yesterday in Europe. J Headache Pain 15:33
18. Rao GN, Kulkarni GB, Gururaj G, Stovner LJ, Steiner TJ (2015) The burden attributable to headache disorders in India: estimates from a community-based study in Karnataka State. J Headache Pain 16:94
19. Rao GN, Kulkarni GB, Gururaj G, Rajesh K, Subbakrishna DK, Steiner TJ, Stovner LJ (2012) The burden of headache disorders in India: methodology and questionnaire validation for a community-based survey in Karnataka State. J Headache Pain 13:543–550
20. Peters M, Bertolote JM, Houchin C, Kandoura T, Steiner TJ (2007) Translation protocol for hybrid documents. J Headache Pain 8(Suppl 1):S40–S47
21. Headache Classification Subcommittee of the International Headache Society (2004) The International Classification of Headache Disorders: 2nd edition. Cephalalgia 24(Suppl 1):9–160
22. Dean AG, Arner TG, Sunki GG, Friedman R, Lantinga M, Sangam S, Zubieta JC, Sullivan KM, Brendel KA, Gao Z, Fontaine N, Shu M, Fuller G, Smith DC, Nitschke DA, Fagan RF (2007) Epi Info™, a database and statistics program for public health professionals, version 3.5.1. Centers for Disease Control and Prevention, Atlanta
23. Yu S, Liu R, Zhao G, Yang X, Qiao X, Feng J, Fang Y, Cao X, He M, Steiner T (2012) The prevalence and burden of primary headaches in China: a population-based door-to-door survey. Headache 52:582–591
24. Andrée C, Stovner LJ, Steiner TJ, Barré J, Katsarava Z, Lainez JM, Lair M-L, Lanteri-Minet M, Mick G, Rastenyte D, Ruiz de la Torre E, Tassorelli C, Vriezen P, Lampl C (2011) The Eurolight project: the impact of primary headache disorders in Europe. Description of methods. J Headache Pain 12:541–549
25. Ayzenberg I, Katsarava Z, Sborowski A, Chernysh M, Osipova V, Tabeeva G, Yakhno N, Steiner TJ (2012) The prevalence of primary headache disorders in Russia: a countrywide survey. Cephalalgia 32:373–381
26. Linde M, Steiner TJ, Chisholm D (2015) Cost-effectiveness analysis of interventions for migraine in four low- and middle-income countries. J Headache Pain 16:15
27. World Health Organization, Lifting The Burden (2011) Atlas of headache disorders and resources in the world 2011. WHO, Geneva

8

The prevalence of primary headache disorders in Ethiopia

Mehila Zebenigus[1], Redda Tekle-Haimanot[2], Dawit K. Worku[3], Hallie Thomas[4] and Timothy J. Steiner[4,5*]

Abstract

Background: Knowledge of the epidemiology of primary headache disorders in sub-Saharan Africa (SSA) remains very limited. We performed a population-based survey in rural and urban areas of Ethiopia, using methods similar to those of an earlier study in Zambia and tested in multiple other countries by *Lifting The Burden*.

Methods: In a cross-sectional survey we visited households unannounced in four regions of Ethiopia: the mostly urban populations in Addis Ababa and its environs and rural populations of selected districts in Oromia, Amhara and South Nations Nationalities and People's Regions States (SNNPRS). We used cluster-randomized sampling: within clusters we randomly selected households, and one adult member (18–65 years old) of each household. The HARDSHIP structured questionnaire, translated into the local languages, was administered face-to-face by trained interviewers. Demographic enquiry was followed by diagnostic questions based on ICHD-II criteria.

Results: From 2,528 households approached, 2,385 of 2,391 eligible members (1,064 [44.7%] male, 596 [25.0%] urban) consented to interview (participating proportion 99.8%). Headache in the preceding year was reported by 1,071 participants (44.9% [95% CI: 42.4–46.3]; males 37.7%, females 49.9%), and headache yesterday by 170 (7.1% [6.2–8.2]; males 45 [4.1%], females 125 [9.2%]). Adjusted for gender, age and habitation (urban/rural), 1-year prevalence of migraine was 17.7%, of tension-type headache (TTH) 20.6%, of all headache on ≥15 days/month 3.2%, and of probable medication-overuse headache (pMOH) 0.7%. The adjusted prevalence of headache yesterday was 6.4%. Very few cases (1.6%) were unclassifiable. All headache disorders were more common in females. TTH was less common in urban areas (OR: 0.3; $p < 0.0001$), but pMOH was very strongly associated (OR: 6.1; $p < 0.0001$) with urban dwelling. Education was negatively associated with migraine (OR: 0.5–0.7; $p < 0.05$) but (at university level) positively with pMOH (OR: 2.9; $p = 0.067$). Income above ETB 500/month showed similar associations: negatively with migraine (OR: 0.8; $p = 0.035$), positively with pMOH (OR: 2.1; $p = 0.164$).

Conclusions: Findings for migraine and TTH in Ethiopia were quite similar to those from Zambia, another SSA country; pMOH was much less prevalent but, as in Zambia, essentially an urban problem. Primary headache disorders are at least as prevalent in SSA as in high-income western countries.

Keywords: Epidemiology, Prevalence, Headache, Migraine, Tension-type headache, Medication-overuse headache, Ethiopia, Sub-Saharan Africa, Global Campaign against Headache

Background

Knowledge of headache prevalence and headache-attributed burden is improving worldwide. Better methodology is being applied to population-based studies [1, 2] and a number of national surveys have been completed within the Global Campaign against Headache [3, 4] in world regions where information was lacking. It is now recognised that headache disorders, especially tension-type headache (TTH) and migraine, are among the most common medical conditions [1, 2] and collectively the third highest cause of years of life lost to disability (YLDs) [5, 6].

Sub-Saharan Africa (SSA) has been one of the large geographical areas devoid of data. The few studies of headache prevalence, including one in Ethiopian textile mill workers [7], have mostly been in select sub-populations

* Correspondence: t.steiner@imperial.ac.uk
[4]Department of Neuroscience, Norwegian University of Science and Technology (NTNU), Edvard Griegs Gate, NO-7491 Trondheim, Norway
[5]Division of Brain Sciences, Imperial College London, London, UK
Full list of author information is available at the end of the article

rather than population-based [7–15], with estimates varying considerably but generally far lower than global means [16]. The consequent perception that headache disorders were relatively uncommon in SSA, and not of significant public-health concern, was reversed after the completion of a survey in Zambia [17, 18]. This study, supported by *Lifting The Burden* (LTB), a UK-registered non-governmental organization conducting the Global Campaign in official relations with the World Health Organization (WHO) [19], reported highly prevalent migraine (22.9%), TTH (22.8%) and probable medication-overuse headache (pMOH) (7.1%) [17]. These were associated with heavy disability burden and lost productivity, calling for action and recognition within public health policy [18].

This study in Ethiopia, also supported by LTB as a project within the Global Campaign against Headache, used very similar methods to the survey in Zambia. Its aims were to add to knowledge regarding primary headache disorders in SSA and discover whether the findings in Zambia would be replicated. The purposes were to inform health policy-makers in Ethiopia and to inform future global estimates undertaken by the Global Burden of Disease project (GBD) [20]. Here we report 1-year prevalences of headache, migraine, TTH, all causes of headache on ≥15 days/month and pMOH, and point (1-day) prevalence of headache ("headache yesterday"). Disability and other aspects of burden attributable to these disorders will be described elsewhere.

Methods

Ethics

Approvals were obtained from the Ethics Review Committee of the Department of Neurology, and the Institutional Review Board and Research and Publication Committee of the College of Health Sciences of Addis Ababa University, and from the Regional Health Bureau of each Region where the survey was undertaken.

Informed consent was obtained from participants before enrolment. Personal data were anonymised during analysis and dissemination.

Study design

This was a cross-sectional questionnaire-based survey of adults aged 18-65 years. It was designed in accordance with published guidelines [1]. We selected and engaged with participants by calling at households unannounced. We used cluster-randomized sampling, randomly selecting households within clusters and one adult member of each biologically-unrelated family within a household.

Survey sites

The main study was conducted in four Regions of Ethiopia: the mostly urban populations in Addis Ababa and its environs and rural populations of selected districts from Oromia, Amhara and South Nations Nationalities and People's Regions States (SNNPRS).

The population distribution of Ethiopia was 17% urban, 83% rural (2011 data [21]). In order to have sufficient numbers for urban/rural comparisons, we oversampled the urban population (25%). Addis Ababa held close to 50% of the urban population of Ethiopia [22]; therefore we aimed to take half the urban sample there and the remainder equally from the other three selected Regions. Rural respondents came equally from the latter three Regions.

Selection and training of interviewers

In Addis Ababa, the interviewer was a nurse from the Department of Neurology, Addis Ababa University, College of Health Sciences. In the other three Regions, interviewers were nurses from health centres in urban areas and Health Extension Workers from health stations in rural areas (the latter are young women with at least grade-10 education and one year of didactic and practical training in health care; their primary charge is to promote health through education, screening, prevention and selective clinical interventions [23]). All interviewers attended a 3-day training session at their respective health-service facilities, including clinical aspects of headache disorders and the theoretical and practical aspects of the study design and purpose, and were then assessed in supervised interviews.

Questionnaire

We used a culturally modified version of the structured Headache-Attributed Restriction, Disability, Social Handicap and Impaired Participation (HARDSHIP) questionnaire [2], translated according to LTB's translation protocol for lay documents [24] into two local languages: Oromo for the Oromia Region and Amharic for the remaining three Regions. We piloted the questionnaire for acceptability first in Addis Ababa in the original English, translated at point of application by the interviewer, then in the translated versions in a total sample of 160 from all Regions (40 urban, 120 rural), using a mixture of convenience and purposive sampling. We modified questions accordingly. These participants were not included in the study results.

The questionnaire was composed of five parts: personal and demographic enquiry, and headache screening questions, which were addressed to all respondents; these were followed in those screening positively by diagnostic questions based on ICHD-II [25], enquiry into burden and questions on selected comorbidities. The screening question for headache was: "In the last year, have you had headache?" Participants who answered "no" were classified as headache-free; those who answered "yes" were asked if all their headaches were of one or more types and, if more than one, to focus in the subsequent questions on the one that was most bothersome. The point prevalence of headache was estimated by asking: "Did you have a headache yesterday?"

Main study

This was completed during April and May 2014.

In each Region, Ethiopian nationals aged 18–65 years were randomly sampled by cold-calling door-to-door. We randomly selected a zone (study area) within each Region and a district within each zone. The sampling procedure was designed to accommodate multiple families living in single dwelling-places in unplanned settlements. In each district the interviewer randomly selected a block or circumscribed area of dwellings and, within that block or area, one or more dwellings. In each selected dwelling, the interviewer first identified the number of families living there, in one or more households (defined as sharing a kitchen). Each biologically unrelated family within a dwelling was included, but only one participant was selected from each family. Where a member of one family in a dwelling was a first- or second-degree relative of a member of another family also within that dwelling, the two families were considered as one.

The female head of each family was asked to list all adult family members living within that dwelling. From this list, one person was randomly selected. Only this person was included in the sample. If present, he or she was immediately asked the demographic and screening questions; if not, the female head-of-family answered these questions on behalf of the participant. In either case, if the screening question was answered negatively the interview was complete at that point. If the screening question was answered positively, and the selected respondent was present, the full interview continued; if the selected respondent was not present, an appointment was made for the interviewer to return for this purpose.

Where the door to a selected dwelling was not answered at first visit, two further attempts were made before the dwelling was excluded and replaced by another according to the sampling algorithm.

Every selected respondent was included unless withholding consent, failing to be available on two occasions for which an appointment had been made, or unable to comprehend the questions. As the survey proceeded, DKW checked each questionnaire and discarded those that were incomplete for essential information. Excluded respondents were replaced from other households, since sampling was continued until the requisite number was achieved.

Diagnosis

Interviewers did not make diagnoses: these were derived algorithmically during analysis [2]. We first separated participants reporting headache on ≥15 days/month; we described these as a separate group, because they cannot be fully diagnosed by questionnaire. Those among this group who also reported regular use of headache medication on >3 days/week were considered to have pMOH. To all others, the algorithm applied ICHD-II criteria in the order: migraine, TTH, probable migraine, probable TTH [1, 25]. Cases of migraine and probable migraine, and of TTH and probable TTH, were combined for prevalence estimation and further analyses. Remaining cases were unclassified.

Quality control

To ensure completeness of data collection, each interviewer checked responses to questionnaires before ending each visit. The principal investigator made random unannounced checks, in the field, of the interviewers' work-quality. The interviewers were told that this might occur at any time.

Data entry and management

Data from questionnaires were entered into a secure database. Before entry, the forms were scrutinised for accuracy, completeness, inconsistencies, wrong entries, illegible markings and missed entries. Two epidemiologists from Addis Ababa University entered the data independently, with cross-checking. Mismatches were fewer than 0.5%, and resolved by referring to the original forms.

Statistics and analysis

We aimed for a sample size of 2,000 according to published guidelines [26]. For planning purposes we anticipated a 20% non-participation proportion and a requirement to visit 2,400 households.

We analysed age as a categorical variable (18–25, 26–35, 36–45, 46–55, 56–65 years). We classified marital status as single, married, widowed or divorced, educational level as illiterate (none), primary (grades 1–7), secondary (grades 8–12) or higher (college or university), employment status as unemployed or as unskilled, skilled or professional work. We categorised income per capita per month as ≤ ETB 500 or > ETB 500 (at the time of the survey, USD 1.00 = ETB 18.93, so this was approximately USD 1.00/day).

We used descriptive summaries for sociodemographic and clinical characteristics. We estimated prevalences as proportions (%). We measured headache frequency in days/month, multiplying by 12 to estimate days/year, and expressed this as a mean ± standard deviation (SD). We used chi-squared and Fisher's exact tests in comparisons of proportions and distributions. We used logistic regression analysis to examine associations between demographic variables and prevalence, calculating odds ratios (ORs) with 95% confidence intervals (CIs). We regarded $p < 0.05$ as significant.

Analyses were performed using SPSS/PC version 20.0 software packages for statistical analysis (SPSS, INC, Chicago, IL) and Excel Professional Plus 2010 Version 14.0.7166.5000.

Results

From 2,528 households approached, 2,461 biologically unrelated participants were successfully interviewed of whom 2,385 met the entry criteria and were included in the analysis (exclusions were aged >65 years). There were 61 household refusals in the urban study area and none in the rural areas; these were not counted as non-participants since we had not established the presence of anyone eligible [1]. There were 6 refusals by selected respondents, 2 (0.3%) in the urban area and 4 (0.2%) in the rural areas. The overall participating proportion was 99.8%.

The sociodemographic characteristics of participants are displayed in Table 1. Females (55.7%) outnumbered males (44.3%); the expected ratio was 50.3:49.7 [21] (chi-squared = 27.628; $p < 0.0001$). The age distribution of our sample reasonably matched that of the national population except for under-representation in the 18–25 age group (estimated expected proportion 27% based on 2011

Table 1 Demographic characteristics of the study sample

	All n (%)	Rural n (%)	Urban n (%)	p^a
Total	2,385	1,789 (75.0)	596 (25.0)	–
Gender				
Female	1,328 (55.7)	970 (54.2)	358 (60.1)	
Male	1,057 (44.3)	819 (45.8)	238 (39.9)	0.0133[b]
Age (years)				
18–25	583 (24.4)	399 (22.3)	184 (30.9)	<0.0001[c]
26–35	873 (36.7)	648 (36.2)	225 (37.8)	
36–45	452 (19.0)	351 (19.6)	101 (16.9)	
46–55	325 (13.6)	264 (14.8)	61 (10.2)	
56–65	152 (6.4)	127 (7.1)	25 (4.2)	
Marital status				
Single	1,597 (67.0)	1,317 (73.6)	280 (47.0)	<0.0001[c]
Married	480 (20.1)	239 (13.4)	241 (40.4)	
Widowed	104 (4.4)	63 (3.5)	41 (6.9)	
Divorced	204 (8.6)	170 (9.5)	34 (5.7)	
Educational level				
None (illiterate)	947 (39.7)	876 (49.0)	71 (11.9)	<0.0001[c]
Primary	756 (31.7)	602 (33.7)	154 (25.8)	
Secondary	449 (18.8)	235 (13.1)	214 (35.9)	
Higher	233 (9.8)	76 (4.2)	157 (26.3)	
Employment				
Housewife	829 (34.8)	723 (40.4)	106 (17.8)	<0.0001[c]
Student	219 (9.2)	141 (7.9)	78 (13.1)	
Employed (non-farmer)	598 (25.1)	230 (12.9)	368 (61.7)	
Farmer	660 (27.7)	659 (36.8)	1 (0.2)	
Unemployed	47 (2.0)	8 (0.4)	39 (6.5)	
Retired	32 (1.3)	28 (1.6)	4 (0.7)	
Income per month (ETB)[d]				
≤ 500	958 (40.5)	887 (49.7)	71 (12.3)	<0.0001[b]
> 500	1,405 (59.5)	897 (50.3)	508 (87.7)	

[a]comparing distributions between rural and urban participants; [b]Fisher's exact test; [c]chi-squared test; [d]results missing for 22 participants; ETB: Ethiopian birr (at the time of the study, USD 1.00 = ETB 18.93; therefore ETB 500/month was approximately USD 1/day)

data [21]; chi-squared = 7.903; $p = 0.0049$), which occurred in the rural sample. Because we deliberately over-sampled the urban population, our sample (25:75) did not match the national urban/rural distribution (17:83 [21]; chi-squared = 107.895; $p < 0.0001$). Adjustments to observed prevalences were therefore necessary for habitation as well as age and gender, which, accordingly, are reported below. Rural participants were not only significantly older than urban ($p < 0.0001$) but also poorer ($p < 0.0001$) and less well educated ($p < 0.0001$), with almost half (49.0%) being illiterate.

Prevalence overall and by age, gender and habitation is set out in Table 2. In total, 1,071 participants (44.9% [95% CI: 42.4–46.3]; males 37.7%, females 49.9%) reported headache in the preceding year. Table 2 shows both the observed prevalences of each headache type, and adjusted values for gender, age and habitation. TTH was the most prevalent (observed: 20.7% [definite: 15.5%; probable: 5.2%]; adjusted: 20.6%), slightly ahead of migraine (observed: 19.0% [definite 10.8%; probable 8.2%]; adjusted: 17.7%). All causes of headache on ≥15 days/month were 3.2% and pMOH 0.7% (both adjusted). There were 38 cases (1.6%) of unclassified headache. Headache on the day prior to the interview (headache yesterday) was reported by 170 participants (7.1% [6.2–8.2]; males 45 [4.1%], females 125 [9.2%]; prevalence adjusted for gender, age and habitation: 6.4%).

All headache types were more common in females, migraine by about 3:2 ($p < 0.0001$ [Fisher's exact]). For TTH ($p = 0.3596$), pMOH (by about 2:1; $p = 0.1863$) and other headache on ≥15 days/month (also by about 3:2; $p = 0.0613$), differences were not significant. Headache yesterday was reported more than twice as commonly by females ($p < 0.0001$). Age relationships were generally rather flat, although pMOH and other headache on ≥15 days/month tended to become more prevalent with advancing age, and this was reflected in headache yesterday. TTH was most common (31.6%) in the oldest age group (56–65 years) and least common (16.0%) in the youngest (≤25 years). TTH was more common in rural areas ($p < 0.0001$), but the opposite was true of pMOH ($p < 0.0001$) and numerically of other headache on ≥15 days/month ($p = 0.5667$); consequently, headache yesterday was reported more often by urban than rural dwellers, although the difference was not significant ($p = 0.1189$).

We used logistic regression analysis to look at associations of migraine, TTH and pMOH with habitation and socioeconomic indicators (Table 3). This analysis confirmed a strong negative association between urban dwelling and TTH (OR: 0.3; $p < 0.0001$), but a very powerful positive association (OR: 6.1; $p < 0.0001$) of urban dwelling with pMOH. Education to any level was associated with reduced migraine prevalence, and above primary level with reduced TTH prevalence; however, education to secondary level and especially above (OR: 2.9; $p = 0.067$) appeared to raise the odds of pMOH, although these associations were not significant. These findings were in line with associations with income: migraine was less prevalent (OR: 0.8; $p = 0.035$) and pMOH more prevalent (OR: 2.1; not significant) in those with incomes above ETB 500/month.

Table 2 Observed 1-year prevalence (% [95% confidence intervals]) by gender, age and habitation, overall and by headache type, and adjusted values for gender, age and habitation

	Migraine ($n = 452$)	TTH ($n = 493$)	pMOH ($n = 21$)	Other headache on ≥15d/m ($n = 67$)	Any headache yesterday ($n = 170$)
All ($N = 2{,}385$)	19.0 [17.4–20.6]	20.7 [19.1–22.3]	0.9 [0.5–1.3]	2.8 [2.2–3.6]	7.1 [6.2–8.2]
Gender					
Male ($n = 1{,}057$)	14.1 [12.0–16.2]	19.8 [17.4–22.2]	0.6 [0.2–1.3]	2.1 [1.4–3.2]	4.1 [2.9–5.3]
Female ($n = 1{,}328$)	22.8 [20.5–25.1]	21.4 [19.2–23-6]	1.1 [0.7–1.9]	3.4 [2.5–4.5]	9.2 [7.7–10.8]
Age (yr)					
18–25 ($n = 583$)	18.4 [15.3–21.6]	16.0 [13.0–19.0]	1.0 [0.4–2.3]	2.1 [1.1–3.6]	6.2 [4.5–8.5]
26–35 ($n = 873$)	20.4 [17.7–23.1]	20.8 [18.1–23.5]	0.7 [0.3–1.2]	1.9 [1.0–2.8]	6.8 [5.3–8.6]
36–45 ($n = 452$)	18.1 [14.6–21.7]	23.9 [20.0–27.8]	0.9 [0.3–2.3]	2.2 [0.9–3.6]	8.2 [6.0–11.1]
46–55 ($n = 325$)	19.4 [15.1–23.7]	19.1 [14.8–23.4]	1.5 [0.6–3.7]	5.2 [3.2–8.3]	8.6 [6.0–12.2]
56–65 ($n = 152$)	14.5 [8.9–20.1]	31.6 [24.2–39.0]	1.3 [0.1–5.0]	2.6 [0.8–6.8]	6.6 [3.5–11.8]
Habitation					
Rural ($n = 1{,}789$)	18.6 [16.8–20.4]	24.4 [22.4–26.4]	0.4 [0.2–0.8]	2.7 [2.0–3.6]	6.7 [5.6–7.9]
Urban ($n = 596$)	20.0 [16.8–23.2]	9.4 [7.1–11.7]	2.4 [1.4–3.9]	3.2 [2.0–5.0]	8.6 [6.6–11.1]
Adjusted for gender, age and habitation	17.7%	20.6%	0.7%	2.5%	6.4%

TTH tension-type headache, *pMOH* probable medication-overuse headache, *d/m*: days/month

Table 3 Logistic regression analysis of associations with each diagnosis adjusting for gender, age and all variables listed

	Migraine		Tension-type headache		pMOH	
	OR	*p*	OR	*p*	OR	*p*
Habitation						
Rural	reference		reference		reference	
Urban	1.1 [0.9–1.4]	0.466	0.3 [0.2–0.4]	<0.0001	6.1 [2.5–15.3]	<0.0001
Education						
None	reference		reference		reference	
Primary	0.5 [0.4–0.6]	<0.0001	1.0 [0.8–1.3]	0.908	0.5 [0.1–2.1]	0.367
Secondary	0.6 [0.4–0.8]	0.000	0.6 [0.5–0.8]	0.003	1.8 [0.6–5.5]	0.284
College or University	0.7 [0.5–1.0]	0.042	0.4 [0.4–0.8]	0.006	2.9 [0.9–9.4]	0.067
Employment						
Employed (non-farming)	reference		reference		numbers too small to calculate	
Housewife	2.8 [2.1–3.7]	<0.0001	3.0 [2.2–4.2]	<0.0001		
Student	0.3 [0.2–0.4]	<0.0001	0.4 [0.2–0.6]	<0.0001		
Farmer	1.2 [0.9–1.7]	0.159	2.7 [2.0–3.8]	<0.0001		
Unemployed	0.05 [0.0–0.1]	<0.0001	0.05 [0.02–0.1]	<0.0001		
Retired	0.02 [0.001–0.1]	<0.0001	0.2 [0.1–0.3]	<0.0001		
Income per month (ETB)						
≤ 500	reference		reference		reference	
> 500	0.8 [0.7–1.0]	0.035	1.0 [0.8–1.2]	0.806	2.1 [0.7–5.7]	0.164

pMOH probable medication-overuse headache, *OR* odds ratio with 95% confidence interval in parenthesis, *ETB* Ethiopian birr (at the time of the study, USD 1.00 = ETB 18.93; therefore ETB 500/month was approximately USD 1/day)

Discussion

This study was the first population-based survey using established methodology [1] and questionnaire [2] to estimate the prevalence of primary headache disorders in Ethiopia. Minimising potential biases, it included diverse regions, employed an appropriate mix of cluster-sampling and simple random sampling, applied ICHD-II diagnostic criteria [25] and had a very high participating proportion (99.8%). It found that headache disorders were highly prevalent in this country: 1-year prevalence of any headache was 44.9%; adjusted for gender, age and habitation (urban/rural), the 1-year prevalence of migraine was 17.7%, of TTH 20.6%, of all causes of headache on ≥15 days/month 3.2%, and of pMOH 0.7%. There was a very small proportion (1.6%) of unclassified headache. TTH (OR: 0.3) was less prevalent among the urban population, but urban dwelling was very strongly associated (OR: 6.1) with pMOH. Education was associated with reduced migraine prevalence (OR: 0.5–0.7) but a tendency to raised odds of pMOH (OR: 2.9 [$p = 0.067$] at university level). Income above ETB 500/month (approximately USD 1/day) showed associations in expected alignment with these.

This was the second such study within the Global Campaign against Headache to be conducted in SSA: the first was in Zambia, and showed not dissimilar overall results with regard to both migraine (gender- and habitation-adjusted 1-year prevalence 22.9%) and TTH (22.8%) [17]. TTH was the most prevalent headache in Ethiopia, but only by a small margin, and not so in Zambia [17]; we speculate that this may have been due to cultural under-reporting of infrequent episodic TTH in both countries. These findings confirm that, contrary to earlier estimates from Benin [12], Tanzania [8, 11, 13] and, indeed, Ethiopia [7, 27]), primary headache is at least as common in SSA as in the rest of the world [16]. In Zambia, TTH was less common among the university-educated (OR: 0.22) but migraine was more prevalent (OR: 2.1) [17]. However, the principal difference between the countries was in pMOH: 0.7% in Ethiopia, 7.1% in Zambia [17]. Nevertheless, in Ethiopia as in Zambia, pMOH was very much a problem in the urban population rather than rural (Zambia is far more urbanised [40%] [28] than Ethiopia [17%] [21]).

Migraine prevalence in an Ethiopian rural community was previously estimated at only 3% [27], far lower than our 17.7% for an urban/rural mix. In the earlier study, the focus was on chronic recurrent headache (with a reported overall prevalence of 4.7%), which might attract priority in the context of the other challenges of daily life in rural Ethiopia. The screening question was "Do you have recurrent headache", and the survey stopped when participants answered "No" to this question. It is highly likely that people with occasional headache (the majority with headache) were excluded. In addition, the diagnostic questionnaire would diagnose migraine only when all ICHD-I criteria were met (*ie*, excluding probable migraine). These factors together would sufficiently explain the difference between 3 and 17.7%.

Headache yesterday was reported much less frequently in Ethiopia (6.4% adjusted) than Zambia (19.1% adjusted [17, 18]). The reasons are clear: not only pMOH but all causes of headache on ≥15 days/month (key drivers of headache yesterday) were much more common in Zambia, and highly associated with urban dwelling in a more urbanised population. Headache yesterday is equivalent to 1-day prevalence, and can be predicted from the 1-year prevalence of all headache (45.2%) and mean headache frequency in days/month in those affected (4.2). The latter divided by 30 gives the probability of headache on any particular day among those with headache (in this case 0.14); predicted 1-day prevalence is the product of this and 1-year prevalence (*ie*, 6.3%). The observed prevalence of headache yesterday (7.1%) was close to this, which affirms the veracity of these findings. It also demonstrates one benefit of epidemiological enquiry into headache yesterday.

The strengths of this study have been mentioned above. Its principal limitation was that we surveyed in only two languages, while there are over 80 active languages in Ethiopia [29]. Oromo and Amharic are the most widely used: according to 2014 census data, Oromo is spoken by 33.8% of the total population, Amharic by 29.3% [29]. This suggests we can claim to represent a majority (63%) but not all of the population. The logistic difficulties and resource implications associated with each additional language would not have justified including even one more (other key languages: Somali [6.3%], Tigrinya [5.9%], Sidamo [4.8%], Wolaytta [2.2%], Gurage [2.0%] and Afar [1.7%] [29]). We also could not validate the diagnostic questionnaire in the two languages. This would have required at least one of the very few headache experts in the country to take time out from the health service in order to re-interview a subset of participants in the field; we could not justify this. The questionnaire already had a record of successful use in many countries and cultures [2, 17, 18, 30–35].

What are the implications of these findings? For Ethiopia, they show that, far from being relatively uncommon, as past research has indicated, headache disorders are highly prevalent. Since headache disorders are the third greatest cause of disability globally [5, 6], with migraine the principal contributor and MOH also important, it is very probable that they are also in Ethiopia. Data are needed to confirm this, and will be reported in a future publication. However, migraine prevalence in Ethiopia (17.7%) is 20% higher than the estimated global mean reported in GBD 2010 (14.7%) [36]. While pMOH is less common overall (0.7%) than the estimated global mean (about 1.5% [37]), its prevalence in the Ethiopian urban population (2.4%) exceeds it by about 60%. MOH is the result of a form of mistreatment. It is fostered wherever limited access to health care, and limited expertise in management of headache disorders among the health-care providers who are available, lead to a culture, unrestrained by effective public health-education, of recourse to analgesics obtained over-the-counter (OTC). Escalating use is then a behaviour typically leading to MOH everywhere. However, this is obviously dependent on ready access to OTC drugs – both availability, and the means to buy them. It is this, almost certainly, that explains why pMOH is selectively an urban problem, here in Ethiopia as it is in Zambia [17]. Whatever health care is provided for headache in Ethiopia, public education regarding the risk of MOH is needed, and could be provided to the urban population at relatively low cost [38].

There are also implications for the Global Burden of Disease project itself [20]. SSA is a large and populous area of the world: as population-based data from SSA increasingly convincingly demonstrate that headache disorders are very common here, and are incorporated into future iterations of GBD, estimates of headache-attributed burden will rise not only in SSA but globally.

Conclusions

Findings for migraine and TTH in Ethiopia, showing high prevalence of the former, were quite similar to those from Zambia, another SSA country. While pMOH was much less prevalent, it was as in Zambia essentially an urban problem. Primary headache disorders are at least as common in Ethiopia as in high-income western countries, and this study offers confirmation that this is true of the SSA region.

Abbreviations

CI: Confidence interval; d/m: days/month; ETB: Ethiopian birr; GBD: Global Burden of Disease; HARDSHIP: Headache-Attributed Restriction, Disability, Social Handicap and Impaired Participation questionnaire; ICHD: International Classification of Headache Disorders; LTB: *Lifting The Burden*; MOH: Medication-overuse headache; OR: Odds ratio; pMOH: Probable MOH; SD: Standard deviation; SNNPRS: South Nations Nationalities and People's Regions States; SSA: Sub-Saharan Africa; TTH: Tension-type headache; USD: United States dollar; WHO: World Health Organization; YLD: Year of life lost to disability

Acknowledgements

We are grateful to Belachew Degefe, formerly of the Department of Neurology, Addis Ababa University, for assistance in proposal development, acquiring permits and the pilot study. We thank the Regional Health Bureaux, the Department of Neurology at Addis Ababa University, the data collectors and data-entry clerks, and all the people who were interviewed for this study.

Funding

The study was supported by *Lifting The Burden*, a UK-registered non-governmental organization conducting the Global Campaign against Headache in official relations with the World Health Organization.

Authors' contributions

TJS conceived the study and drafted the protocol and study questionnaire, which were subsequently refined by TJS, MZ and RT-H in discussion. RT-H provided supervision in Ethiopia. MZ and DKW were responsible for performance of the study, with MZ acting as principal investigator in the field. HT and TJS carried out the statistical analysis. MZ and TJS drafted the manuscript. All authors reviewed and approved the final version.

Competing interests

TJS is a Director and Trustees of *Lifting The Burden*. The authors declare that they have no competing interests.

Author details

[1]Department of Neurology, School of Medicine, College of Health Science, Addis Ababa University, Addis Ababa, Ethiopia. [2]Department of Internal Medicine, School of Medicine, College of Health Science, Addis Ababa University, Addis Ababa, Ethiopia. [3]Department of Internal Medicine, Bahir Dar University, Bahir Dar, Ethiopia. [4]Department of Neuroscience, Norwegian University of Science and Technology (NTNU), Edvard Griegs Gate, NO-7491 Trondheim, Norway. [5]Division of Brain Sciences, Imperial College London, London, UK.

References

1. Stovner LJ, Al Jumah M, Birbeck GL, Gururaj G, Jensen R, Katsarava Z, Queiroz LP, Scher AI, Tekle-Haimanot R, Wang SJ, Steiner TJ (2014) The methodology of population surveys of headache prevalence, burden and cost: principles and recommendations from the global campaign against headache. J Headache Pain 15:5
2. Steiner TJ, Gururaj G, Andrée C, Katsarava Z, Ayzenberg I, Yu S-Y, Al Jumah M, Tekle-Haimanot R, Birbeck GL, Herekar A, Linde M, Mbewe E, Manandhar K, Risal A, Jensen R, Queiroz LP, Scher AI, Wang SJ, Stovner LJ (2014) Diagnosis, prevalence estimation and burden measurement in population surveys of headache: presenting the HARDSHIP questionnaire. J Headache Pain 15:3
3. Steiner TJ (2004) Lifting the burden: the global campaign against headache. Lancet Neurol 3:204–5
4. Steiner TJ (2005) *Lifting The Burden*: the global campaign to reduce the burden of headache worldwide. J Headache Pain 6:373–7
5. Vos T, Barber RM, Bell B, Bertozzi-Villa A, Biryukov S, Bolliger I, Charlson F, Davis A, Degenhardt L, Dicker D, Duan L, Erskine H, Feigin VL, Ferrari AJ, Fitzmaurice C, Fleming T, Graetz N, Guinovart C, Haagsma J, Hansen GM, Hanson SW, Heuton KR, Higashi H, Kassebaum N, Kyu H, Laurie E, Liang X, Lofgren K, Lozano R, MacIntyre MF et al (2015) Global, regional, and national incidence, prevalence, and years lived with disability for 301 acute and chronic diseases and injuries in 188 countries, 1990–2013: a systematic analysis for the global burden of disease study 2013. Lancet 386:743–800
6. Steiner TJ, Birbeck GL, Jensen RH, Katsarava Z, Stovner LJ, Martelletti P (2015) Headache disorders are third cause of disability worldwide. J Headache Pain 16:58
7. Takele GM, Tekle Haimanot R, Martelletti P (2008) Prevalence and burden of primary headache in Akaki textile mill workers, Ethiopia. J Headache Pain 9: 119–28
8. Dent W, Spiss H, Helbok R, Matuja W, Scheunemann S, Schmutzhard E (2004) Prevalence of migraine in a rural area in South Tanzania: a door-to-door survey. Cephalalgia 24:960–6
9. Quesada-Vazquez AJ, Rodriguez-Santana N (2006) The prevalence of primary headaches in the working population at a psychiatric hospital in Zimbabwe. Rev Neurol 43:129–31
10. Ojini FI, Okubadejo NU, Danesi MA (2009) Prevalence and clinical characteristics of headache in medical students of the University of Lagos, Nigeria. Cephalalgia 29:472–7
11. Winkler A, Stelzhammer B, Kerschbaumsteiner K, Meindl M, Dent W, Kaaya J, Matuja W, Schmutzhard E (2009) The prevalence of headache with emphasis on tension-type headache in rural Tanzania: a community-based study. Cephalalgia 29:1317–25
12. Houinato D, Adoukonou T, Ntsiba F, Adjien C, Avode DG, Preux PM (2010) Prevalence of migraine in a rural community in south Benin. Cephalalgia 30:62–7
13. Winkler A, Dent W, Stelzhammer B, Kerschbaumsteiner K, Meindl M, Kaaya J, Matuja W, Schmutzhard E (2010) Prevalence of migraine headache in a rural area of northern Tanzania: a community-based door-to-door survey. Cephalalgia 30:582–92
14. Dent W, Stelzhammer B, Meindl M, Matuja WBP, Schmutzhard E, Winkler AS (2011) Migraine attack frequency, duration, and pain intensity: disease burden derived from a community-based survey in northern Tanzania. Headache 51:1483–92
15. Gelaye B, Peterlin BL, Lemma S, Tesfaye M, Berhane Y, Williams MA (2013) Migraine and psychiatric comorbidities among sub-Saharan African adults. Headache 53:310–21
16. Stovner LJ, Hagen K, Jensen R, Katsarava Z, Lipton RB, Scher AI, Steiner TJ, Zwart J A (2007) The global burden of headache: a documentation of headache prevalence and disability worldwide. Cephalalgia 27:193–210
17. Mbewe E, Zairemthiama P, Yeh HH, Paul R, Birbeck GL, Steiner TJ (2015) The epidemiology of primary headache disorders in Zambia: a population-based door-to-door survey. J Headache Pain 16:30
18. Mbewe E, Zairemthiama P, Paul R, Birbeck GL, Steiner TJ (2015) The burden of primary headache disorders in Zambia: national estimates from a population-based door-to-door survey. J Headache Pain 16:36
19. Steiner TJ, Birbeck GL, Jensen R, Katsarava Z, Martelletti P, Stovner LJ (2011) The global campaign, World Health Organization and *Lifting The Burden*: collaboration in action. J Headache Pain 12:273–4
20. Institute of Health Metrics and Evaluation. Global Burden of Disease (GBD). http://www.healthdata.org/gbd. Accessed 15 Jun 2016.
21. Index Mundi. Ethiopia Demographics Profile (2014). http://www.indexmundi.com/ethiopia/demographics_profile.html. Accessed 15 Jun 2016.
22. Central Statistical Agency, Government of Ethiopia. Population and Housing Census Report-Country (2007). http://www.csa.gov.et/newcsaweb/images/documents/surveys/Population%20and%20Housing%20census/ETH-pop 2007/survey0/data/Doc/Reports/National_Statistical.pdf. Accessed 15 Jun 2016.
23. Koblinsky M, Tain F, Gaym A, Karim A, Carnell M, Tesfaye S (2010) Responding to the maternal health care challenge: the Ethiopian health extension program. Ethiopian J Health Development 24(s1):105–9
24. Peters M, Bertolote JM, Houchin C, Kandoura T, Steiner TJ (2007) Translation protocol for lay documents. J Headache Pain 8(Suppl 1):S43–4
25. Headache Classification Subcommittee of the International Headache Society (2004) The international classification of headache disorders: 2nd edition. Cephalalgia 24(Suppl 1):9–160
26. Jaykaran Charan J, Biswas T (2013) How to calculate sample size for different study designs in medical research? Indian J Psychol Med 35:121–6
27. Tekle Haimanot R, Seraw B, Forsgren L, Ekbom K, Ekstedt J (1995) Migraine, chronic tension-type headache, and cluster headache in an Ethiopian rural community. Cephalalgia 15:482–8
28. Central Statistical Office, Zambia. Available at http://www.zamstats.gov.zm/. Accessed 17 Jun 2016.
29. Paul LM, Simons GF, Fennig CD (eds) (2016) Ethnologue: Languages of the World, 19th edn. SIL International. Online version at, Dallas, Texas, http://www.ethnologue.com/country/ET/languages. Accessed 17 Jun 2016
30. Yu SY, Cao XT, Zhao G, Yang XS, Qiao XY, Fang YN, Feng JC, Liu RZ, Steiner TJ (2011) The burden of headache in China: validation of diagnostic questionnaire for a population-based survey. J Headache Pain 12:141–6
31. Ayzenberg I, Katsarava Z, Mathalikov R, Chernysh M, Osipova V, Tabeeva G, Steiner TJ (2011) The burden of headache in Russia: validation of the diagnostic questionnaire in a population-based sample. Eur J Neurol 18:454–9
32. Rao GN, Kulkarni GB, Gururaj G, Kavita R, Subbakrishna DK, Steiner TJ, Stovner LJ (2012) The burden of headache disorders in India: Methodology and questionnaire validation for a community-based survey in Karnataka State. J Headache Pain 13:543–50
33. Herekar AD, Herekar AA, Ahmad A, Uqaili UL, Ahmed B, Effendi J, Alvi SZ, Steiner TJ (2013) The burden of headache disorders in Pakistan: methodology of a population-based nationwide study, and questionnaire validation. J Headache Pain 14:73
34. Manandhar K, Risal A, Steiner TJ, Holen A, Koju R, Linde M (2014) Estimating the prevalence and burden of major disorders of the brain in Nepal: methodology of a nationwide population-based study. J Headache Pain 15:52
35. Andrée C, Stovner LJ, Steiner TJ, Barré J, Katsarava Z, Lainez JM, Lantéri- Minet M, Mick G, Rastenyte D, Ruiz de la Torre E, Tassorelli C, Vriezen P, Lampl C (2011) The Eurolight project: the impact of primary headache disorders in Europe. Description of methods. J Headache Pain 12:541–9

36. Vos T, Flaxman AD, Naghavi M, Lozano R, Michaud C, Ezzati M, Shibuya K, Salomon JA, Abdalla S, Aboyans V, Abraham J, Ackerman I, Aggarwal R, Ahn SY, Ali MK, Alvarado M, Anderson HR, Anderson LM, Andrews KG, Atkinson C, Baddour LM, Bahalim AN, Barker-Collo S, Barrero LH, Bartels DH, Basáñez MG, Baxter A, Bell ML, Benjamin EJ, Bennett D et al (2012) Years lived with disability (YLDs) for 1160 sequelae of 289 diseases and injuries 1990–2010: a systematic analysis for the global burden of disease study 2010. Lancet 380:2163–96
37. Westergaard ML, Hansen EH, Glumer C, Olesen J, Jensen RH (2014) Definitions of medication-overuse headache in population-based studies and their implications on prevalence estimates: a systematic review. Cephalalgia 34:409–25
38. Linde M, Steiner TJ, Chisholm D (2015) Cost-effectiveness analysis of interventions for migraine in four low- and middle-income countries. J Headache Pain 16:15

9

The association of headache frequency with pain interference and the burden of disease is mediated by depression and sleep quality, but not anxiety, in chronic tension type headache

María Palacios-Ceña[1,2], Juan J. Fernández-Muñoz[3], Matteo Castaldo[2,4,5], Kelun Wang[2], Ángel Guerrero-Peral[6], Lars Arendt-Nielsen[2] and César Fernández-de-las-Peñas[1,2*]

Abstract

Background: A better understanding of potential relationship between mood disorders, sleep quality, pain, and headache frequency may assist clinicians in determining optimal therapeutic programs. The aim of the current study was to analyze the effects of sleep quality, anxiety, depression on potential relationships between headache intensity, burden of headache, and headache frequency in chronic tension type headache (CTTH).

Methods: One hundred and ninety-three individuals with CTTH participated. Headache features were collected with a 4-weeks headache diary. The Hospital Anxiety and Depression Scale was used for assessing anxiety and depression. Headache Disability Inventory evaluated the burden of headache. Pain interference was determined with the bodily pain domain (SF-36 questionnaire). Sleep quality was assessed with Pittsburgh Sleep Quality Index. Path analyses with maximum likelihood estimations were conducted to determine the direct and indirect effects of depression, anxiety, and sleep quality on the frequency of headaches.

Result: Two paths were observed: the first with depression and the second with sleep quality as mediators. Direct effects were noted from sleep quality, emotional burden of disease and pain interference on depression, and from depression to headache frequency. The first path showed indirect effects of depression from emotional burden and from sleep quality to headache frequency (first model $R^2 = 0.12$). Direct effects from the second path were from depression and pain interference on sleep quality and from sleep quality on headache frequency. Sleep quality indirectly mediated the effects of depression, emotional burden and pain interference on headache frequency (second model $R^2 = 0.18$).

Conclusions: Depression and sleep quality, but not anxiety, mediated the relationship between headache frequency and the emotional burden of disease and pain interference in CTTH.

Keywords: Tension type headache, Sleep quality, Depression, Anxiety

* Correspondence: cesar.fernandez@urjc.es
[1]Department Physical Therapy, Occupational Therapy, Rehabilitation, and Physical Medicine, University Rey Juan Carlos, Alcorcón, Spain
[2]Center for Sensory-Motor Interaction (SMI), Department of Health Science and Technology, School of Medicine, Aalborg University, Aalborg, Denmark
Full list of author information is available at the end of the article

Background

Tension type headache is a common headache disorder with a global prevalence of 42% [1] and has a large socio-economic impact [2]. The general costs in Europe in 2010 for primary headaches were €13.8 billion [3]. In fact, in the Global Burden of Disease Study, it was found that tension type headache was the second most prevalent disorder in the world [4].

Current research regarding the pathogenesis of tension type headache is focused on altered nociceptive pain processing and its role on chronification [5]. It appears that among the clinical features of headache, the frequency of attacks is the most relevant outcome since higher frequency of attacks is associated with higher sensitization [6]. In addition, emotional factors, such as depression or anxiety, and poor sleep quality can also play a role in the sensitization process by increasing excitability of the nociceptive firing [7, 8]. Chiu et al. reported that poor sleep quality and depression were independently associated with reduced pain thresholds, supporting this assumption [9].

There is evidence suggesting that subjects with tension type headache exhibit co-morbid anxiety, depression [10] and sleep insomnia [11]. Interestingly, depression and anxiety are more associated to the headache frequency than to headache diagnosis [12]. Further, poor sleep quality is usually considered a risk factor for progression from the episodic to the chronic form of tension type headache [13]. It seems that the severity and the prevalence of sleep problems increase proportionally to the frequency of the headaches [14]. It is therefore conceivable that both depression and sleep quality can interact at different levels by promoting higher frequency of headaches. Additionally, individuals with tension type headache and comorbid psychiatric disorders often exhibit affective temperament dys-regulation and suicidal behaviors, which may also contribute to this chronification process [15].

In fact, poor sleep quality has been related to higher levels of depression and pain intensity [16] and lower functioning [17] in patients with chronic pain. A better understanding of the potential relationship between mood disorders, i.e., depression and anxiety, and sleep quality with the frequency of headaches in individuals with tension type headache could assist clinicians for determining better therapeutic programs and hence for preventing evolution to the chronic form of the disease. However, no study has investigated potential direct and indirect effects of these variables with headache frequency at the same time in this headache condition. Since depression and sleep disturbances are associated with the frequency of headaches, we included individuals with chronic tension type headache (CTTH). Therefore, the purpose of the current study was to determine the direct and indirect effects of sleep quality, anxiety or depression on the potential relationships between headache intensity, burden of the condition, pain interference and headache frequency in individuals with CTTH. We hypothesized that mood disorders, i.e., depression and anxiety, and poor sleep quality would mediate the association between headache and related-disability with the frequency of headaches.

Methods

Participants

Consecutive patients with a diagnosis of tension type headache were recruited from different university-based hospitals from September 2014 to July 2016. Patients were recruited during routine medical visit. Diagnosis was conducted according to the criteria of the International Classification of Headache Disorders, third edition (ICHD-III beta, 2013) down to third-digit level (code 2.3) by an expert neurologist in the diagnosis and management of headaches [18]. To be included, patients had to describe all the pain features of TTH: bilateral location, pressing and tightening pain, moderate intensity (≤6 on a 10-points numerical pain rate scale, NPRS) and no aggravation of pain during physical activity. Patients should also report neither more than one of photophobia, phonophobia or mild nausea and neither moderate nor severe nausea nor vomiting as requested by the ICHD-III diagnostic criteria [18]. Headache attacks had to be present from at least 3 months with a frequency higher than 15 days per month [18].

Participants were excluded if they presented: 1, patients with epidosic headaches; 2, other primary/secondary headaches including medication overuse headache as defined by the ICHD-III; 3, history of neck or head trauma (i.e., whiplash injury); 4, systemic degenerative diseases, e.g., rheumatoid arthritis, lupus erythematous; 5, diagnosis of fibromyalgia syndrome; 6, receiving anesthetic blocks within the previous 6 months; 7, physical treatment in the neck and/or head received the previous 6 months; 8, abuse of caffeine or other stimulating substances; or, 9, pregnancy.

All participants read and signed a consent form prior to their participation. The local Ethics Committee approved the study (URJC 23/2014, HUFA 14/104, Aalborg N20140063, CESU 5/2015) which took place at three countries (Spain, Denmark, Italy).

Headache clinical outcomes - headache diary

A headache diary over 4 weeks was used to substantiate the diagnosis and to record the headache clinical features [19, 20]. On this diary, patients registered the frequency of headaches (days per week), the headache intensity on an 11points numerical pain rate scale [21] (NPRS; 0: no pain, 10: the maximum pain), and the duration of each headache attack (hours per day). The main outcome in this study was the frequency of headaches.

Hospital Anxiety and Depression Scale (HADS)

The HADS is a 14 item self-report screening scale, seven items for anxiety (HADS-A) and seven for depression (HADS-D), developed to indicate the presence of anxiety and depressive symptoms [22]. Each item scores on a Likert scale (0–3) giving a maximum subscale score of 21 points for each subscale [23]. The HADS has shown good validity and internal consistency (Cronbach's α: 0.84) for being used in subjects with headache [24].

Sleep quality

Sleep quality was assessed with the Pittsburgh Sleep Quality Index (PSQI) [25]. This questionnaire assesses sleep quality over a 1-month period by including 19 self-rated questions and five questions answered by bedmates or roommates. Items use varying response categories recording usual bed time, usual wake time, number of actual hours slept, and number of minutes to fall asleep. All questions are answered on a Likert-type scale (0–3). The sum of all answered for the components yields one global score (0–21) where higher score indicates worse sleep quality. Buysse et al. reported that the PSQI has good internal consistency (α: 0.83) and test-retest reliability (r: 0.85) [26]. A total score > 8.0 has been found to be indicative of poor sleep quality [27].

Headache Disability Inventory (HDI)

The HDI assesses the burden of headache using 25 items that inquire about the perceived impact of headache on emotional functioning and daily life activities [28]. Possible answers for each item are YES (4 points), SOMETIMES (2 points) and NO (0 points). Thirteen items asses the emotional component of headache (HDI-E, maximum score: 52) and the remaining 12 items assess the physical component (HDI-P, maximum score: 48). A higher score suggests a greater burden of headache for each subscale. The HDI has exhibited good stability at short ($r = 0.93$-0.95) and long ($r = 0.76$-0.83) term follow-ups [29].

Pain interference

To determine the interference of pain, we used the bodily pain domain of the health-related quality of life Medical Outcomes Study Short Form 36 (SF-36) questionnaire [30]. After summing the Likert-scaled items of this domain, it is categorized from 0 (lowest level of pain) to 100 (highest level of pain) [31]. Lower scores represent higher interference of pain.

Statistical analysis

Means and confidence intervals were calculated to describe the outcomes. The Kolmogorov-Smirnov test revealed that all data had a normal distribution ($P > 0.05$). To determine the relationship between the dependent measure (the frequency of headaches) and the independent outcomes (headache intensity, headache duration, HDI-E, HDI-P, sleep quality, pain interference, HADS-D and HADS-A), different Pearson product–moment correlation coefficients were first assessed.

Since anxiety was not significantly associated with the frequency of headaches, we conducted two different path analyses with depression and sleep quality as independent measures, since both were associated with headache frequency. Two path analyses with maximum likelihood estimations were conducted to evaluate the potential direct and indirect effects of independent variables on the association between headache frequency with headache intensity, headache duration, sleep quality, HDI-E, HDI-P, interference of pain, and HADS-D using AMOS computer program [32]. A path model analysis is a regression model extension relating independent, intermediary and dependent variables [33]. In the hypothesized model, the frequency of headache was the dependent variable; headache intensity, headache duration, HDI-E, HDI-P, and interference of pain were the independent outcomes, and sleep quality and depression (HADS-D) were intermediary variables. In a path analysis, single arrows indicate causation between intermediary and dependent variable. Further, arrows also connect the error terms with their respective intermediary variables. Double arrows indicate correlation between pairs of independent variables. The path coefficient is a standardized regression coefficient (beta) showing the direct effect of an independent variable (pain interference) on a dependent (headache frequency) variable. These path coefficients may be used to decompose correlations into direct and indirect effects, corresponding to direct and indirect paths reflected within the arrows in the model. Indirect effects occur when the relationship between two variables (e.g. headache frequency and interference of pain) is mediated by one or more variables (i.e., depression or sleep quality).

In the first model, headache intensity, sleep, HDI-E, HDI-P and pain interference were identified as predictors of depression. Likewise, depression was specified as a predictor of headache frequency. In the second model, headache intensity, HDI-E, HDI-P, HADS-D and pain interference were identified as predictors of sleep quality, and sleep quality was also specified as predictor of the frequency of headaches.

The evaluation of each model data was based on several recommended indexes. AMOS provides several fit of them that are largely independent of the sample size: chi-square statistic (X^2) [34, 35]; the goodness of fit index (GFI) and adjusted goodness of fin index (AGFI) whose value reference is at 90 to consider an acceptable model [36], and the comparative fin index (CFI) which accepted adequate value is over 0.90 [37]. Finally, within parsimony adjustment indices, the errors of the root mean square approximation (RMSEA) whose values < 0.08 are good to accept the model [38] were also calculated. Missing data were treated with maximum likelihood imputation.

Results

Clinical data of the sample

A total of 250 individuals with headache were screened for possible eligibility criteria. Finally, 193 (73% women) satisfied all eligibility criteria of CTTH, agreed to participate and signed the informed consent. The remaining 57 were excluded for the following reasons: co-morbid migraine ($n = 27$), episodic tension type headache ($n = 10$), previous whiplash ($n = 10$), fibromyalgia ($n = 5$) and medication overuse headache ($n = 5$). Seventy-five (38%) of the patients were taking prophylactic drugs (i.e., amitriptyline) on a regular basis. Demographic data and outcome measure scores are listed in Table 1.

Correlation analysis

Table 1 summarizes the Pearson's correlation coefficients and the descriptive analysis between all variables. Significant positive correlations were found between the frequency of headaches with headache intensity, headache duration, sleep quality, HDI-E, HDI-P and HADS-D: the greater the headache intensity, the longer the headache duration, the worse the quality of sleep, the higher the emotional or physical component of the headache and the higher the depression, the higher the frequency of headache attacks. Further, headache frequency was negatively associated with pain interference: the lower the bodily pain score, i.e., the higher the inference of pain, the higher the frequency of headaches.

First path analysis - depression as mediator

The hypothesized model fit the data was excellent, with $X^2 = 3.14$ $X^2/df = 5$, Goodness of Fit Index (GFI): 0.96; Adjusted Goodness of Fit Index (AGFI): 0.91; Comparative Fit Index (CFI): 0.97, and Normal Fit Index (NFI): 0.97. Further, Root Mean Square Error of Approximation (RMSEA) was 0.07. Figure 1 displays all the parameter estimates (standardized solution).

According to the direct effects, significant paths were noted from sleep quality (B = 0.25; $P < 0.01$), HDI-E (B = 0.16; $P < 0.01$) and pain interference (B = −0.04; $P < 0.05$) on depression. Likewise, a significant path was also indicated from depression (B = 0.71; $P < 0.01$) on headache frequency. The direct effects from HDI-P (B = 0.15; $P =$ 0.133) and headache intensity (B = 0.15; $P = 0.166$) on depression were not significant. The amount of depression explained by all predictors in this model was $R^2 = 0.42$.

Further, the path analysis included an indirect effect from HDI-E to headache frequency, exerted through depression (B = 0.13, $P < 0.01$), and from the sleep quality to headache frequency, also exerted through depression (B = 0.06, $P <$ 0.01). The indirect effect of depression on the remaining outcomes was not statistically related to headache frequency: pain interference (B = −0.04, $P > 0.05$), headache intensity (B = 0.02, $P > 0.05$), and HDI-P (B = −0.04, $P > 0.05$). Overall, the amount of headache frequency explained by all predictors in this first model was $R^2 = 0.12$.

Second path analysis - sleep quality as mediator

The hypothesized model fit the data was also excellent, with $X^2 = 4.42$ $X^2/df = 5$, Goodness of Fit Index (GFI): 0.97; Adjusted Goodness of Fit Index (AGFI): 0.84; Comparative Fit Index (CFI): 0.96, and Normal Fit Index (NFI): 0.96. In addition, Root Mean Square Error of Approximation (RMSEA) was 0.07. Figure 2 displays all the parameter estimates (standardized solution).

According to the direct effects, significant paths were observed from depression (B = 0.29; $P < 0.01$) and pain interference (B = −0.03; $P < 0.01$) on sleep quality. A significant path was also indicated from sleep quality (B = 0.48; $P < 0.01$) on headache frequency. The rest direct effects were not significant. The amount of sleep quality explained by predictors in this model was $R^2 = 0.42$.

Table 1 Demographic variables and pearson-product moment correlation matrix for each study variable

	Mean	95% CI	1	2	3	4	5	6	7	8
1. Headache frequency (days/month)	18.1	17.5–18.7								
2. Headache intensity (0–10)	5.9	5.5–6.3	.145*							
3. Headache duration (hours/attack)	7.3	6.6-8.0	.249**	n.s						
4. Pittsburg Questionnaire (0–21)	17.1	15.8–18.4	.223**	.177**	.165*					
5. HDI-E (0–52)	18.7	17.0–20.4	.341**	.212**	.350**	.328**				
6. HDI-P (0–48)	22.5	20.9–24.1	.235**	.165*	.237**	.232**	.828**			
7. Bodily Pain (0–100)	51.2	47.9–54.6	-.245**	-.165*	n.s.	-.350**	-.409**	-.442**		
8. HADS-D (0–21)	8.0	7.5–8.6	.274**	.227**	.313**	.426**	.538**	.405**	-.389**	
9. HADS-A (0–21)	10.0	9.3-10.7	n.s.	n.s	n.s	n.s	n.s	n.s	n.s	.208**

95% CI: 95% confidence interval
HDI Headache Disability Inventory (*E* Emotional, *P* Physical), *HADS* Hospital Anxiety and Depression Scale (*D* Depression, *A* Anxiety)
*$P < 0.05$; **$P < 0.01$

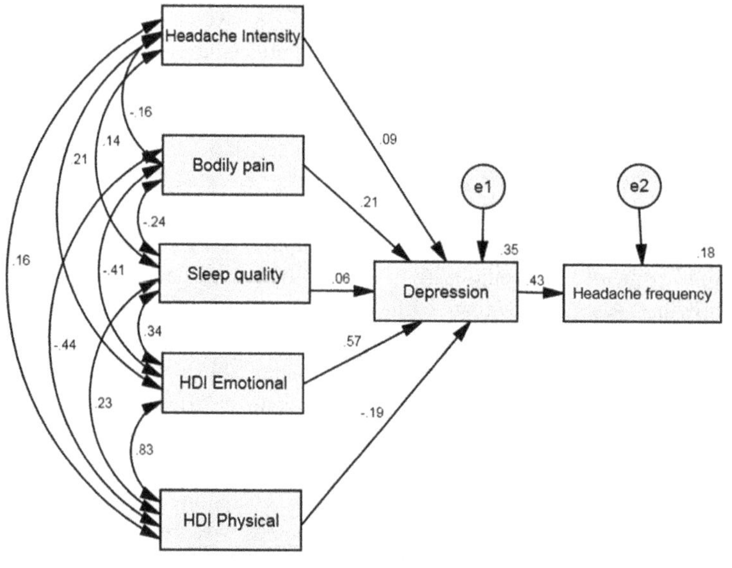

Fig. 1 Path analyses to headache frequency from headache intensity, sleep quality, bodily pain, and burden of headache (physical and emotional) with depression as the mediating variable. Standardized direct path coefficients are presented. Data from *double arrows* represent correlations between the variables whereas data from *single arrows* represent standardized regression weights (parameter estimates). e1 and e2: error terms for each variable

The path analysis model also included several indirect effects of sleep quality from depression (B = 0.06; $P <$ 0.01), HDI-E (B = 0.04; $P < 0.01$) and pain interference (B = −0.04; $P < 0.01$) on headache frequency. The indirect effects of sleep quality on the remaining predictors were not significantly related to the frequency of headache attacks: headache intensity (B = 0.01; $P > 0.05$) and HDI-P (B = −0.02; $P > 0.05$). Overall, the amount of headache frequency explained by all predictors in this second model was $R^2 = 0.18$.

Discussion

This is the first study investigating the indirect effects of depression, anxiety and sleep quality on headache frequency in individuals with tension type headache. We observed that depression and sleep quality, but not

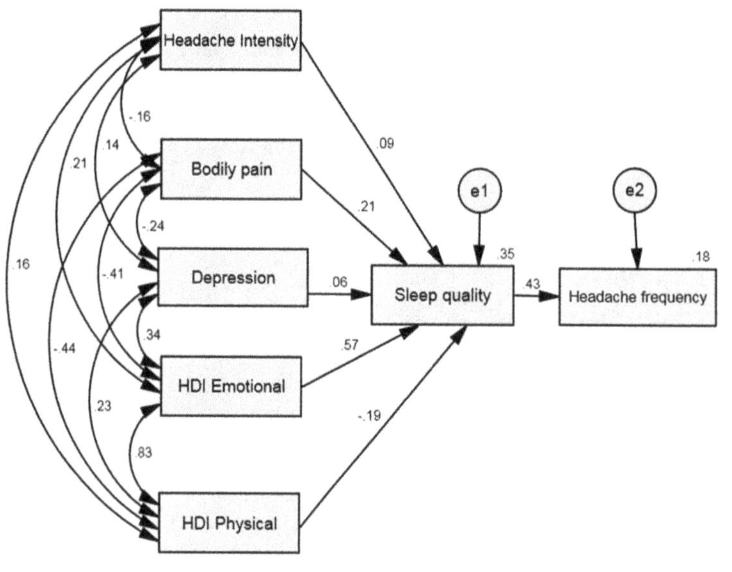

Fig. 2 Path analyses to headache frequency from headache intensity, depression, bodily pain, and burden of headache (physical and emotional) with sleep quality as the mediating variable. Standardized direct path coefficients are presented. Data from *double arrows* represent correlations between the variables, where data from *single arrows* represents the standardized regression weight (parameter estimates). e1 and e2: error terms for each variable

anxiety, mediated the relationship between the frequency of headaches with the emotional burden of condition and pain interference in subjects with CTTH. These results support the assumption that headache frequency is related to the emotional burden of the condition but with an indirect mediator effect of depression and sleep quality; whereas the relation with interference of pain is only mediated by sleep quality.

The findings from this study show, firstly, and in accordance with prior literature, that depression and sleep quality are factors associated with the frequency of headaches in CTTH [12, 14]. The study also demonstrated that depressive levels and sleep quality mediated the relationship between the emotional burden of headache and the frequency of attacks. Thus, while a small amount of variance (12% or 18%) within the relationship between the emotional burden of condition and headache frequency was indirectly mediated by depression or sleep quality, respectively, the relationships with other variables were also significant (although attenuated). This suggests that the emotional burden of headache may contribute to the frequency of headaches via other factors. For instance, emotional stress is associated with increased mechanical pain hypersensitivity [7]; therefore, it is possible that a higher emotional burden of headache (stressful situation) can contribute to the excitability of the central nervous system and therefore increasing the frequency of headache attacks. Similarly, poor sleep quality and depression are also associated with increased sensitivity [9]; therefore, a synergistic effect may occur in headache sufferers who do not sleep well under stressful emotional situations. In fact, sleep deficiency is associated with more severe headaches [39] which would explain why sleep quality, but not depression, also mediated the relationship between the pain interference (i.e., bodily pain domain) and headache frequency. Finally, other aspects not assessed in the current study may also be involved in these interactions.

Depression and anxiety have a significant impact on quality of life and increase the burden on patients with headache [40]; however in the current study depression, but not anxiety, was found to have a significant indirect effect on headache frequency. Although current methodology does not allow determining the mechanisms involved in the mediating relationship of depression on headache frequency; it has been previously suggested that depression predominantly contributes to chronic pain via supra-spinal mechanisms and emotional modulation of pain [41].

The indirect effect of sleep quality on the frequency of headaches was slightly higher than depression, which agrees with previous research supporting a correlation between sleep quality and the frequency of headaches [13]. In addition, in the second path revealed that sleep quality also mediated the relationship between pain interference and the frequency of headaches, suggesting that different indirect effects are involved on each model. However, whether poor sleep quality leads to headache or conversely is unclear since underlying mechanisms of both conditions are shared by common pathogenic mechanisms [13].

Uncertainty over biological mechanisms in these interactions exists, however our results have clinical implications. Since emotional stress and poor sleep quality are the most common triggers for tension type headache [42, 43], proper management of their associated factors seems to be relevant. In fact, emotional stress, depression, and sleep are of clinical interest because they represent modifiable risk factors implicated in the chronicity of headaches [44]. Our study found an interaction between depression, the emotional burden of headache, sleep quality and frequency of headaches in subjects with CTTH. Therefore, proper copying management of stressful emotional events per se may not be the primary mechanism of action for decreasing the frequency of headache attacks in CTTH. Rather, the mechanism may be a reduction of depressive symptoms, or an alteration in the relationship between sleep quality and these emotional factors. In fact, current findings would suggest that management of patients with CTTH should include therapeutic interventions targeted to decrease the emotional burden of headache (copying strategies or cognitive behavioral techniques), to decrease depressive symptoms (i.e., psychological approaches) and to improve sleep quality.

Although strengths of this study include a large sample size and the inclusion of CTTH patients according to the most updated diagnostic criteria, the use of diagnostic diaries and the use of standardized instruments; our study has its limitation due to the fact that we included a sample consisted mainly of CTTH patients referred to a tertiary headache center and thus not representative of the general population. Additionally, the impact of daily medications to prevent headache was not considered in the path models. However, since 38% of our sample was taking preventive drugs and because headache history and headache features were comparable to previous studies, our study sample was probably fairly representative for a patient group encountered in a clinical setting. Second, the study is cross-sectional and causal relations are thus impossible to ascertain. Third, it should be noted that the HADS is a screening rather than diagnostic instrument for depression and anxiety symptoms with a tendency to underestimate prevalence of both disorders [45]. In fact, we should note that anxiety and depression levels observed in our sample of CTTH were low; therefore, it is possible that the interactions found in the current study maybe different in subjects with higher levels of anxiety or depression.

Conclusions

This study found that a significant amount of variance in the relationship between headache frequency and the emotional burden of condition was indirectly mediated by depression and sleep quality, but not anxiety, in individuals with CTTH. Further, sleep quality also mediated the relationship between pain interference and the frequency of headaches. Our results would suggest that depressive symptoms and sleep quality play a relevant role in the chronicity of pain in individuals with CTTH. Future longitudinal studies will help to determine the clinical implications of these findings.

Abbreviations

CFI: Comparative fin index; CTTH: Chronic tension type headache; GFI: Goodness of fit index; HADS: Hospital Anxiety and Depression Scale; HDI: Headache Disability Inventory; ICHD3: International Classification of Headache Disorders, third edition; NPRS: Numerical pain rate scale; PSQI: Pittsburgh Sleep Quality Index; RMSEA: Root mean square approximation

Author contributions

All authors contributed to the study concept and design. JJFM and CFdlP did the main statistical analysis and interpretation of data. MPC and CFdlP contributed to draft the report. LAN obtained funding. LAN, KW, MC, and AG provided administrative, technical, and material support. LAN and CFdlP supervised the study. All authors revised the text for intellectual content and have read and approved the final version of the manuscript.

Competing interests

The authors declare that they have no competing interests.

Disclosures

Financial disclosure statements have been obtained, and no conflicts of interest have been reported by the authors or by any individuals in control of the content of this article.

Author details

[1]Department Physical Therapy, Occupational Therapy, Rehabilitation, and Physical Medicine, University Rey Juan Carlos, Alcorcón, Spain. [2]Center for Sensory-Motor Interaction (SMI), Department of Health Science and Technology, School of Medicine, Aalborg University, Aalborg, Denmark. [3]Department of Psychology, Universidad Rey Juan Carlos, Alcorcón, Spain. [4]Master in Sport Physiotherapy, University of Siena, Siena, Italy. [5]Poliambulatorio Fisiocenter, Collecchio, Parma, Italy. [6]Headache Unit. Hospital Clínico Universitario de Valladolid, Valladolid, Spain.

References

1. Ferrante T, Manzoni GC, Russo M, Camarda C, Taga A, Veronesi L et al (2013) Prevalence of tension-type headache in adult general population: the PACE study and review of the literature. Neurol Sci 34:S137–S138
2. Dowson A (2015) The burden of headache: global and regional prevalence of headache and its impact. Int J Clin Pract Suppl 182:3–7
3. Raggi A, Leonardi M (2015) Burden and cost of neurological diseases: a European North–south comparison. Acta Neurol Scand 132:16–22
4. Global Burden of Disease Study (2013) Collaborators (2015) Global, regional, and national incidence, prevalence, and years lived with disability for 301 acute and chronic diseases and injuries in 188 countries, 1990–2013: a systematic analysis for the Global Burden of Disease Study 2013. Lancet 386: 743–800
5. de Tommaso M, Fernández-de-las-Peñas C (2016) Tension type headache. Curr Rheumatol Rev 12:1–13
6. Buchgreitz L, Lyngberg AC, Bendtsen L, Jensen R (2006) Frequency of headache is related to sensitization: A population study. Pain 123:19–27
7. Cathcart S, Petkov J, Winefield AH, Lushington K, Rolan P (2010) Central mechanisms of stress-induced headache. Cephalalgia 30:285–295
8. de Tommaso M, Delussi M, Vecchio E, Sciruicchio V, Invitto S, Livrea P (2014) Sleep features and central sensitization symptoms in primary headache patients. J Headache Pain 15:64
9. Chiu YH, Silman AJ, Macfarlane GJ, Ray D, Gupta A, Dickens C, Morriss R, McBeth J (2005) Poor sleep and depression are independently associated with a reduced pain threshold. Results of a population based study. Pain 115:316–321
10. Beghi E, Bussone G, D'Amico D et al (2010) Headache, anxiety and depressive disorders: the HADAS study. J Headache Pain 11:141–150
11. Uhlig BL, Engstrøm M, Ødegård SS, Hagen KK, Sand T (2014) Headache and insomnia in population-based epidemiological studies. Cephalalgia 34:745–751
12. Zwart JA, Dyb G, Hagen K, Ødegård KJ, Dahl AA, Bovim G et al (2003) Depression and anxiety disorder associated with headache frequency: The Nord-Trøndelag Health Study. Eur J Neurol 10:147–152
13. Rains JC, Davis RE, Smitherman TA (2015) Tension-type headache and sleep. Curr Neurol Neurosci Rep 15:520
14. Sancisi E, Cevoli S, Vignatelli L, Nicodemo M, Pierangeli G, Zanigni S, Grimaldi D, Cortelli P, Montagna P (2010) Increased prevalence of sleep disorders in chronic headache: a case–control study. Headache 50:1464–1472
15. Serafini G, Pompili M, Innamorati M, Gentile G, Borro M, Lamis DA, Lala N, Negro A, Simmaco M, Girardi P, Martelletti P (2012) Gene variants with suicidal risk in a sample of subjects with chronic migraine and affective temperamental dysregulation. Eur Rev Med Pharmacol Sci 16:1389–1398
16. Naughton F, Ashworth P, Skevington SM (2007) Does sleep quality predict pain-related disability in chronic pain patients? The mediating roles of depression and pain severity. Pain 127:243–252
17. Baldwin CM, Ervin AM, Mays MZ, Robbins J, Shafazand S, Walsleben J et al (2010) (2010) Sleep disturbances, quality of life, and ethnicity: the Sleep Heart Health Study. J Clin Sleep Med 6:176–183
18. ICHD-III (2013) International classification of headache disorder: Headache Classification Subcommittee of the International Headache Society, 3nd edition. Cephalalgia 33:629–808
19. Phillip D, Lyngberg AC, Jensen R (2007) Assessment of headache diagnosis: a comparative population study of a clinical interview with a diagnostic headache diary. Cephalalgia 27:1–8
20. Jensen R, Tassorelli C, Rossi P, Allena M, Osipova V, Steiner T, Sandrini G, Olesen J, Nappi G, Basic Diagnostic Headache Diary Study Group (2011) A basic diagnostic headache headache diary (BDHD) is well accepted and useful in the diagnosis of headache. a multicentre European and Latin American study. Cephalalgia 31:1549–1560
21. Jensen MP, Turner JA, Romano JM, Fisher L (1999) Comparative reliability and validity of chronic pain intensity measures. Pain 83:157–162
22. Zigmond AS, Snaith RP (1983) The hospital anxiety and depression scale. Acta Psychiatr Scand 67:361–370
23. Herrmann-Lingen C, Buss U, Snaith RP (2011) Hospital Anxiety and Depression Scale – Deutsche version (HADS-D). Verlag Hans Huber, Bern
24. Juang KD, Wang SJ, Lin CH, Fuh JL (1999) Use of the Hospital Anxiety and Depression Scale as a screening tool for patients with headache. Zhonghua Yi Xue Za Zhi (Taipei) 62:749–755
25. Cole JC, Dubois D, Kosinski M (2007) Use of patient-reported sleep measures in clinical trials of pain treatment: a literature review and synthesis of current sleep measures and a conceptual model of sleep disturbance in pain. Clin Ther 29:2580–2588
26. Buysse DJ, Reynolds CF, Monk TH, Berman SR, Kupfer DJ (1989) The Pittsburgh sleep quality index: a new instrument for psychiatric practice and research. Psychiatry Res 28:193–213
27. Carpenter JS, Andrykowski MA (1998) Psychometric evaluation of the Pittsburgh sleep quality index. J Psychosom Res 45:5–13
28. Jacobson GP, Ramadan NM, Norris L, Newman CW (1994) The Henry Ford hospital headache disability inventory. Neurology 44:837–842
29. Jacobson GP, Ramadan NM, Norris L, Newman CW (1995) Headache disability inventory (HDI): short-term test-retest reliability and spouse perceptions. Headache 35:534–539
30. Ware JE, Sherbourne CD (1992) The MOS 36-item short-form health survey (SF-36). I. Conceptual framework and item selection. Med Care 30:473–483
31. McHorney CA, Ware JE, Raczek AE (1993) The MOS 36-Item Short-Form Health Survey (SF-36): II. Psychometric and clinical tests of validity in measuring physical and mental health constructs. Med Care 31:247–263
32. Abuckle JL, Wothke W (1999) Amos 4.0 users guide. Small waters, Chicago
33. Duncan O (1966) Path analysis: sociological examples. Am J Sociology 72:1–12

34. Jöreskog KG, Sörbom D (1979) Advanced in factor analysis and structural equation models. M.A. Abl, Cambridge
35. Saris WE, Stronkhorst H (1984) Casual modelling in non-experimental research: an introduction to the LISREL approach. Sociometric Research Foundation, Amsterdam
36. Hu L, Bentler PM (1999) Cut-off criteria for fit indexes in covariance structure analysis: conventional criteria versus new alternatives. Structural Equation Mod 6:1–55
37. Bentler PM (1990) Comparative fit indices in structural models. Psychological Bull 107:238–246
38. Steiger JH, Lind C (1980) Statistically based tests for the number of common factors, Paper presented at the annual meeting of the Psychometric Society, Iowa City, IA
39. Houle TT, Butschek RA, Turner DP, Smitherman TA, Rains JC, Penzien DB (2012) Stress and sleep duration predict headache severity in chronic headache sufferers. Pain 153:2432–2440
40. Zebenholzer K, Lechner A, Broessner G, Lampl C, Luthringshausen G, Wuschitz A, Obmann SM, Berek K, Wöber C (2016) Impact of depression and anxiety on burden and management of episodic and chronic headaches - a cross-sectional multicentre study in eight Austrian headache centres. J Headache Pain 17:15
41. Terry EL, DelVentura JL, Bartley EJ, Vincent AL, Rhudy JL (2013) Emotional modulation of pain and spinal nociception in persons with major depressive disorder (MDD). Pain 154:2759–2768
42. Wang J, Huang Q, Li N, Tan G, Chen L, Zhou J (2013) Triggers of migraine and tension-type headache in China: a clinic-based survey. Eur J Neurol 20: 689–696
43. Haque B, Rahman KM, Hoque A, Hasan AT, Chowdhury RN, Khan SU, Alam MB, Habib M, Mohammad QD (2012) Precipitating and relieving factors of migraine versus tension type headache. BMC Neurol 12:82
44. Rains JC (2008) Chronic headache and potentially modifiable risk factors: screening and behavioral management of sleep disorders. Headache 48:32–39
45. Steel Z, Marnane C, Iranpour C, Chey T, Jackson JW, Patel V, Silove D (2014) The global prevalence of common mental disorders: a systematic review and meta-analysis 1980–2013. Int J Epidemiol 43:476–493

10

Copeptin for risk stratification in non-traumatic headache in the emergency setting

Claudine Angela Blum[1,3*], Bettina Winzeler[1], Nicole Nigro[1], Philipp Schuetz[3], Silke Biethahn[2], Timo Kahles[2], Cornelia Mueller[1], Katharina Timper[1,9], Katharina Haaf[2], Janina Tepperberg[2], Margareth Amort[4], Andreas Huber[5], Roland Bingisser[6], Peter Stephan Sándor[7], Krassen Nedeltchev[2], Beat Müller[3], Mira Katan[8†] and Mirjam Christ-Crain[1†]

Abstract

Background: In the emergency setting, non-traumatic headache is a benign symptom in 80% of cases, but serious underlying conditions need to be ruled out.
Copeptin improves risk stratification in several acute diseases. Herein, we investigated the value of copeptin to discriminate between serious secondary headache and benign headache forms in the emergency setting.

Methods: Patients presenting with acute non-traumatic headache were prospectively enrolled into an observational cohort study. Copeptin was measured upon presentation to the emergency department. Primary endpoint was serious secondary headache defined by a neurologic cause requiring immediate treatment of the underlying disease. Secondary endpoint was the combination of mortality and hospitalization within 3 months. Two board-certified neurologist blinded to copeptin levels verified the endpoints after a structured 3-month-telephone interview.

Results: Of the 391 patients included, 75 (19%) had a serious secondary headache. Copeptin was associated with serious secondary headache (OR 2.03, 95%CI 1.52–2.70, $p < 0.0001$). Area under the curve (AUC) for copeptin to identify the primary endpoint was 0.70 (0.63–0.76). After adjusting for age > 50, focal-neurological abnormalities, and thunderclap onset of symptoms, copeptin remained an independent predictive factor for serious secondary headache (OR 1.74, 95%CI 1.26–2.39, $p = 0.001$). Moreover, copeptin improved the AUC of the multivariate logistic clinical model (p-LR-test < 0.001).
Even though copeptin values were higher in patients reaching the secondary endpoint, this association was not significant in multivariate logistic regression.

Conclusions: Copeptin was independently associated with serious secondary headache as compared to benign headaches forms. Copeptin may be a promising novel blood biomarker that should be further validated to rule out serious secondary headache in the emergency department.

Keywords: Headache, Head pain, Emergency, Biomarker, Copeptin, Vasopressin

* Correspondence: claudineblum@yahoo.com; claudine.blum@ksa.ch
[†]Equal contributors
[1]Division of Endocrinology, Department of Internal Medicine, University Hospital Basel, Basel, Switzerland
[3]Internal Medicine, Medical University Clinic, Kantonsspital Aarau, Tellstrasse, CH-5001 Aarau, Switzerland
Full list of author information is available at the end of the article

Background

Headache has a high prevalence in the general population and presents an important public health problem [1].

Non-traumatic headache has a prevalence of 0.5 to 4.5% in patients presenting to the emergency department (ED), and it remains a major diagnostic challenge [2–5]. The majority of these patients have benign headache. However, in 3.8 – 20% of headache patients, a headache secondary to a potentially life-threatening condition is diagnosed with immediate implications for therapeutic interventions. These include subarachnoidal hemorrhage, cerebral aneurysm, intracranial bleeding, sinus vein thrombosis, temporal arteriitis, or meningitis [2, 5–7]. It has been shown by various authors that red flags like age >50 years, focal-neurological signs, thunderclap onset of symptoms or altered mental status have a remarkable negative predictive value around 0.98–0.99, however with varying sensitivities (between 0.39 and 100%) and specificities (between 65 and 98%) [7–11]. To improve the differentiation of benign headaches from secondary, potentially serious headache forms, various clinical algorithms which include these red flags have been proposed, but they are only inconsistently applied in clinical practice [7, 12]. Therefore, the use of biomarkers has potential merits as diagnostic tools.

Only few biomarkers have been investigated in headache, [13–22] and except D-dimer in specific vascular etiologies, [14, 17] they have not found their way into emergency algorithms. To our knowledge, there is no data on biomarkers for discriminating between serious secondary and benign headache forms.

Copeptin is a hypothalamic stress hormone that mirrors the individual stress level even more subtly than circulating cortisol [23]. In its function as a stress hormone, copeptin serves as a prognostic marker in various acute disease states, such as cerebrovascular event, myocardial infarction or pneumonia [24]. Apparently, copeptin allows tapping an endogenous information system of our body that, through mechanisms still poorly understood, assesses the severity of damage [25].

We herein prospectively evaluated the use of copeptin for discriminating between benign headache forms and serious secondary headache, and the degree of association with serious secondary headache.

Methods

Study design and participants

This multicenter observational study was performed at the ED of two tertiary care hospitals in northern Switzerland from October 2010 to March 2013.

All patients with current non-traumatic headache as a chief complaint presenting to the ED or as an emergency to the medical or neurological walk-in clinic of the two tertiary centers were eligible and screened.

Exclusion criteria were trauma within 7 days, chronic headache defined as > 3 months duration, age < 18 years, missing informed consent, and inability to comply with study procedures due to insufficient knowledge of the German language.

Chronic headache with an acute exacerbation was not an exclusion criterion.

Clinical variables

Recruitment was during 24 h and on weekdays and weekends.

After informed consent was given by the patient, baseline data were assessed by questionnaire at the time of the acute presentation. This included medical history, age, gender, body mass index, ethnicity and country of origin, past medical history, smoking history, current medication, alcohol and coffee consumption (units per day), and substance abuse. Clinical headache presentation and headache history was assessed by detailed standardized, validated questionnaire containing the International Classification of Headache Disorders (ICHD) [26] and included depression screening by Primary Care Evaluation of Mental Disorders (PRIME-MD) questionnaire [27] and categorization by a validated, diagnostic algorithm into one of four clinical scenarios (Thunderclap headache, meningitis, new or worsening headache, headache similar to previous episodes) as described by Grimaldi et al. [7]. Disease severity, quality of daily living, and interference of symptoms with quality of life was assessed using the standardized, validated migraine disability assessment (MIDAS) [28].

Clinical items assessed by the treating physician were recorded at the time of the acute presentation and included physical examination, neurological assessment, Glasgow Coma Scale, blood pressure, pulse rate, and body temperature.

Blood sampling and assays

Blood samples for copeptin measurement were drawn on admission in the emergency department and were either obtained from an indwelling venous catheter or by venous puncture. Blood samples were immediately centrifuged and stored in the refrigerator. Apart from blood sampling for study purposes, routine blood sampling was performed at the discretion of the treating physicians and was performed in 354 (91%) patients.

At ED discharge, the diagnostic work-up was recorded, including neuroimaging, lumbar puncture and additional disease-specific evaluations in secondary headaches.

Blood Plasma was frozen at –70 °C. Copeptin levels were measured by batch analysis with a commercial chemiluminescence sandwich immunoassay (B.R.A.H.M.S LUMItest CT-proAVP, B.R.A.H.M.S AG, Hennigsdorf/ Berlin, Germany), as described in detail elsewhere, with a lower detection limit of the assay of 0.4 pmol/L and the functional assay sensitivity (<20% interassay CV) of < 1 pmol/L) [29, 30]. The treating physicians and the study team were blinded to copeptin levels at all times.

Follow-up

At 3 months, a structured follow-up telephone interview was performed to assess course and outcome of the disease. The earliest possible contact was 14 days before this time point. If the patient was not reached until 4 weeks after the scheduled interview, his primary care physician was contacted for follow-up information. If the patient had consulted the hospital since study inclusion and no other data was available, this date was taken as time of last follow-up. To minimize loss of follow-up, the study team tried to re-contact the patient until the last scheduled follow-up interview in June 2013. The final headache diagnosis and the judgement whether the headache had been serious or not was made in each patient after the follow-up interview by two independent physicians by chart review and verified by a board-certified neurologist. Disagreements between study physicians were resolved by a final adjudication of an independent neurologist. They were all blinded to copeptin levels.

Outcomes

The objective of this study was to evaluate copeptin as a marker for risk stratification in non-traumatic headache, namely for ruling out serious secondary causes of headache. The primary endpoint was serious secondary headache as opposed to benign headache.

Our hypothesis was that based on previous studies on copeptin in other diseases, [29, 31–34] a cutoff of ≤ 5 pmol/l would have a sensitivity of ≥ 97% for ruling out serious secondary headache causes, and that a cutoff of ≥ 20 pmol/l would have a specificity of ≥90% for the presence of serious secondary NTH.

The secondary endpoint was the combined endpoint of death or hospitalization of any cause within 3 months.

Headache was defined according to the International Headache Society as pain located above the orbitomeatal line. A serious secondary headache was defined as a headache with a neurologic cause as listed in the ICHD-II criteria [9] requiring subsequent treatment of the underlying disease or condition, which, if left untreated, would have the potential risk of permanent damage or death(see also Appendix). All other patients with an uneventful 3-month follow-up were diagnosed with benign headache.

Our gold standard for the final diagnosis of headache was the clinical diagnosis according to ICHD-II criteria after 3 months, verified by a board-certified neurologist. Headaches which clearly belonged to the primary headache entities but did not fulfill the full diagnostic criteria were classified as "primary headache, not classified", e.g. a first episode of migraine, which did not yet fulfill the criterion of at least 3 episodes.

As this study was started before the current version ICHD3-beta was in place, we continued to use the ICHD-II classification for consistency throughout the whole study.

Analysis

Discrete variables are summarized as counts (percentage), and continuous variables as medians and interquartile ranges(IQRs). Frequency comparison was done by chi-square test. Two-group comparisons of continuous variables were performed using Student's *t*-test or the Mann–Whitney-U test, depending on their distribution. Receiver operating characteristic (ROC) curve for copeptin was calculated, and the area under the ROC curve (AUC) was used to assess the discriminatory potential of copeptin to accurately identify patients with serious secondary headache [35]. Further, we calculated logistic regression models to estimate the magnitude of the association between copeptin and the pre-specified endpoints. To assess the independence of this association from other risk scores and important outcome predictors (chosen from the published literature) we calculated multivariable regression models and added all parameters based on their association in the univariate models (p-value cut off for further evaluation was <0.05). This included age > 50 years, sudden onset of headache, an abnormal neurological examination, [11] clinical scenario 4 (history of previous similar headache) for the clinical model (multivariate model 1), [7] D-dimer, fibrinogen, leukocytes and C-reactive protein [13, 36] for the laboratory model (multivariate model 2). To avoid overfitting, we calculated two final models, thus no more than one variable per ten events were included in these final two models. In addition, we compared the ROC curves based on the logistic models with and without copeptin using the likelihood ratio test [37]. All statistical tests were 2-tailed. $p < 0.05$ was considered significant. STATA 12.1 (StataCorp LP, College Station, TX, USA) was used for data analysis.

Sample size considerations

Based on the patient numbers from previous years, about 400 patients per year were estimated to be eligible for this study. With an estimated informed consent rate of 90–95% and an estimated loss of follow-up of 5–10%, 360 patients were estimated to complete the study. According to pre-existing literature, 10–20% of these 360 patients would present with serious non-traumatic headache, thus 50–60 patients would reach the primary endpoint. Based on the literature and pilot data [25], a mean copeptin difference of 15 pmol/L (SD of 30 pmol/L) between these groups was expected. This difference would be detected with a power of 80%.

Results

Characteristics of study subjects

From October 2010 to March 2013, 398 patients were enrolled into the CoHead-Study (see Fig. 1 for study flow chart). The 3-month telephone interviews were terminated in July 2013. 7 patients were lost to follow-up and were therefore not included in the analysis.

Baseline characteristics are shown in Table 1. Median age was 41 (IQR 30–57), 146 patients (37%) were men. Median headache duration was 3 days (IQR 0.5–7); median pain strength on Visual Analogue Scale (VAS) was 8 (IQR 6–9). At discharge, a primary headache form was diagnosed in 219 (56%) patients, and secondary headache in 172 (44%) patients, of which 75 (19.2%) were classified as serious.

The group of serious secondary headache was heterogeneous: 8 patients (2%) had subarachnoidal hemorrhage, 7 (1.8%) sinus vein thrombosis, 10 (2.6%) intracranial bleeding, and 7 (1.8%) had viral meningitis (detailed diagnoses are shown in Table 2).

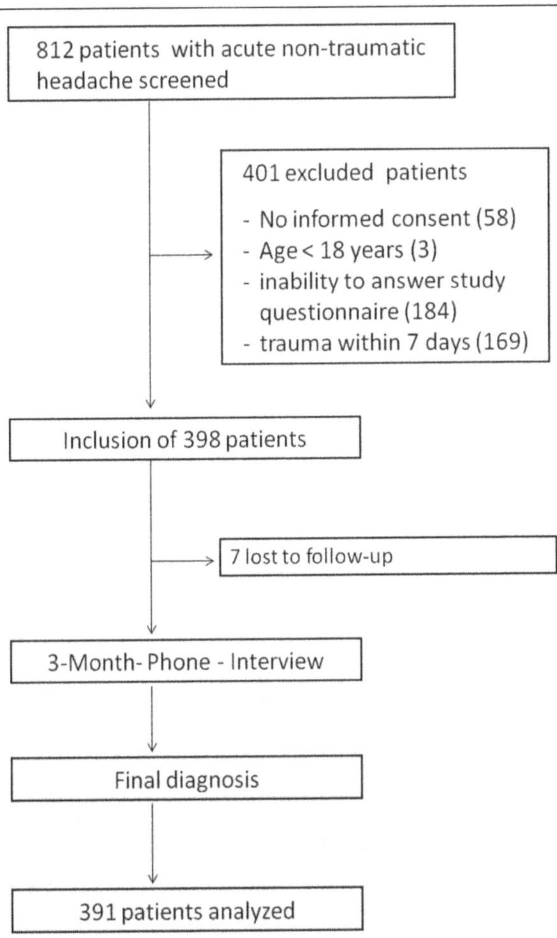

Fig. 1 STROBE study flow diagram

Median time to follow-up was 99 days (IQR 91–118; range 9–632). Two patients (0.5%) died during follow-up. Both had initially presented with serious secondary headache: one with subarachnoidal bleeding and one with bacterial meningitis. Hospitalization rate was 94 patients (24.0%), of which 61 (15.6%) were hospitalized immediately following study inclusion.

Main results

Association of copeptin with serious secondary headache

Copeptin levels were higher in serious secondary headache forms as compared to all other headache forms (median 6.44 pmol/L (IQR 3.97–11.29) vs. 3.89 pmol/L (IQR 2.59–6.10)($p < 0.0001$), see Fig. 2). The AUC for copeptin to detect serious secondary headache was 0.70 (95% confidence interval (CI) 0.63–0.76). At the predefined rule-out cutoff for serious secondary headache of 5.0 pmol/L, copeptin had a sensitivity of 64.4%; at the predefined rule-in cutoff of 20 pmol/L, copeptin had a specificity of 95.3% to rule in a serious secondary headache. At the cutoff of 2.5 pmol/L, copeptin had a sensitivity of 91.8% to rule out serious secondary headache, i.e. a negative predictive value of 0.93. For different copeptin cutoffs, see Table 3.

In univariate analysis, copeptin was associated with serious secondary headache with an OR of 2.03 (95%CI 1.52–2.70, $p < 0.0001$). Other strong predictors were age >50 years (OR 2.83, 95%CI 1.69–4.74, $p < 0.0001$), an abnormal neurological exam (OR 3.50, 95%CI 1.99–6.14, $p < 0.0001$), and thunderclap onset of symptoms (OR 4.23, 95%CI 2.38–7.52, $p < 0.0001$; for detailed results of the univariate analysis, see Table 4a).

We included the strongest clinical risk factors from the univariate analysis along with copeptin in a multivariate model. After adjustment, copeptin remained independently associated with serious secondary headache (OR 1.74, 95%CI 1.26–2.39, $p = 0.001$). The clinical factors age > 50 years (OR 2.25, 95%CI 1.28–3.96), male gender (OR 1.84, 95%CI 1.27–3.52), focal-neurological findings (OR 2.63, 95%CI 1.99–6.14), and thunderclap onset (OR 2.89, 95%CI 2.38–7.52) also remained associated with serious secondary headache (for detailed values, see Table 4b).

Moreover, copeptin improved the AUC of the multivariate logistic clinical model (model without copeptin: AUC 0.735 (95%CI 0.664–0.807), model with copeptin: AUC 0.7544 (95% CI0.683–0.825), p-LR-test < 0.001).

In a second multivariate model, laboratory values including fibrinogen, leukocytes and copeptin were assessed. Only copeptin remained associated with serious secondary headache (OR 1.80, 95%CI 1.33–2.44, $p < 0.0001$; for detailed values, see Table 4c).

Table 1 Baseline characteristics[a]

Baseline characteristics	All patients (*n* = 391)	Benign headache (*n* = 316)	Serious secondary headache (*n* = 75)
Age (years)	41 (30 – 57)	39 (28 – 54)	56 (40 – 66)
Male sex	146 (37.3%)	107 (33.9%)	39 (52.0%)
Comorbidities			
Hypertension	51 (13.0%)	36 (11.4%)	15 (20.0%)
Coronary heart disease	17 (4.3%)	8 (2.5%)	9 (12.0%)
Atrial fibrillation	2 (0.5%)	1 (0.3%)	1 (1.3%)
Cerebrovascular ischemic disease	2 (0.5%)	0	2 (2.7%)
Chronic obstructive lung disease	1 (0.3%)	1 (0.3%)	0
Multiple sclerosis	2 (0.5%)	2 (0.6%)	0
Chronic pain syndrome	7 (1.8%)	6 (1.9%)	1 (1.3%)
Depression	17 (4.3%)	16 (5.1%)	1 (1.3%)
Epilepsy	9 (2.3%)	3 (0.9%)	6 (8.0%)
Associated headache symptoms			
Nausea	214 (54.7%)	178 (56.3%)	36 (48.0%)
Vomiting	106 (27.1%)	83 (26.3%)	23 (30.7%)
Visual aura	124 (31.7%)	107 (33.9%)	17 (22.7%)
Photophobia	190 (48.6%)	160 (50.6%)	30 (40.0%)
Thunderclap onset headache	67 (17.1%)	39 (12.3%)	28 (37.3%)
Nuchal rigidity	10 (2.6%)	6 (1.9%)	4 (5.3%)
Scenario[b]			
1: Worst headache ever	67 (17.1%)	39 (12.3%)	28 (37.3%)
2: fever/neck stiffness	26 (6.6%)	21 (6.6%)	5 (6.7%)
3: recent worsening	169 (43.2%)	141 (44.6%)	28 (37.3%)
4: history of previous similar headache	112 (28.6%)	99 (31.3%)	13 (17.3%)
5: none of the above	17 (4.3%)	16 (5.1%)	1 (1.3%)
Clinical findings			
Systolic blood pressure (mmHg)	134 (121 – 148)	131 (120 – 145)	139 (125 – 159)
Diastolic blood pressure (mmHg)	80 (71–88)	80 (70 – 87)	78 (73 – 89)
Temperature (°C)	37 (36.7–37.4)	37.0 (36.7–37.4)	37.1 (36.7–37.4)
Headache duration (days)	3 (0.5–7)	2 (1 – 7)	3 (1 – 6)
Visual Analogue Scale (0–10) for pain at ED	8 (6 – 9)	8 (6 – 9)	8 (5 – 10)
Focal-neurological finding	74 (18.9%)	46 (14.6%)	28 (37.3%)
Immediate hospitalization	61 (15.6%)	39 (12.3%)	22 (29.3%)

[a]data are shown as median (IQR) or n (%)
[b]clinical scenarios according to Grimaldi et al. [7]
Scenario 1 (worst headache ever): thunderclap-onset headache suggestive for subarachnoidal bleeding
Scenario 2 (fever/neck stiffness): potential meningitis
Scenario 3 (recent worsening) corresponds to tumor or temporal arteriitis
Scenario 4 (history of previous similar headache) corresponds to a primary headache form

Association of copeptin with mortality or hospitalization

In the 94 (24.0%) patients reaching the composite endpoint death or hospitalization of any cause within 3 months, copeptin values were higher as compared to patients without these events (median 6.44 pmol/L(IQR 3.97–11.29) vs. 3.89 (IQR 2.59–6.01; $p = 0.0006$). The AUC for the composite endpoint was 0.62 (95%CI 0.56-0.68). In univariate logistic regression analysis, copeptin was a predictor for the composite endpoint (OR 1.45, 95%CI 1.12–1.88, $p = 0.005$).

Other strong predictors were age > 50 years (OR 2.77, 95%CI 1.72–4.46), an abnormal neurologic exam (OR 4.23, 95%CI 2.47–7.24), thunderclap onset of headache (OR 3.04, 95%CI 1.75–5.29), clinical scenario 4 (history

Table 2 Headache classification

Headache classification ($n = 391$)	n (%)
Primary headache	219 (56.0)
- Primary headache, not classified	38 (9.7)
- Migraine	114 (29.1)
- Tension-type headache	51 (13.0)
- Cluster headache	4 (1.0)
- Trigeminus neuralgia	6 (1.5)
- Medication overuse headache	6 (1.5)
Secondary headache	172 (44.0)
- Not serious[a]	97 (24.8)
- Serious:	75 (19.2)
- Subarachnoidal bleeding	8 (2.0)
- Sinus vein thrombosis	7 (1.8)
- Intracerebral bleeding	10 (2.6)
- Cerebral tumor	6 (1.5)
- Cerebral ischemia	6 (1.5)
- Dissection of carotid artery	4 (1.0)
- Temporal arteriitis	3 (0.8)
- Bacterial meningitis	1 (0.3)
- Viral meningoencephalitis	7 (1.8)
- Neuroinflammatory disease[b]	4 (1.0)
- Chronic subdural hematoma	5 (1.3)
- High intracranial pressure	3 (0.8)
- Low intracranial pressure	3 (0.8)
- Hypertensive urgency	1 (0.3)
- Associated with epileptic seizure	5 (1.3)
- Herpes zoster with cranial nerve affection	1 (0.3)
- Acute glaucoma	1 (0.3)

[a]31 systemic infections, 2 electrolyte disorders, 23 headaches due to teeth, facial skin or otorhinolaryngologic aetiology, 6 cases of arterial hypertension, 5 muscular headaches, 4 psychosomatic causes, 1 medication side effect, 1 multifactorial headache. 4 residual post-traumatic headaches, 8 hypoliquorrhea syndromes where no measures were necessary, 1 residual postoperative headache, 7 mild viral meningitis without detection of any pathogen, 1 pseudotumor cerebri without necessity of intervention, 1 patient each with headache secondary to Bell's palsy, Tolosa Hunt syndrome, and polyneuritis cranialis
[b]Neuritis vestibularis, Miller-Fisher syndrome, clinically isolated syndrome, and retrobulbar neuritis

of previous similar headache; OR 0.56, 95%CI 0.32–0.97), and C-reactive protein (OR 1.31, 95%CI 1.07–1.60; see also Table 4a). After inclusion of the significant clinical predictors from the univariate analysis along with copeptin in a multivariate model, only age >50 (OR 2.34, 95% CI 1.41–3.89), focal-neurological findings (OR 3.41, 95% CI 1.94–6.02) and thunderclap onset (OR 2.21, 95% CI 1.18–4.15) remained associated with the composite endpoint death or hospitalization, but not copeptin (for detailed values, see Table 4b). In the second multivariate model, C-reactive protein (OR 1.27, 95%CI 1.04–1.56) but not copeptin (OR 1.39 (95%CI 1.0–1.94), $p = 0.05$), remained associated with death or hospitalization, (For detailed values, see Table 4c).

Limitations

We are aware of potential limitations.

First, we included patients with headache irrespective of the underlying cause or disease. This leads to an inhomogeneous case mix with small numbers of each underlying cause, both in benign and in serious secondary headaches. However, using broad inclusion criteria reduces selection bias and, arguably, represents the true clinical population admitted to an emergency setting with acute headache.

Second, our gold standard for the final diagnosis of headache was the clinical diagnosis according to ICHD criteria after 3 months, verified by a board-certified neurologist. We abstained from brain imaging due to organizational and monetary restraints. In patients without brain imaging, there remains a small risk that a cerebral pathology may have been missed. However, we considered it to be rather unlikely that a clinically relevant cerebral pathology would remain unnoticed at 3 months. Moreover this would have introduced a bias towards the null hypothesis thus underestimating the real association.

Third, even though we aimed to recruit 24 h per day and 7 days per week, sampling error is possible, as patients arriving at night might have been missed by the staff on duty. Furthermore, this cohort represents an emergency department population and not the general headache patient.

Fourth, as copeptin rises after a stress stimulus independent from its cause, potential confounding factors have to be ruled out, such as hypoxia or hypovolemia, and inflammatory states [38–40].

Discussion

Our main finding is that copeptin was higher in serious secondary headaches requiring subsequent treatment of the underlying disease, as compared to benign headache forms. Importantly, after adjusting for the classical clinical risk factors age >50, sudden onset of headache and abnormal neurological exam [11], copeptin remained an independent risk factor for serious secondary headache. However, the initial hypothesis that copeptin would rule out serious secondary headache at the predefined cutoff of 5.0 pmol/L and rule in serious secondary headache at 20 pmol/L with a high sensitivity and specificity could "as is" not be confirmed. But at a lower cutoff level of 2.5 pmol/L, copeptin had a sensitivity of > 90%.

The most commonly postulated mechanism for the early copeptin elevation in acute illness is that copeptin reflects the activation of the hypothalamus-pituitary-adrenal axis at the hypothalamic level [41]. Copeptin

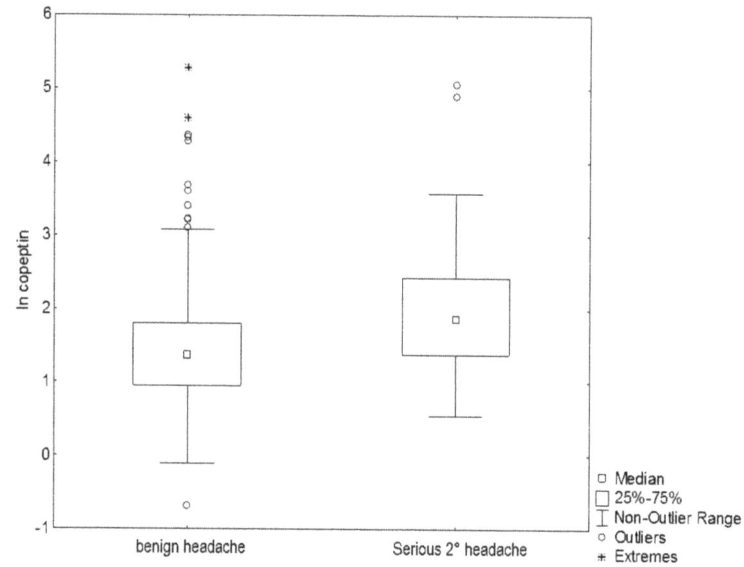

Fig. 2 Boxplot of copeptin values

promptly rises in different physical stress situations, correlating with the magnitude of stress [41–43]. Consequently, copeptin has been shown to be useful for an early rule out of acute myocardial infarction [29] and for prognosis in acute ischemic stroke [31]. We now show that copeptin may also be a promising marker for ruling out serious secondary headaches.

In acute headache with its high burden of disease [44], no biomarker has been established in clinical routine to improve discrimination between serious secondary and benign headache forms, even though fast and early identification of serious secondary headaches at the ED is crucial and has remained an unmet clinical need [2]. Algorithms based on clinical features do exist, but are inconsistently applied; [2] thus, there is room for improvement. Some biomarkers have been explored when specific causes of secondary headache were suspected, such as D-dimers for ruling-out sinus vein thrombosis [14]. Furthermore, there have been efforts for biomarker-guided treatment in migraine, for example by predicting treatment response to triptans by measuring levels of calcitonin gene-related peptide or neurokinin A [22]. Based on our data, copeptin seems to have potential as a biomarker in unselected patients presenting with acute non-traumatic headache to the emergency department.

Table 3 Sensitivity and Specificity of copeptin to predict serious secondary headache at different cutoffs

Copeptin value	Sensitivity (%)	Specificity (%)
2.5 pmol/l	91.8	23.3
5.0 pmol/l	64.4	66.7
10.0 pmol/l	27.4	89.9
20.0 pmol/l	12.3	95.3
30.0 pmol/l	5.5	96.5

However, as copeptin rises after stress independent from its cause, potential confounding factors have to be ruled out, especially extra-neurologic causes such as systemic inflammation. Further studies seem warranted which analyze the influence of stress and pain itself on copeptin values before copeptin may be introduced into clinical decision-making.

Interestingly, male gender was independently associated with serious secondary headache in multivariate analysis. We attribute this finding to the fact that primary headache, especially migraine, is more frequent in women [45].

Even though copeptin has been shown to predict adverse outcome in various diseases [46, 47], there was only a trend for the association with the combined endpoint of death or hospitalization in this study after adjusting for all other relevant risk factors. Copeptin was not associated with mortality or hospitalization in multivariate analysis. When looking only at mortality, copeptin levels were higher in nonsurvivors as compared to survivors. However, due to the very small number of nonsurvivors ($n = 2$), this finding needs further evaluation in larger cohorts.

Copeptin seems therefore not to be an ideal marker to identify patients in need for hospitalization, probably because there are other factors contributing to hospitalization which are not sufficiently reflected by copeptin levels, such as psychosocial factors (e.g., need for nursing care, patients' fears of worsening or uncontrollable pain), comorbidities, or organizational reasons (observation until further investigations were performed, i.e. at night and on week-ends).

Table 4 Main results: univariate and multivariate analysis of primary and secondary endpoint*

a. Univariate analysis of primary and secondary endpoint

	Serious secondary headache			Composite endpoint mortality or hospitalization		
Predictors	OR	95%CI	*p*	OR	95%CI	*p*
Copeptin (ln[a])	2.03	1.52–2.70	<0.0001	1.45	1.12.1.88	0.005
Age > 50	2.83	1.69–4.74	<0.0001	2.77	1.72–4.46	<0.0001
Male gender	2.12	1.27–3.52	0.004	1.41	0.88–2.27	0.150
Focal-neurological symptoms	3.50	1.99–6.14	<0.0001	4.23	2.47–7.24	<0.0001
Thunderclap onset	4.23	2.38–7.52	<0.0001	3.04	1.75–5.29	<0.0001
Scenario 4*	0.46	0.24–0.87	0.018	0.56	0.32–0.97	0.040
D-Dimer (ln[a])	1.50	1.00–2.27	0.052	1.28	0.87–1.89	0.205
Fibrinogen (ln[a])	2.95	1.10–7.89	0.031	2.29	0.91–5.80	0.080
C-reactive protein (ln[a])	1.06	0.87–1.30	0.544	1.31	1.07–1.60	0.010
Leukocyte count (ln[a])	2.04	1.01–4.13	0.046	0.63	0.34–1.16	0.136

b. Multivariate model 1: Copeptin and clinical variables

	Serious secondary headache			Composite endpoint mortality or hospitalization		
Predictors	OR	95%CI	Predictors	OR	95%CI	*p*
Copeptin (ln[a])	1.73	1.26–2.40	0.001	1.23	0.91–1.65	0.173
Age > 50	2.25	1.28–3.96	0.005	2.34	1.41–3.89	0.001
Male gender	1.84	1.04–3.26	0.035			
Focal-neurological symptoms	2.63	1.40–4.92	0.003	3.41	1.94–6.02	<0.0001
Thunderclap onset	2.90	1.49–5.65	0.002	2.21	1.18–4.15	0.013
Scenario 4[b]	0.73	0.35–1.50	0.388	0.81	0.43–1.51	0.503

c. Multivariate model 2: Copeptin and laboratory variables[a]

	Serious secondary headache**			Composite endpoint mortality or hospitalization***		
Predictors	OR	95%CI	*p*	OR	95%CI	*p*
Copeptin (ln)	1.80	1.33–2.44	<0.0001	1.39	1.0–1.94	0.050
Fibrinogen (ln)	1.22	0.93–1.61	0.158			
Leukocyte count (ln)	1.78	0.82–3.83	0.143			
C-reactive protein (ln)				1.27	1.04–1.56	0.021

*$n = 75$ events for the primary endpoint, $n = 94$ events for the secondary endpoint
[a]All laboratory values were transformed by natural logarithm (ln)
[b]Scenario 4 of Grimaldi et al. [7]: previous headache history presenting with a similar episode
For model 2, we performed a subgroup analysis of **$n = 327$ and ***$n = 279$ patients with available values of fibrinogen, leukocyte count, and C-reactive protein

The greatest potential of copeptin in the studied setting is to rule out serious headache forms by its high negative predictive value with a similar accuracy as the clinical rule based on "red flags". We speculate that the reason lies in the non-specific and prompt elevation of copeptin in stress situations. Besides the underlying disease in secondary headache forms, pain itself as a stress stimulus may have contributed to the increase in copeptin levels. This would explain why some individual patients with migraine also had very high copeptin values. So far, there is only data on copeptin levels in relation to chest pain but not to other pain stimuli. In chest pain, copeptin levels are higher in acute myocardial infarction than in extracardiac chest pain [29]. Thus, if pain stimuli are rather small and other relevant stress stimuli are lacking, low copeptin levels should accurately identify benign headache forms.

Conclusion

Copeptin was independently associated with serious secondary headache as compared to benign headaches forms. Copeptin may be a promising novel blood biomarker for risk stratification in patients with non-traumatic headache.

Appendix

Definition of serious secondary NTH

A serious NTH will require subsequent treatment of the underlying disease or condition. If untreated, the patient faces the risk of permanent damage or death.

The following diagnoses were selected from the list of secondary NTH in the ICHD-II criteria [9] as meeting the above criterion:

- [G44.81] Headache attributed to cranial or cervical vascular disorder, i.e. the following:

Headache attributed to
- ischaemic stroke or transient ischaemic attack
- non-traumatic intracranial haemorrhage
- unruptured vascular malformation
- vasculitis
- cerebral venous thrombosis (CVT)
- other intracranial vascular disorder
- Headache or facial or neck pain attributed to arterial dissection

- [G44.813] Headache attributed to arterial hypertension, i.e. the following:

Headache attributed to
- phaeochromocytoma
- hypertensive crisis without hypertensive encephalopathy
- hypertensive encephalopathy
- pre-eclampsia
- eclampsia
- other

- [G44.82] Headache attributed to non-vascular intracranial disorder, i.e. the following:

- high cerebrospinal fluid pressure
- idiopathic intracranial hypertension (IIH)
- intracranial hypertension secondary to metabolic, toxic or hormonal causes
- intracranial hypertension secondary to hydrocephalus
- low cerebrospinal fluid pressure
- epileptic seizure
- other non-vascular intracranial disorder

- [G44.82] Headache attributed to non-infectious inflammatory disease, i.e. the following:

Headache attributed to
- neurosarcoidosis
- aseptic (non-infectious) meningitis
- lymphocytic hypophysitis
- other non-infectious inflammatory disease

- [G44.822] Headache attributed to intracranial neoplasm
- [G44.4 or G44.83] Headache attributed to a substance or its withdrawal, i.e. the following:

- Carbon monoxide-induced headache
- Cocaine-induced headache
- Other

- [G44.821] Headache attributed to intracranial infection
- [G44.84] Headache or facial pain attributed to disorder of cranium, neck, eyes, ears, nose, sinuses, teeth, mouth or other facial or cranial structures, i.e. the following:

- Headache attributed to acute glaucoma
- Other

- [G44.847, G44.848 or G44.85] Cranial neuralgias and central causes of facial pain, i.e. the following:

- Optic neuritis
- Head or facial pain attributed to acute herpes zoster
- other

Abbreviations

AUC: Area under the curve; CI: Confidence interval; ED: Emergency Department; ICHD: International Classification of Headache Disorders; IQR: Interquartile range; ROC: Receiver operating characteristic; VAS: Visual analogue scale

Acknowledgements

We gratefully thank the staff of the emergency departments of all participating hospitals in supporting this study. Furthermore, we thank the many supporting doctors, nurses, medical students and laboratory personnel at all participating centers, especially Prof. Ulrich W. Buettner, Vreni Wyss, Martha Kaeslin Meyer, Renate Hunziker, Uzma Mirza, and Jasmin Martin.

Funding

MCC, CB, MK: This study was supported by a grant by the Swiss National Foundation (PP0P3_123346) to MCC and to MK (PZ00P3_142422), the Nora van Meeuwen Häfliger Stiftung and the Gottfried Julia Bangerter-Rhyner Stiftung, and a grant to CB from the Vizerektorat of the University Basel. BM, CB and PhS: Research funds from the Department of Endocrinology, Diabetology and Metabolism, the Medical University Clinic, the W&W Fund of the Kantonsspital Aarau, and the "Argovia Professorship" of the Medical Faculty of the University of Basel.

Authors' contributions

CB, PhS, KT, MA, BM, MK and MCC designed the study and wrote the protocol. PeS, KN and RB made substantial contributions to the protocol design. CB, BW, NN, KN, BM, and MCC coordinated the study. CB, NN, BW, RB, KT, CM, KH, JT, SB, TK and MA recruited patients for the study. CB, NN, BW, KT, KH, JT, MK, MCC, SB, PhS, PeS, KN, BM, HA, and KH participated in data gathering and evaluation. CB, MK and MCC analyzed the data and drafted the manuscript. BW, NN, PhS, SB, TK, CM, KT, KH, JT, MA, HA, RB, PeS, KN, and BM critically revised the manuscript. All authors read and approved the final manuscript.

Competing interests

MCC, PhS, MK and BM received speaker honoraria, consultant fees and unrestricted research grant for projects unrelated to this study from Thermofisher AG, the manufacturer of the Copeptin assay. RB has received honoraria for presentations, unrestricted grants for research and for educational purposes from Boehringer-Ingelheim, AstraZeneca, Bayer, and ThermoFisher AG unrelated to this study.
CB, BW, NN, SB, TK, CM, KT, KH, JT, MA, AH, PeS, and NK declare no competing interests.

Author details

[1]Division of Endocrinology, Department of Internal Medicine, University Hospital Basel, Basel, Switzerland. [2]Department of Neurology, Medical University Clinic, Kantonsspital Aarau, Aarau, Switzerland. [3]Internal Medicine, Medical University Clinic, Kantonsspital Aarau, Tellstrasse, CH-5001 Aarau, Switzerland. [4]Clinic of Neurology, University Hospital Basel, Basel, Switzerland. [5]Center of Laboratory Medicine, Kantonsspital Aarau, Aarau, Switzerland. [6]Emergency Department, University Hospital Basel, Basel, Switzerland. [7]Neurology, RehaClinic AG, Bad Zurzach, Switzerland. [8]Clinic of Neurology, University Hospital Zürich, Zürich, Switzerland. [9]Max-Planck-Institute for Metabolism Research, Cologne, Germany.

References

1. Schuetz P, Christ-Crain M, Wolbers M, Schild U, Thomann R, Falconnier C, Widmer I, Neidert S, Blum CA, Schonenberger R, Henzen C, Bregenzer T, Hoess C, Krause M, Bucher HC, Zimmerli W, Muller B, Pro Hsg (2007) Procalcitonin guided antibiotic therapy and hospitalization in patients with lower respiratory tract infections: a prospective, multicenter, randomized controlled trial. BMC Health Serv Res 7:102
2. Locker T, Mason S, Rigby A (2004) Headache management–are we doing enough? An observational study of patients presenting with headache to the emergency department. Emerg Med J 21:327–332
3. Morgenstern LB, Huber JC, Luna-Gonzales H, Saldin KR, Grotta JC, Shaw SG, Knudson L, Frankowski RF (2001) Headache in the emergency department. Headache 41:537–541
4. Stevenson RJ, Dutta D, MacWalter RS (1998) The management of acute headache in adults in an acute admissions unit. Scott Med J 43:173–176
5. Ang SH, Chan YC, Mahadevan M (2009) Emergency department headache admissions in an acute care hospital:why do they occur and what can we do about it? Ann Acad Med Singapore 38:1007–1010
6. Ramirez-Lassepas M, Espinosa CE, Cicero JJ, Johnston KL, Cipolle RJ, Barber DL (1997) Predictors of intracranial pathologic findings in patients who seek emergency care because of headache. Arch Neurol 54:1506–1509
7. Grimaldi D, Nonino F, Cevoli S, Vandelli A, D'Amico R, Cortelli P (2009) Risk stratification of non-traumatic headache in the emergency department. J Neurol 256:51–57
8. Cortelli P, Cevoli S, Nonino F, Baronciani D, Magrini N, Re G, De Berti G, Manzoni GC, Querzani P, Vandelli A (2004) Evidence-based diagnosis of nontraumatic headache in the emergency department: a consensus statement on four clinical scenarios. Headache 44:587–595
9. Headache Classification Subcommittee of the International Headache Society (2004) The International Classification of Headache Disorders: 2nd edition. Cephalalgia 24 Suppl 1:9–160
10. Holle D, Obermann M (2013) The role of neuroimaging in the diagnosis of headache disorders. Ther Adv Neurol Disord 6:369–374
11. Locker TE, Thompson C, Rylance J, Mason SM (2006) The utility of clinical features in patients presenting with nontraumatic headache: an investigation of adult patients attending an emergency department. Headache 46:954–961
12. Breen DP, Duncan CW, Pope AE, Gray AJ, Al-Shahi Salman R (2008) Emergency department evaluation of sudden, severe headache. QJM 101:435–443
13. Loder E, Harrington MG, Cutrer M, Sandor P, De Vries B (2006) Selected confirmed, probable, and exploratory migraine biomarkers. Headache 46: 1108–1127
14. Kosinski CM, Mull M, Schwarz M, Koch B, Biniek R, Schlafer J, Milkereit E, Willmes K, Schiefer J (2004) Do normal D-dimer levels reliably exclude cerebral sinus thrombosis? Stroke 35:2820–2825
15. Guldiken S, Guldiken B, Demir M, Kabayel L, Ozkan H, Turgut N, Hunkar R, Kat S (2011) Soluble CD40 ligand and prolactin levels in migraine patients during interictal period. J Headache Pain 12:355–360
16. Arulmani U, Maassenvandenbrink A, Villalon CM, Saxena PR (2004) Calcitonin gene-related peptide and its role in migraine pathophysiology. Eur J Pharmacol 500:315–330
17. Meng R, Wang X, Hussain M, Dornbos D 3rd, Meng L, Liu Y, Wu Y, Ning M, Ferdinando SB, Lo EH, Ding Y, Ji X (2014) Evaluation of plasma D-dimer plus fibrinogen in predicting acute CVST. Int J Stroke 9:166–173
18. Egea-Guerrero JJ, Revuelto-Rey J, Murillo-Cabezas F, Munoz-Sanchez MA, Vilches-Arenas A, Sanchez-Linares P, Dominguez-Roldan JM, Leon-Carrion J (2012) Accuracy of the S100beta protein as a marker of brain damage in traumatic brain injury. Brain Inj 26:76–82
19. Blyth BJ, Farhavar A, Gee C, Hawthorn B, He H, Nayak A, Stocklein V, Bazarian JJ (2009) Validation of serum markers for blood–brain barrier disruption in traumatic brain injury. J Neurotrauma 26:1497–1507
20. Teepker M, Munk K, Mylius V, Haag A, Moller JC, Oertel WH, Schepelmann K (2009) Serum concentrations of s100b and NSE in migraine. Headache 49:245–252
21. Forcelini CM, Dantas DC, Luz C, Santin R, Stein AT, Barros HM, Barea LM (2011) Analysis of leukocytes in medication-overuse headache, chronic migraine, and episodic migraine. Headache 51:1228–1238
22. Durham P, Papapetropoulos S (2013) Biomarkers associated with migraine and their potential role in migraine management. Headache 53:1262–1277
23. Widmer IE, Puder JJ, Konig C, Pargger H, Zerkowski HR, Girard J, Muller B (2005) Cortisol response in relation to the severity of stress and illness. J Clin Endocrinol Metab 90:4579–4586
24. Katan M, Muller B, Christ-Crain M (2008) Copeptin: a new and promising diagnostic and prognostic marker. Crit Care 12:117
25. Katan M, Christ-Crain M (2010) The stress hormone copeptin: a new prognostic biomarker in acute illness. Swiss Med Wkly 140:w13101
26. Friedman BW, Hochberg ML, Esses D, Grosberg B, Corbo J, Toosi B, Meyer RH, Bijur PE, Lipton RB, Gallagher EJ (2007) Applying the International Classification of Headache Disorders to the emergency department: an assessment of reproducibility and the frequency with which a unique diagnosis can be assigned to every acute headache presentation. Ann Emerg Med 49:409–419, 419 e401-409
27. Marlow RA, Kegowicz CL, Starkey KN (2009) Prevalence of depression symptoms in outpatients with a complaint of headache. J Am Board Fam Med 22:633–637
28. Lipton RB, Stewart WF, Sawyer J, Edmeads JG (2001) Clinical utility of an instrument assessing migraine disability: the Migraine Disability Assessment (MIDAS) questionnaire. Headache 41:854–861
29. Reichlin T, Hochholzer W, Stelzig C, Laule K, Freidank H, Morgenthaler NG, Bergmann A, Potocki M, Noveanu M, Breidthardt T, Christ A, Boldanova T, Merki R, Schaub N, Bingisser R, Christ M, Mueller C (2009) Incremental value of copeptin for rapid rule out of acute myocardial infarction. J Am Coll Cardiol 54:60–68
30. Morgenthaler NG, Struck J, Alonso C, Bergmann A (2006) Assay for the measurement of copeptin, a stable peptide derived from the precursor of vasopressin. Clin Chem 52:112–119
31. Katan M, Fluri F, Morgenthaler NG, Schuetz P, Zweifel C, Bingisser R, Muller K, Meckel S, Gass A, Kappos L, Steck AJ, Engelter ST, Muller B, Christ-Crain M (2009) Copeptin: a novel, independent prognostic marker in patients with ischemic stroke. Ann Neurol 66:799–808
32. Zweifel C, Katan M, Schuetz P, Siegemund M, Morgenthaler NG, Merlo A, Mueller B, Christ-Crain M (2010) Copeptin is associated with mortality and outcome in patients with acute intracerebral hemorrhage. BMC Neurol 10:34
33. Kruger S, Ewig S, Kunde J, Hanschmann A, Marre R, Suttorp N, Welte T (2009) C-terminal provasopressin (copeptin) in patients with community-acquired pneumonia–influence of antibiotic pre-treatment: results from the German competence network CAPNETZ. J Antimicrob Chemother 64:159–162
34. Seligman R, Papassotiriou J, Morgenthaler NG, Meisner M, Teixeira PJ (2008) Copeptin, a novel prognostic biomarker in ventilator-associated pneumonia. Crit Care 12:R11
35. Hanley JA, McNeil BJ (1982) The meaning and use of the area under a receiver operating characteristic (ROC) curve. Radiology 143:29–36
36. Jensen MB, Chacon MR, Sattin JA, Aleu A, Lyden PD (2008) The promise and potential pitfalls of serum biomarkers for ischemic stroke and transient ischemic attack. Neurologist 14:243–246

37. Vickers AJ, Cronin AM, Begg CB (2011) One statistical test is sufficient for assessing new predictive markers. BMC Med Res Methodol 11:13
38. L'Abate P, Wiegert S, Struck J, Wellmann S, Cannizzaro V (2013) Determinants of plasma copeptin: a systematic investigation in a pediatric mechanical ventilation model. Respir Physiol Neurobiol 185:222–227
39. Morgenthaler NG, Muller B, Struck J, Bergmann A, Redl H, Christ-Crain M (2007) Copeptin, a stable peptide of the arginine vasopressin precursor, is elevated in hemorrhagic and septic shock. Shock 28:219–226
40. Muller B, Morgenthaler N, Stolz D, Schuetz P, Muller C, Bingisser R, Bergmann A, Tamm M, Christ-Crain M (2007) Circulating levels of copeptin, a novel biomarker, in lower respiratory tract infections. Eur J Clin Invest 37:145–152
41. Katan M, Morgenthaler N, Widmer I, Puder JJ, Konig C, Muller B, Christ-Crain M (2008) Copeptin, a stable peptide derived from the vasopressin precursor, correlates with the individual stress level. Neuro Endocrinol Lett 29:341–346
42. Aliberti S, Di Pasquale M, Zanaboni AM, Cosentini R, Brambilla AM, Seghezzi S, Tarsia P, Mantero M, Blasi F (2012) Stratifying risk factors for multidrug-resistant pathogens in hospitalized patients coming from the community with pneumonia. Clin Infect Dis 54:470–478
43. Riquelme R, Jimenez P, Videla AJ, Lopez H, Chalmers J, Singanayagam A, Riquelme M, Peyrani P, Wiemken T, Arbo G, Benchetrit G, Rioseco ML, Ayesu K, Klotchko A, Marzoratti L, Raya M, Figueroa S, Saavedra F, Pryluka D, Inzunza C, Torres A, Alvare P, Fernandez P, Barros M, Gomez Y, Contreras C, Rello J, Bordon J, Feldman C, Arnold F, Nakamatsu R, Riquelme J, Blasi F, Aliberti S, Cosentini R, Lopardo G, Gnoni M, Welte T, Saad M, Guardiola J, Ramirez J (2011) Predicting mortality in hospitalized patients with 2009 H1N1 influenza pneumonia. Int J Tuberc Lung Dis 15:542–546
44. Torres A, Blasi F, Peetermans WE, Viegi G, Welte T (2014) The aetiology and antibiotic management of community-acquired pneumonia in adults in Europe: a literature review. Eur J Clin Microbiol Infect Dis 33:1065–1079
45. Buse DC, Loder EW, Gorman JA, Stewart WF, Reed ML, Fanning KM, Serrano D, Lipton RB (2013) Sex differences in the prevalence, symptoms, and associated features of migraine, probable migraine and other severe headache: results of the American Migraine Prevalence and Prevention (AMPP) Study. Headache 53:1278–1299
46. Charles PG, Whitby M, Fuller AJ, Stirling R, Wright AA, Korman TM, Holmes PW, Christiansen KJ, Waterer GW, Pierce RJ, Mayall BC, Armstrong JG, Catton MG, Nimmo GR, Johnson B, Hooy M, Grayson ML (2008) The etiology of community-acquired pneumonia in Australia: why penicillin plus doxycycline or a macrolide is the most appropriate therapy. Clin Infect Dis 46:1513–1521
47. Ananda-Rajah MR, Charles PG, Melvani S, Burrell LL, Johnson PD, Grayson ML (2008) Comparing the pneumonia severity index with CURB-65 in patients admitted with community acquired pneumonia. Scand J Infect Dis 40:293–300
48. von Elm E, Altman DG, Egger M, Pocock SJ, Gotzsche PC, Vandenbroucke JP (2007) The Strengthening the Reporting of Observational Studies in Epidemiology (STROBE) statement: guidelines for reporting observational studies. PLoS Med 4:e296

11

Primary headache disorders in the adult general population of Pakistan

A. A. Herekar[1,2], A. Ahmad[1,3], U. L. Uqaili[1,3], B. Ahmed[1,4], J. Effendi[1,3], S. Z. Alvi[1,5], M. A. Shahab[6], U. Javed[7], A. D. Herekar[1,8], Rafiq Khanani[9] and T. J. Steiner[10,11*]

Abstract

Background: The large geographical gaps in our knowledge of the prevalence and burden of headache disorders include almost all of Eastern Mediterranean Region (EMR). We report a nationwide population-based study in Pakistan, an EMR country with the sixth largest population in the world, conducted as a project within the Global Campaign against Headache.

Methods: We surveyed six locations from the four provinces of Pakistan: Punjab, Sindh, Khyber Pakhtunkhwa and Baluchistan. We randomly selected and visited rural and urban households in each. One adult member (18–65 years) of each household, also randomly selected, was interviewed by a trained non-medical interviewer from the same location using a previously-validated structured questionnaire translated into Urdu, the national language. We estimated 1-year prevalences of the headache disorders of public-health importance and examined their associations with demographic variables using multivariate analysis.

Results: There were 4223 participants (mean age 34.4 ± 11.0 years; male 1957 [46.3%], female 2266 [53.7%]; urban 1443 [34.2%], rural 2780 [65.8%]). Participation proportion was 89.5%. Headache in the previous year was reported by 3233 (76.6% [95% CI: 75.3–77.8%]). The age- and gender-adjusted 1-year prevalence of migraine was 22.5% [21.2–23.8%] (male 18.0% [16.8–19.2%], female 26.9% [25.6–28.2%]), of tension-type headache (TTH) 44.6% [43.1–46.1%] (male 51.2% [49.7–52.7%], female 37.9% [36.4–39.4%]), of probable medication-overuse headache 0.7% [0.5–1.0%] (male 0.7% [0.5–1.0%], female 0.8% [0.5–1.1%]) and of other headache on ≥15 days/month 7.4% [6.6–8.2%] (male 4.4% [3.8–5.0%], female 10.4% [9.5–11.3%]). Migraine was more prevalent in females by a factor of 3:2 although this association barely survived ($P = 0.039$) after correcting for other factors. TTH was more prevalent in males by about 4:3 ($P = 0.026$). All headache and migraine were age-related, peaking in the age group 40–49 years; TTH peaked a decade earlier. Higher education ($P = 0.004$) and income ($P = 0.001$) were negatively associated with prevalence of migraine.

Conclusion: With three quarters of its population affected, headache disorders must be on the public-health agenda of Pakistan. Worldwide, these disorders are the third leading cause of disability; information from specific enquiry into the burden attributable to headache disorders in this country is needed to inform health policy and priority-setting, and will be reported soon.

Keywords: Headache disorders, Migraine, Tension-type headache, Medication-overuse headache, Epidemiology, Prevalence, Population-based survey, Eastern Mediterranean Region, Pakistan, Global campaign against headache

* Correspondence: t.steiner@imperial.ac.uk
[10]Department of Neuroscience, Norwegian University of Science and Technology (NTNU), Edvard Griegs Gate, NO-7491 Trondheim, Norway
[11]Division of Brain Sciences, Imperial College London, London, UK
Full list of author information is available at the end of the article

Background

Headache disorders affect almost half the world's population, according to a survey of the published literature conducted nine years ago [1]. Tension-type headache (TTH) and migraine are the major contributors in terms of prevalence, being the second and third most common disorders in the world [2]. In 2013, migraine was recognised as the sixth-highest cause of disability in the world [3]. Also important in public-health terms, because of the burdens they impose at individual level, are the group of disorders characterized by headache on ≥15 days/month; these include medication-overuse headache (MOH), not itself a primary headache disorder but, in almost all cases, a *sequela* due to mismanagement of either migraine or TTH [4]. MOH is the 18th-highest cause of disability in the world [3].

Large geographical gaps in our knowledge of the prevalence and burden of headache disorders have been evident from the various surveys [1, 2, 5, 6]. In a continuing endeavour to fill these, *Lifting The Burden* (LTB), a United Kingdom-based non-governmental organisation conducting the Global Campaign against Headache [7] in official relations with the World Health Organization [8], has been supporting population-based studies in many parts of the world: among others, in Russia in Eastern Europe [9], in China in the Western Pacific Region [10] and in India [11] and Nepal [12] in South East Asia. Over 2.5 billion people live in these countries, where knowledge was virtually absent. In the Eastern Mediterranean Region is another large geographical knowledge gap; the countries include Pakistan, with the sixth largest population in the world [13] and characterised by economic and political instability and, in parts, by geographical inaccessibility.

We report here the prevalence results of a nationwide cross-sectional population-based survey in Pakistan. It was conducted as part of the series of similar studies within the Global Campaign against Headache, and following the standardized methodology developed by LTB for such studies [14]. It is the first to be published from the Region. Its two purposes were to contribute to knowledge of the global burden of headache [3] and to provide evidence for national health policy in Pakistan.

Methods

The detailed methodology has been published previously [15]. Here the methods are summarized.

Ethics

The Ethics Review Board of the Dow University of Health Sciences approved the study protocol. All participants were informed about the nature and purpose of the survey and gave their consent to taking part. Data protection legislation was complied with.

Survey

We conducted the survey in six locations purposively selected from the four provinces of Pakistan to represent the national population: Lahore and Multan (Punjab), Karachi and Sukkur (Sindh), Abbottabad (Khyber Pakhtunkhwa) and Gwadar (Baluchistan). Rural and urban households randomly selected in each location were visited unannounced by a team of 12 trained non-medical interviewers recruited from, and therefore familiar with, the same locations. One randomly-selected adult member (18–65 years) of each household was interviewed using LTB's structured HARDSHIP questionnaire translated into Urdu, the national language. This questionnaire, used in similar studies conducted in other countries [16], included demographic enquiry, screening and diagnostic questions for headache. Additionally, weight and height were measured, and body mass index (BMI) calculated.

Diagnosis

Diagnoses were not made by the interviewers, but subsequently by diagnostic algorithm [16], applied to the most bothersome headache if a participant reported more than one type of headache. The diagnostic questions had been validated earlier in a Pakistani population [15]. Cases were removed for individual review of medication use when headache was reported on ≥15 days/month, and diagnosed either as probable MOH (pMOH) or other headache on ≥15 days/month. All remaining cases (episodic headache) were classified by applying modified ICHD-II criteria in hierarchical sequence: first definite migraine, then definite TTH, then probable migraine and finally probable TTH. Cases falling into none of these categories were unclassified. During subsequent analysis, definite and probable migraine were combined, as were definite and probable TTH, for generating prevalence estimates for migraine and TTH. The correctness of this approach has been argued [14].

Data management

Data from completed questionnaires were entered into SPSS version 16.0. We applied full double data-entry by two operators working independently, subsequently eliminating errors by reference to the original forms.

Statistics

We planned a total sample size of 4149. In calculating this we assumed a headache prevalence of 50% and applied a confidence level of 99% and confidence interval (CI) of 2%.

Data analysis was conducted using Stata/SE 12.0 and SPSS v 23. Continuous variables were summarized as means and standard deviations (SDs), and categorical variables as numbers and percentages.

We categorised age as 18–29, 30–39, 40–49, 50–59 or 60–65 years; marital status as "single", "married" or "divorced, widowed or separated"; habitation as "urban" or "rural"; educational level as "none", "some schooling" (up to high school) or "college" (including university); income level as "poor" or "not poor" ("poor" meaning below the poverty line [30th population income percentile, or income per quarter of < PKR 9,000 or USD 90] [17]); BMI according to the WHO classification [18] as "underweight" (<18.5), "normal" (18.5–24.9), "overweight" (25.0–29.9), "obese" (30–39.9) or "morbidly obese" (>40).

We used chi-squared to compare distributions between categorical variables. We calculated headache prevalences as percentages with 95% CIs. We performed bivariate analyses, calculating odds ratios (ORs) with 95% CIs, to look for associations between headache types (migraine, TTH or all headache on ≥15 days/month) and demographic variables. In subsequent multivariate logistic regression analyses, we calculated Exp(B) with 95% CIs taking prevalence of each headache type as the dependent variable and gender, age, marital status, habitation, education level, income, province and BMI as factors. Model-fitting statistics indicated a good fit (chi-squared = 501.98, df = 60, $P <$ 0.001). In the principal (prevalence) and bivariate association analyses we set statistical significance at $P < 0.05$; in the multivariate analysis, because of multiple comparisons we set it at $P < 0.02$.

Quality assurance

We applied preventative, detective and corrective quality assurance procedures as described elsewhere [15]. During the data verification process, irregularities in data collection were identified in one location, Multan, and rectified, which necessitated discarding the original (fraudulent) data and repeating the survey in this location (a full account of this has been published elsewhere [19]). The results reported here include the data from the second survey in Multan.

Results

The survey was completed by 4223 participants (1957 [46.3%] male, 2266 [53.7%] female) aged 18–65 years (mean 34.4 ± 11.0), of whom 1443 (34.2%) lived in urban and 2780 (65.8%) in rural areas. The participation proportion was 89.5% overall, with regional variation between 69% and >99%. The sample was generally well matched to the population of all Pakistan for gender, age and urban/rural habitation according to figures from Pakistan's last census (1998) [20], albeit with males and the over-50 age groups slightly under-represented. Most participants (72.1%) were married, 26.0% were unmarried and only 1.9% were divorced, separated or widowed; the latter two groups were also slightly under-represented. During bivariate analysis, prevalences were adjusted for age and gender by weighting according to population data [20] since these were likely to be influencing factors.

Observed prevalences of all headache and of the specific headache types, overall and by gender, are shown in Table 1. Headache of any sort ("all headache") in the past year was reported by 3233 participants, an observed 1-year prevalence of 76.6%. There was no difference between males and females. TTH was by far the most prevalent headache disorder (44.7%), but migraine was also very common, reported by over one fifth (22.9%) of participants. Headache on ≥15 days/month was reported by almost one in 12 participants (8.1%), of whom a small minority (0.7%) were diagnosed as pMOH. Only 37 cases (0.9%) were unclassifiable, similar numbers in each gender (Table 1). Migraine was more prevalent in females in a ratio of 3:2 ($P < 0.001$), pMOH and other headache on ≥15 days/month about two-fold (the latter significantly [$P < 0.001$] but the former not). TTH, on the other hand, was more prevalent in males by a factor of about 4:3 ($P < 0.001$) (Table 1).

Relationships with age are shown in Fig. 1 and Table 2. The curves for all headache and migraine show prevalence increasing to a peak during the age range 40–49 years, then declining; prevalence of TTH peaked 10 years earlier but remained high in the 5th decade. The observed prevalence of pMOH increased steadily with age, although numbers were too small to show a significant relationship.

Table 3 shows the bivariate analyses. Married participants had more overall headache (OR = 1.8) and migraine (OR = 1.5) than those who were single. Participants who were divorced, widowed or separated also had more headache (OR = 1.9), migraine (OR = 1.8) and headache on ≥15 days/month (OR = 2.5), but less TTH (OR = 0.7) than single participants. No significant associations emerged between marital status and pMOH.

Urban dwelling was weakly positively associated with migraine (OR = 1.2) and more strongly with other headache on ≥15 days/month (OR = 1.8) but negatively with TTH (OR = 0.7) (Table 3).

Increasing educational level was negatively associated with migraine and other headache on ≥15 days/month, and positively with TTH (Table 3). Accordingly, being not poor was negatively associated with migraine (OR = 0.8) and strongly so with other headache on ≥15 days/month (OR = 0.4), and with all headache (OR = 0.7), but positively with TTH (OR = 1.3) (Table 3).

BMI was calculated for 3889 participants (for 334, either height or weight was not recorded). Only a little over half of participants (2,152; 55.5%) were of normal weight: over 40% were overweight (1156; 29.8%) or obese (417; 10.7%) and nine participants were morbidly obese. The extremes (underweight and obese) were negatively associated with all headache and TTH but positively with migraine; obesity was also positively associated with headache on ≥15 days/month (Table 3).

Table 1 Observed and age- and gender-adjusted 1-year prevalences of all headache and headache types

Headache type	Observed overall (N = 4223) (%) [95% CI]	Age-adjusted (%) [95% CI]		Age- and gender-adjusted (N = 4223) (%) [95% CI]
		Males (n = 1957)	Females (n = 2266)	
All headache	76.6 [75.3–77.9]	75.4 [74.1–76.7]	76.8 [75.5–78.1]	76.1 [74.8–77.4]
Migraine	22.9 [21.6–24.2]	18.0 [16.8–19.2]	26.9 [25.6–28.2]	22.5 [21.2–23.8]
Tension-type headache	44.7 [43.2–46.2]	51.2 [49.7–52.7]	37.9 [36.4–39.4]	44.6 [43.1–46.1]
Probable medication-overuse headache	0.7 [0.5–1.0]	0.7 [0.5–1.0]	0.9 [0.6–1.2]	0.8 [0.5–1.1]
Other headache on ≥15 days/month	7.4 [6.6–7.9]	4.4 [3.8–5.0]	10.4 [9.5–11.3]	7.4 [6.6–8.2]
Unclassifiable	0.9 [0.6–1.2]	1.2 [0.9–1.5]	0.8 [0.5–1.1]	1.0 [0.7–1.3]

CI confidence interval. Adjusted for age and gender in SPSS v23 by weighting in accordance with the formula Weight = proportion in population/proportion in sample, taking population data from [20]

In multivariate analysis (Table 4), the positive association between female gender and migraine barely survived ($P > 0.02$), but the association with headache on ≥ 15 days/month remained strongly significant, as did the negative association with TTH. Age 40–49 years remained positively associated with migraine, and an association emerged with headache on >15 days/month, while ages 30–49 were positively associated with TTH. Migraine was confirmed as more prevalent among married participants, but otherwise there were no associations with marital status. No associations with area of habitation survived. Some schooling was positively associated with TTH whereas college education continued to be strongly negatively associated with migraine. No other associations with educational level survived. Being poor remained strongly associated with both migraine and headache on ≥15 days/month, but the negative association with TTH did not survive. There were regional variations: relative to the Punjab, migraine was much less common in Khyber Pakhtunkhwa and TTH was less common in all other regions, but especially in Khyber Pakhtunkhwa; on the other hand, headache on ≥15 days/month was more common in Sindh and Baluchistan. Being underweight and being obese each remained negatively associated with TTH, but no other associations with BMI survived.

Discussion

This first-ever nationwide population-based study of the prevalence of headache disorders in Pakistan (indeed, in any country in the Eastern Mediterranean Region) has revealed much headache in the country. The overall 1-year prevalence of 76.6% is substantially higher than the reported global average of 46% [1]. At 22.9% and 44.7%, the prevalences of migraine and TTH each greatly exceed their respective global estimates of 14.7% and 20.7% from the Global Burden of Disease Survey 2010 [2]. Headache on ≥15 days/month is highly prevalent (8.1%), although only 0.7% of the adult population have pMOH.

With 4223 participants, a participation proportion of 89.5%, a representative sample and a well-performing diagnostic instrument [15], these estimates from Pakistan have low margins of uncertainty. The key methodological limitation was that we could not reach most slum-dwellers,

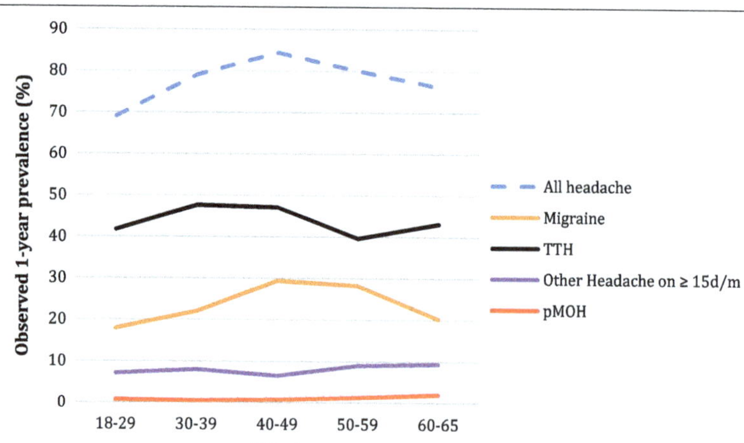

Fig. 1 Observed 1-year prevalences of headache types by age (TTH: tension-type headache; d/m: days/month; pMOH: probable medication-overuse headache)

Table 2 Observed prevalences of migraine and tension-type headache, by age and gender

Age group (years)	One-year prevalence % (n)			
	Male		Female	
	Migraine	TTH	Migraine	TTH
18–29	15.3% (110)	47.4% (342)	20.1% (164)	36.8% (300)
30–39	17.8% (74)	53.0% (220)	24.6% (162)	44.5% (293)
40–49	20.6% (90)	59.2% (258)	38.3% (164)	34.8% (149)
50–59	20.7% (60)	47.9% (139)	36.4% (96)	30.7% (81)
60–65	19.4% (24)	47.6% (59)	22.1% (15)	35.3% (24)

TTH tension-type headache

who are inevitably excluded from household surveys while making up an estimated 45.5% of the urban population according to some statistics [21]. These are people below the poverty line, in whom, if the association with poverty holds (see below), headache will be common.

This study was one of a series being conducted by LTB in pursuit of the Global Campaign against Headache. While several of these are not yet completed or fully analyzed, the careful enquiry incorporated into the methodology of these studies is finding that headache prevalences have in the past been significantly underestimated. For example, very similar findings have emerged from India, a country which shares Pakistan's genetic, environmental and cultural composition: the 1-year prevalence in Karnataka State of all headache was 63.9%, of migraine 25.2% (with a 4:3 female preponderance)

Table 3 Bivariate analyses† to demonstrate potential associations between headache types and demographic factors, habitation and body mass index

Variable ($N = 4223$)	Odds ratios (95% confidence intervals)				
	All headache ($n = 3233$)	Migraine ($n = 967$)	Tension-type headache ($n = 1887$)	Probable MOH ($n = 30$)	Other headache on ≥15 d/m ($n = 312$)
Age					
18–29 years ($n = 1537$)	Reference	Reference	Reference	Reference	Reference
30–39 years ($n = 1074$)	1.8 (1.5–2.1)*	1.3 (1.1–1.6)*	1.3 (1.1–1.5)*	0.7 (0.2–2.1)	1.1 (0.9–1.5)
40–49 years ($n = 865$)	2.5 (2.1–3.1)*	1.8 (1.4–2.3)*	1.2 (1.1–1.5)*	1.1 (0.4–3.0)	0.9 (0.7–1.3)
50–59 years ($n = 554$)	1.9 (1.5–2.4)*	1.8 (1.4–2.3)*	0.9 (0.8–1.1)	2.0 (0.7–5.2)	1.3 (0.9–1.8)
60–65 years ($n = 193$)	1.5 (1.1–2.1)*	1.2 (0.8–1.7)	1.1 (0.8–1.4)	3.3 (1.0–10.5)*	1.4 (0.8–2.3)
Marital status ($N = 4182$; missing 41)					
Single ($n = 1309$)	Reference	Reference	Reference	Reference	Reference
Married ($n = 2637$)	1.8 (1.5–2.1)*	1.5 (1.3–1.8)*	1.1 (1.0–1.3)	1.8 (0.7–4.5)	1.1 (0.8–1.4)
Divorced, widowed or separated ($n = 236$)	1.9 (1.4–2.7)*	1.8 (1.3–2.5)*	0.7 (0.5–0.9)*	-	2.5 (1.6–3.7)*
Habitation ($N = 4223$)					
Rural ($n = 2780$)	Reference	Reference	Reference	Reference	Reference
Urban ($n = 1443$)	1.0 (0.9–1.2)	1.2 (1.0–1.4)	0.7 (0.6–0.8)*	1.9 (0.9–4.2)	1.8 (1.4–2.3)*
Educational level ($N = 3263$; missing 960)					
None ($n = 600$)	Reference	Reference	Reference	Reference	Reference
Some schooling ($n = 2454$)	1.2 (1.0–1.4)	0.5 (0.4–0.7)*	2.2 (1.8–2.6)*	1.2 (0.4–3.6)	0.6 (0.4–0.8)*
College ($n = 209$)	0.6 (0.4–0.8)*	0.5 (0.3–0.7)*	1.5 (1.1–2.1)*	-	0.4 (0.2–0.8)*
Income level ($N = 3606$; missing 617)					
Poor ($n = 1127$)	Reference	Reference	Reference	Reference	Reference
Not poor ($n = 2479$)	0.7 (0.6–0.9)*	0.8 (0.7–0.9)*	1.3 (1.1–1.5)*	0.8 (0.3–1.7)	0.4 (0.3–0.5)*
Body mass index ($N = 3889$; missing 334)					
Normal ($n = 2152$)	Reference	Reference	Reference	Reference	Reference
Underweight ($n = 155$)	0.6 (0.4–1.0)*	1.7 (1.1–2.5)*	0.4 (0.3–0.7)*	1.8 (0.4–8.2)	1.2 (0.6–2.1)
Overweight ($n = 1156$)	1.0 (0.8–1.2)	1.2 (1.0–1.4)	0.9 (0.7–1.0)	0.9 (0.4–2.2)	1.0 (0.7–1.3)
Obese ($n = 417$)	0.6 (0.5–0.8)*	1.6 (1.3–2.1)*	0.4 (0.3–0.5)*	0.3 (0.04–2.1)	1.5 (1.0–2.2)*
Morbidly obese ($n = 9$)	0.2 (0.15–0.25)*	1.6 (1.3–2.1)*	0.4 (0.3–0.5)*	1.1 (0.3–4.0)	0.7 (0.4–1.2)

MOH medication-overuse headache, *d/m* days/month. †Adjusted in SPSS v23 for age and/or gender (as appropriate) by weighting in accordance with the formula Weight = proportion in population/proportion in sample, taking population data from [20]. *$P < 0.05$

Table 4 Multivariate analysis of associations between headache types and demographic and environmental factors and body mass index

Variable	Exp(B) (95% confidence intervals)		
	Migraine ($n = 967$)	Tension-type headache ($n = 1887$)	Headache on ≥15 d/m ($n = 342$)
Gender ($N = 4223$) compared to male ($n = 1957$)			
Female ($n = 2266$)	1.3 (1.01–1.7) $P = 0.039$	0.8 (0.7–0.97) $P = 0.026$	2.0 (1.4–2.9) **$P < 0.001$**
Age ($N = 4223$) compared to 18–29 years ($n = 1507$)			
30–39 years ($n = 1197$)	0.9 (0.6–1.3) $P = 0.522$	1.5 (1.1–2.0) **$P = 0.012$**	1.2 (0.7–2.0) $P = 0.536$
40–49 years ($n = 1101$)	2.0 (1.3–2.9) **$P = 0.001$**	2.4 (1.7–3.4) **$P < 0.001$**	2.0 (1.2–3.5) **$P = 0.015$**
50–59 years ($n = 330$)	1.1 (0.6–2.1) $P = 0.720$	1.4 (0.8–2.3) $P = 0.201$	2.0 (0.9–4.4) $P = 0.076$
60–65 years ($n = 88$)	2.1 (0.7–6.7) $P = 0.201$	2.8 (1.1–7.1) $P = 0.034$	1.8 (0.3–9.4) $P = 0.515$
Marital status ($N = 4182$; missing 41) compared to single ($n = 1089$)			
Married ($n = 3015$)	1.8 (1.2–2.5) **$P = 0.002$**	1.3 (0.9–1.7) $P = 0.115$	1.2 (0.7–2.0) $P = 0.490$
Divorced, widowed or separated ($n = 78$)	0.5 (0.1–1.8) $P = 0.277$	0.8 (0.3–2.0) $P = 0.683$	1.4 (0.5–4.3) $P = 0.568$
Habitation ($N = 4223$) compared to rural ($n = 2780$)			
Urban ($n = 1443$)	1.3 (1.0–1.7) $P = 0.053$	1.1 (0.9–1.3) $P = 0.554$	1.0 (0.7–1.5) $P = 0.895$
Educational level (N = 3277; missing 946) compared to none ($n = 166$)			
Some schooling ($n = 2691$)	0.8 (0.5–1.2) $p = 0.263$	1.8 (1.2–2.9) **$p = 0.011$**	1.3 (0.7–2.4) $p = 0.503$
College ($n = 420$)	0.4 (0.2–0.8) **$p = 0.004$**	1.0 (0.6–1.7) $p = 0.959$	0.9 (0.4–2.0) $p = 0.721$
Income level ($N = 3606$; missing 617) compared to poor ($n = 1127$)			
Not poor ($n = 2479$)	0.5 (0.4–0.7) **$p < 0.001$**	0.8 (0.6–1.01) $p = 0.061$	0.3 (0.2–0.5) **$p < 0.001$**
Province ($N = 4223$) compared to Punjab ($n = 2431$)			
Sindh ($n = 1017$)	1.0 (0.8–1.4) $P = 0.781$	0.7 (0.5–0.9) **$P = 0.002$**	2.2 (1.5–3.4) **$P < 0.001$**
Baluchistan ($n = 201$)	0.5 (0.2–0.9) $P = 0.022$	0.5 (0.3–0.9) **$P = 0.011$**	2.7 (1.2–5.9) **$P = 0.013$**
Khyber Pakhtunkhwa ($n = 574$)	0.2 (0.1–0.3) **$P < 0.001$**	0.4 (0.3–0.6) **$P < 0.001$**	0.5 (0.3–1.1) $P = 0.077$
Body mass index ($N = 3889$; missing 334) compared to normal ($n = 2152$)			
Underweight ($n = 155$)	0.8 (0.4–1.4) $P = 0.412$	0.5 (0.3–0.8) **$P = 0.005$**	1.4 (0.7–2.9) $P = 0.386$
Overweight ($n = 1156$)	1.2 (0.9–1.6) $P = 0.193$	1.0 (0.8–1.3) $P = 1.00$	1.3 (0.8–1.9) $P = 0.298$
Obese or morbidly obese ($n = 426$)	0.9 (0.6–1.4) $P = 0.573$	0.4 (0.3–0.6) **$P < 0.001$**	1.4 (0.8–2.6) $P = 0.249$

Significant associations ($P < 0.02$) are emboldened. *d/m* days/month

and of TTH 35.1% [22]. Also in Nepal, a similar nationwide study found 1-year prevalences of all headache of 84.9%, of migraine 34.1% and of TTH 41.5% [12], and in Russia, another similar study found prevalences of 62.9% for all headache, 20.8% for migraine and 30.8% for TTH [9]. It would therefore be incorrect to suggest, although they are very common in Pakistan, that headache in general and migraine in particular are excessively prevalent in this country. The reality is that these are very common disorders worldwide, to a degree that is only now being recognised. Only in the Far East does evidence persist of lower prevalence: for example, 23.8% for all primary headache and 9.3% for migraine from a similar nationwide study supported by LTB in China [10]. Whether the reasons for this are genetic, environmental or cultural is yet to be ascertained.

The prevalence in Pakistan of all causes of headache on ≥15 days/month (8.1%) is approaching three times the estimated global average of 3% [1], but still not outside the range found by similar studies. It is similar in Nepal (7.4%) [12] and Georgia (7.6%) [23], and appreciably higher in Russia (10.4%) [9], but lower in India (3.0%) [22]. In Russia, but apparently not Georgia, much of this is associated with medication overuse, and therefore reported as pMOH, with prevalences of 7.2% and 0.9% respectively. In India, the prevalence of pMOH is 1.2% [22] and in Nepal it is 2.1% [12] against Pakistan's 0.7%. Pakistan therefore mirrors Georgia – also a lower-middle-income country – in this respect. This level of highly-frequent headache in Pakistan must be a cause of concern, for it signals much public ill health. A cross-sectional survey cannot establish the causes: these require investigation in clinical settings, although, as in Georgia, medication overuse does not appear to be the major factor. Studies elsewhere suggest multiple factors [24], including high consumption of caffeine (which is present in black tea, typically consumed many times a day in Pakistan) and various health-related issues such as asthma, hypothyroidism and hypertension. Pakistan's unrecognized public ill health and disability warrant enquiry into these factors.

There were some associations of interest. As everywhere [1], observed prevalence of migraine was higher in females than in males, reflecting a female predisposition understood to be hormonally determined [25]. However, the ratio was only 1.5:1 (26.9% versus 18.0%) and multivariate analysis found female gender, with Exp(B) = 1.3, to be only barely significant ($P = 0.039$). It may be noted, as a plausible explanation, that the culture of Pakistan expects women's interviews to be conducted in their husbands' presence while, at the same time, discouraging women from expressing pain in front of their husbands (neurologists in Pakistan are familiar with anecdotal accounts of husbands seeking divorce from their wives on account of their "constant complaints" of headache). In other words, migraine may have been somewhat under-reported by women. Speculatively, the same may have occurred, to a greater degree, with TTH, a disorder perhaps more easily hidden than migraine: in contrast to most studies elsewhere, we found in Pakistan a significantly higher prevalence of TTH in males (51.2%) than in females (37.9%), although this difference, with Exp(B) = 0.8, was also barely significant ($P = 0.026$) after correction for other factors. Comment is still needed on why the prevalence of TTH in males (51.2%) is unusually high – more than in India, and even Nepal, where prevalence was again higher in males (44.6%) than females (38.7%) [12]. This finding occurred consistently in every city surveyed except Sukkur (n = 81). The male:-female working ratio is very high in Pakistan [26]; the burden of supporting the entire household falls almost solely on the male. Whether or not this is a relevant factor may emerge in future studies in other mostly patriarchal countries: preliminary results from Saudi Arabia (unpublished) show a similar trend.

Age had differential impacts on headache types and in the genders. For migraine, the trends were slightly different in males and females, with a more significant effect seen in females (Table 2). Migraine in females increased from adolescence (18–29 years) to middle age (30–49), declining slightly in the perimenopausal years (50–59) and sharply decreasing in the postmenopausal age group of 60–65. These trends can be attributed to the well-documented influence on migraine of oestrogen levels [25]. For TTH, prevalence peaked later in males (40–49) than in females (30–39).

The associations with educational level were complex and not easily explained, except to the extent that they matched those of income level (these two factors themselves being strongly correlated, although each retained some independent associations with the probabilities of migraine and TTH in multivariate analysis [Table 4]). Poverty by itself was positively associated with migraine and headache on ≥15 days/month and negatively with TTH, although the last observation did not hold true after multivariate analysis. In general, therefore, it seems migraine is associated with lower socioeconomic status (SES), being significantly less prevalent among the college-educated and not poor. Educational and income levels affect lifestyle, diet, stress and general hardship levels and, of course, general health and access to health care, so that the social causation hypothesis is speculatively invoked to explain this association [27]: lower SES brings stress and other disease mediators that increase the incidence or duration of illness. The association between poverty and headache has been noted elsewhere [9, 23, 28].

The differences between provinces are noteworthy. Punjab and Sindh have more migraine than Khyber Pakhtunkhwa and, probably, Baluchistan, whereas Punjab has more TTH than all other provinces. Yet headache on ≥15 days/month is more common in Sindh and Baluchistan than in Punjab or, especially, Khyber Pakhtunkhwa. These differences are not easily explained. Each province is largely occupied by a different ethnic group: Punjabi, Sindhi, Baloch and Pashtun, although there are many minority groups. Punjab is an agricultural province with warmer weather; it has higher average SES, which appears contradictory to the trend for migraine but in line with that for headache on ≥15 days/month. Khyber Pakhtunkhwa, which has least headache of all types, has more rural dwellings and a colder climate, and much of it is at high altitudes. In Nepal, increasing altitude, at least between sea level and 2,500 m, is correlated with increasing migraine prevalence [12]. Khyber Pakhtunkhwa is also beset by armed conflict and terrorism, which might be expected to increase rather than reduce headache levels. These differences warrant further investigation.

Associations with BMI were also complex, those of migraine and TTH again appearing to be in opposite directions. Such associations have been studied extensively [29–31]. Possible mechanisms to link migraine and headache on ≥15 days/month with obesity have been described [30] and will not be commented on here. From a public-health perspective, it is of interest if obesity is a risk factor for these disorders since it is potentially modifiable (unlike age, gender and poverty). However, the positive association of obesity with migraine did not survive multivariate analysis, whereas the *negative* association with TTH remained strong (Exp(B) 0.4; $P <$ 0.001). Previous studies [32] have been unable to link TTH with BMI. Overall, not much can be made of these findings with respect to BMI, although it might be observed that obesity is quickly becoming a public-health problem in Pakistan [33].

There are limitations to our study. First, all weightings relied on data that are almost twenty years old given that Pakistan's last census was in 1998 [20]. Second, as noted earlier, we could not reach almost 45% of the urban population who were slum-dwelling [21], which potentially introduced a bias. Third, because of the security situation in Pakistan during the conduct of this study, we were unable to access Quetta, the largest city in Baluchistan province, and areas north of Abbotabad in the Khyber Pakhtunkhwa province. The same concern limited us from going into the deep rural population. Whether these restrictions led to appreciable bias is unknown.

What is the importance of these findings to Pakistan? It is clear that headache disorders in this country are extremely prevalent in absolute terms, and high also relative to global means. These facts were not previously known. But Pakistan has many and considerable public-health problems [32], and prevalence alone does not establish a case for priority. In this regard it can be noted that migraine is the sixth highest cause of disability in the world [3] and Pakistan has much more migraine than the world on average. Burden data will be reported in a future publication.

Conclusion

With over three quarters of its population affected, headache disorders must be on the public-health agenda of Pakistan. Worldwide, these disorders are the third leading cause of disability [6]; information from specific enquiry into the burden attributable to headache disorders in this country is needed to inform health policy and priority-setting, and will be reported soon.

Funding

The study was supported by *Lifting The Burden*, a United Kingdom-based non-governmental organization conducting the Global Campaign against Headache in official relations with the World Health Organization.

Authors' contributions

ADH and TJS conceived the study. TJS drafted the protocol and study questionnaire, which were subsequently refined by TJS and ADH in discussion. ADH provided supervision in Pakistan. AAH, AA, ULU, BA, JE, SZA and RK were responsible for conduct of the study in the field, with ADH acting as principal investigator. UJ and MAS carried out the statistical analysis. AAH and TJS drafted the manuscript. All authors reviewed and approved the final version.

Competing interests

TJS is a Director and Trustee of *Lifting The Burden*. There were no other conflicts of interest.

Author details

[1]Headache Research Foundation of Pakistan, Karachi, Pakistan. [2]Department of Surgery, University of Texas at San Antonio, San Antonio, TX, USA. [3]Dow University of Health Sciences, Karachi, Pakistan. [4]Department of Neurology, Center for Movement Disorders and Neurorestoration, University of Florida College of Medicine, Gainesville, FL, USA. [5]Department of Medicine, University of Nevada, Las Vegas, USA. [6]Aga Khan Medical College, Aga Khan Medical University Hospital, Karachi, Pakistan. [7]School of International and Public Affairs, Columbia University, New York, NY, USA. [8]Department of Neurology, Baqai Medical University, Karachi, Pakistan. [9]Department of Pathology and Microbiology Department at Dow University of Health Sciences, Karachi, Pakistan. [10]Department of Neuroscience, Norwegian University of Science and Technology (NTNU), Edvard Griegs Gate, NO-7491 Trondheim, Norway. [11]Division of Brain Sciences, Imperial College London, London, UK.

References

1. Stovner LJ, Hagen K, Jensen R, Katsarava Z, Lipton R, Scher A, Steiner T, Zwart JA (2007) The global burden of headache: a documentation of headache prevalence and disability worldwide. Cephalalgia 27:193–210
2. Vos T, Flaxman AD, Naghavi M, Lozano R, Michaud C, Ezzati M, Shibuya K, Salomon JA, Abdalla S, Aboyans V, Abraham J, Ackerman I, Aggarwal R, Ahn SY, Ali MK, Alvarado M, Anderson HR, Anderson LM, Andrews KG, Atkinson C, Baddour LM, Bahalim AN, Barker-Collo S, Barrero LH, Bartels DH, Basáñez MG, Baxter A, Bell ML, Benjamin EJ, Bennett D et al (2012) Years lived with disability (YLDs) for 1160 sequelae of 289 diseases and injuries 1990–2010: a systematic analysis for the Global Burden of Disease Study 2010. Lancet 380: 2163–2196
3. Global Burden of Disease Study Collaborators (2015) Global, regional, and national incidence, prevalence, and years lived with disability for 301 acute and chronic diseases and injuries in 188 countries, 1990–2013: a systematic analysis for the Global Burden of Disease Study 2013. Lancet 386:743–800
4. Headache Classification Committee of the International Headache Society (2013) The international classification of headache disorders, 3rd edition (beta version). Cephalalgia 33:629–808
5. World Health Organization and Lifting The Burden (2011) Atlas of headache disorders and resources in the world 2011. WHO Press, Geneva
6. Steiner TJ, Birbeck GL, Jensen RH, Katsarava Z, Stovner LJ, Martelletti P (2015) Headache disorders are third cause of disability worldwide. J Headache Pain 16:58
7. Steiner TJ (2004) Lifting the burden: The global campaign against headache. Lancet-Neurology 3:204–205
8. Steiner TJ, Birbeck GL, Jensen R, Katsarava Z, Martelletti P, Stovner LJ (2010) *Lifting The Burden*: the first 7 years. J Headache Pain 11:451–455

9. Ayzenberg I, Katsarava Z, Sborowski A, Chernysh M, Osipova V, Tabeeva G, Yakhno N, Steiner TJ (2012) The prevalence of primary headache disorders in Russia: a countrywide survey. Cephalalgia 32:373–381
10. Yu S, Liu R, Zhao G, Yang X, Qiao X, Feng J, Fang Y, Cao X, He M, Steiner T (2012) The prevalence and burden of primary headaches in China: a population-based door-to-door survey. Headache 52:582–591
11. Rao GN, Kulkarni GB, Gururaj G, Rajesh K, Subbakrishna DK, Steiner TJ, Stovner LJ (2012) The burden of headache disorders in India: methodology and questionnaire validation for a community-based survey in Karnataka State. J Headache Pain 13:543–550
12. Manandhar K, Risal A, Linde M, Steiner TJ (2016) The burden of headache disorders in Nepal: estimates from a population-based survey. J Headache Pain 17:3
13. United Nations Department of Economic and Social Affairs, Population Division (2015) World population prospects: the 2015 revision. Key findings and advance tables (Working Paper No ESA/P/WP241). United Nations, New York
14. Stovner LJ, Al Jumah M, Birbeck GL, Gururaj G, Jensen R, Katsarava Z, Queiroz LP, Scher AI, Tekle-Haimanot R, Wang SJ, Steiner TJ (2014) The methodology of population surveys of headache prevalence, burden and cost: principles and recommendations from the Global Campaign against Headache. J Headache Pain 15:5
15. Herekar AD, Herekar AA, Ahmad A, Uqaili UL, Ahmed B, Effendi J, Alvi SZ, Steiner TJ (2013) The burden of headache disorders in Pakistan: methodology of a population-based nationwide study, and questionnaire validation. J Headache Pain 14:73
16. Steiner TJ, Gururaj G, Andrée C, Katsarava Z, Ayzenberg I, Yu S-Y, Al Jumah M, Tekle-Haimanot R, Birbeck GL, Herekar A, Linde M, Mbewe E, Manandhar K, Risal A, Jensen R, Queiroz LP, Scher AI, Wang SJ, Stovner LJ (2014) Diagnosis, prevalence estimation and burden measurement in population surveys of headache: presenting the HARDSHIP questionnaire. J Headache Pain 15:3
17. The World Bank (2013) Poverty headcount ratio at national poverty lines (% of population)(Pakistan). World Bank, Washington DC, http://data.worldbank.org/indicator/SI.POV.NAHC?locations=PK (last accessed 11 Jan 2017)
18. World Health Organization (2016) Obesity and overweight. Fact sheet 311 (updated June 2016). World Health Organization, Geneva, http://www.who.int/mediacentre/factsheets/fs311/en/ (last accessed 21 Dec 2016)
19. Ahmed B, Ahmad A, Herekar AA, Uqaili UL, Effendi J, Alvi SZ, Herekar AD, Steiner TJ (2014) Fraud in a population-based study of headache: prevention, detection and correction. J Headache Pain 15:37
20. Pakistan Bureau of Statistics (2016) Population census 1998 (updated December 2016). Government of Pakistan, Islamabad, http://www.pbs.gov.pk/population-tables (last accessed 21 Dec 2016)
21. United Nations Statistics Division (2016) Slum population as percentage of urban (Pakistan 2014) (updated February 2016). United Nations, New York, http://data.un.org/Data.aspx?d=MDG&f=seriesRowID%3a710 (last accessed 21 Dec 2016)
22. Kulkarni GB, Rao GN, Gururaj G, Stovner LJ, Steiner TJ (2015) Headache disorders and public ill-health in India: prevalence estimates in Karnataka State. J Headache Pain 16:67
23. Katsarava Z, Dzagnidze A, Kukava M, Mirvelashvili E, Djibuti M, Janelidze M, Jensen R, Stovner LJ, Steiner TJ (2009) Primary headache disorders in the Republic of Georgia: prevalence and risk factors. Neurology 73:1796–1803
24. Bigal ME, Sheftell FD, Rapoport AM, Tepper SJ, Lipton RB (2002) Chronic daily headache: identification of factors associated with induction and transformation. Headache 42:575–581
25. Brandes JL (2006) The influence of estrogen on migraine: a systematic review. JAMA 295:1824–1830
26. World Bank Group (2016) Ratio of female to male labor force participation rate (%) (modeled ILO estimate) (Pakistan). World Bank, Washington DC, http://data.worldbank.org/indicator/SL.TLF.CACT.FM.ZS?locations=PK (last accessed 21 Dec 2016)
27. Stewart WF, Roy J, Lipton RB (2013) Migraine prevalence, socioeconomic status, and social causation. Neurology 81:948–955
28. Winter AC, Berger K, Buring JE, Kurth T (2012) Associations of socioeconomic status with migraine and non-migraine headache. Cephalalgia 32:159–170
29. Bigal ME, Liberman JN, Lipton RB (2006) Obesity and migraine: a population study. Neurology 66:545–550
30. Bigal ME, Lipton RB, Holland PR, Goadsby PJ (2007) Obesity, migraine, and chronic migraine: possible mechanisms of interaction. Neurology 68:1851–1861
31. Keith SW, Wang C, Fontaine KR, Cowan CD, Allison DB (2008) BMI and headache among women: results from 11 epidemiologic datasets. Obesity 16:377–383
32. Bigal ME, Tsang A, Loder E, Serrano D, Reed ML, Lipton RB (2007) Body mass index and episodic headaches: a population-based study. Arch Intern Med 167:1964–1970
33. Nanan DJ (2002) The obesity pandemic – implications for Pakistan. J Pakistan Med Assoc 52:342–346

12

Clinical patterns of primary stabbing headache

Dong Yeop Kim[1†], Mi Ji Lee[1†], Hyun Ah Choi[1], Hanna Choi[2] and Chin-Sang Chung[1*]

Abstract

Background: The clinical features and disease courses of primary stabbing headache (PSH) are diverse. We aimed to identify distinct clinical patterns of PSH.

Methods: We prospectively screened consecutive first-visit patients who presented with stabbing headache at the Samsung Medical Centre Headache Clinic from June 2015 to March 2016. Demographics, headache characteristics, and disease courses were prospectively evaluated. After discerning factors related to the chronicity at the time of presentation, clinical patterns were identified based on the frequency (daily vs. intermittent), clinical course (remitted or not), and total disease duration (<3 or >3 months).

Results: In the 65 patients with PSH included in this study, monophasic ($n = 31$), intermittent ($n = 17$), and chronic daily ($n = 12$) patterns were identified. The median disease durations were 9 days for monophasic PSH, 9 months for chronic daily PSH, and 2 years for intermittent PSH. The features of monophasic PSH were greater severity, single and side-locked locations, more attacks per day, daily occurrence, and good treatment response. Chronic daily PSH was associated with female predominance, longer-lasting stabs, and multiple or migrating locations on bilateral or alternating sides. The characteristics of intermittent PSH included female predominance and sporadic stabs with less intensity.

Conclusions: Our study demonstrated distinct clinical patterns of PSH. In addition to help early recognition of disease, our findings suggest different pathophysiologic mechanisms. Future prospective studies are required to reveal the etiologies of these different PSH patterns and their optimal treatment strategies.

Keywords: Primary stabbing headache, Clinical course, Pattern, Remission, Prognosis

Background

Primary stabbing headache (PSH) is a primary headache disorder characterised by transient and localised pain attacks occurring as either a single stab or series of stabs [1]. Since this disorder was first described as "ophthalmodynia periodica" in 1964, the nomenclature was revised to PSH in the second edition of the International Classification of Headache Disorders (ICHD-2) [2]. The diagnostic criteria for PSH have recently been revised in the ICHD 3rd edition beta version (ICHD-3 beta), particularly regarding the location of the pain and associated symptoms [3]. Most PSH patients have very brief attacks [4–7]. Migraineurs often have PSH, during or independently from migraine attack [8]. PSH is one of indomethacin-responsive headaches. Currently, the pathophysiologic mechanisms of PSH are not fully understood. Although most PSH are idiopathic and benign, secondary causes have been reported [9, 10].

While PSH is common in population-based subjects, a diagnosis of PSH is relatively infrequent in clinic-based studies [4, 5, 11]. Less impact on daily life and self-limiting nature of PSH might be a reason for not visiting a clinic [8]. However, patients visiting a headache clinic may have different features. Variable disease durations and attack frequencies have been reported in different clinic-based cohorts with PSH [5, 12]. To date, the

* Correspondence: cspaul@naver.com
†Equal contributors
[1]Department of Neurology, Samsung Medical Center, Sungkyunkwan University School of Medicine, Seoul, Korea
Full list of author information is available at the end of the article

clinical patterns and related clinical outcomes have not been systematically examined in prospective studies. The identification of clinical patterns is useful for the diagnosis of primary headache disorders [13, 14]. Furthermore, clarifying the clinical characteristics of the different clinical courses can provide insight into the underlying pathophysiology of the disease. In the present study, we aimed to investigate the clinical patterns of PSH and related characteristics.

Methods

Patient selection

We prospectively screened consecutive first-visit patients who presented with stabbing headaches at the Samsung Medical Centre Headache Clinic from October 2015 to December 2016. Patients were screened even when their stabbing headache was not the main purpose of their visit. Of the patients who agreed to participate in this study, those who were diagnosed with ICHD-3 beta 4.7 PSH were included. Patients were excluded if any primary or secondary headache disorders other than PSH were diagnosed at the first or follow-up visits. When the patients reported the persistence of localised stabs in the occipital nerve territory, they were assessed for any tenderness or response to occipital nerve blocks in order to exclude occipital neuralgia. The Samsung Medical Center Institutional Review Board has approved this study.

Evaluations

Before the screening, all patients completed standard questionnaires regarding their demographics, headache characteristics and medical and social histories. When patients were identified to have any headaches of stabbing nature, they were asked to participate this study. Two investigators (M.J.L. and H.A.C.) interviewed all of the patients with a structured questionnaire that was specifically designed for assessing stabbing headaches. The questionnaire included questions on the duration, frequency, onset, evolution, and previous history of stabs; accompanying PSH-specific symptoms, such as allodynia, jolts, and body jabs; and differentiating symptoms, such as skin rash. Premorbid migraine was self-screened with ID-migraine^{TM} and confirmed by the investigators [15]. Physician-diagnosed depression, anxiety, and panic disorders were self-reported by patients. Insomnia was also self-reported. Stress perceptions during the previous 3 months prior to visit were evaluated with numeric rating scales of 0 – 100, modified from Schramm et al. [16]. The patients were followed by the investigators with a follow-up questionnaire that evaluated their clinical outcomes and treatment responses.

The diagnoses of PSH were made based on the ICHD-3 beta criteria for 4.7 Primary Stabbing Headache [1]. Brain or cervical imaging studies were performed when clinically required to exclude secondary causes.

Determination of disease course

Remission was defined as the complete resolution of headaches for more than 14 days for patients with daily PSH and more than twice the average interval of stabs in patients with non-daily PSH. If the patients' symptoms already remitted before the first visit, the clinical course was considered remitted without follow-up. Clinical courses of patients with persistent symptoms were determined when followed up for >14 days. Follow-up was terminated when the patients showed remission. After excluding three patients with <14 days of follow-up, the median duration of follow-up was 60 days (range, 14 – 325). If the patient's symptoms were too infrequent to detect remission (i.e., 2–3 attacks per year) during the follow-up period, the clinical courses were determined at the investigator's discretion. The total duration of disease is presented as the number of days since symptom onset to the last attack regardless of treatment.

Pattern identification

The occurrence pattern and disease course were used to identify the clinical patterns. In patients in remission and total disease durations less than 3 months, the clinical course was considered monophasic. The pattern could not be determined in unremitted patients with total disease durations less than 3 months. Patients with total disease durations over 3 months and daily stabs were characterised with a chronic daily pattern. In patients with a chronic daily pattern, a chronic progressive pattern was identified if the frequency, severity, or extent increased. An intermittent pattern was defined as the non-daily occurrence of stabs, without predefined frequency criteria. Patients with intermittent patterns were diagnosed with clustering or sporadic patterns based on the daily stab occurrence pattern. A clinical pattern was considered distinct if 10 or more patients had a similar course.

Statistical analysis

Chi-square and Fisher's exact tests were used to compare categorical variables among the groups, while Student's t-tests and Mann–Whitney tests were performed for group comparisons of continuous variables according to their distribution. The statistical analyses were performed with SPSS (version 18.0; IBM Corporation, Armonk, NY, USA). Differences were considered significant at a two-tailed p value less than 0.05.

Results

Study subjects

Among the 71 patients screened during the study period, six were excluded because they had diagnoses other than PSH at the baseline or follow-up visit (occipital neuralgia, $n = 1$; trigeminal neuralgia, $n = 2$; postherpetic neuralgia, $n = 1$; active herpes zoster, $n = 1$; and spinal cord tumor, $n = 1$). Finally, a total of 65 patients with PSH were included in the analysis.

Patient characteristics

The demographics and headache characteristics of the study subjects are listed in Table 1. Our study subjects showed a female preponderance (69.2%) and wide range of age (median, 54 years; range, 25–83). The symptoms occurred as a pattern of single (15.4%) or series (84.6%) of stabs. The majority of patients showed a daily occurrence (72.3%), but an intermittent pattern of occurrence on a monthly (12.4%) or yearly (13.8%) basis was also reported. A history of stabbing headache before the index event was reported for 14 (21.5%) patients.

Disease courses

The total disease durations were widely distributed (median, 40 days; range, 1–13,170 days; Fig. 1). When the disease durations were stratified into 2-week strata, two peaks in the lowest and highest strata were observed (Fig. 2). Remission was achieved in 28 (43.1%) patients, while 37 (56.9%) patients showed persistent symptoms. The mode of remission was spontaneous in 17 (45.9%) patients and due to pharmacologic treatment in 20 (54.1%).

Demographics and headache characteristics of study subjects were compared according to the chronicity of the PSH at the time of presentation (Table 2). Patients with acute/subacute PSH ($n = 41$) had a more severe ($p = 0.012$) and side-locked ($p = 0.044$) stabs than patients with chronic PSH (56.0%, $p = 0.068$). Patients with

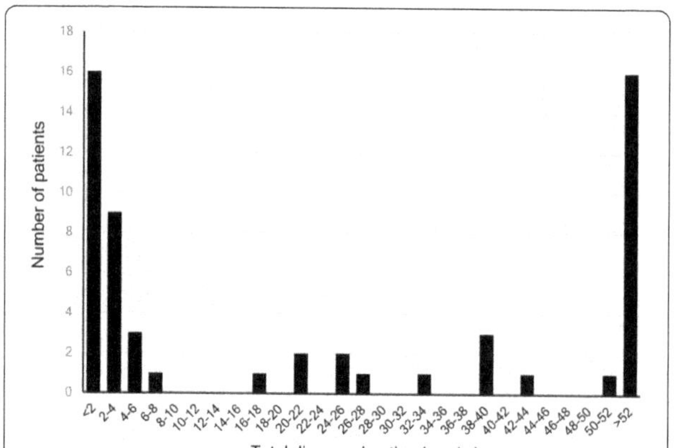

Fig. 1 Distribution of the total disease durations

Table 1 Patient characteristics

Age (y)	54 (25 – 83)
Female sex	45 (69.2%)
Disease duration prior to visit (d)	40 (1 – 13,140)
Follow-up (d)	44 (3 – 325)
Total disease duration (d)	40 (1 – 13,170)
Severity	7 (2 – 10)
Duration (s)	1 (<1 – 60)
Affected territory (not exclusive)	
Occipital nerve	55 (84.6%)
Trigeminal nerve	8 (12.3%)
Multifocal	16 (24.6%)
Side	
Side-locked	45 (69.2%)
Bilateral or alternating	20 (30.8%)
Migrating location	15 (23.1%)
Stab frequency per day	
1 (sporadic stab)	10 (15.4%)
2 – 10	26 (40%)
10 – 30	10 (15.4%)
30 – 100	11 (16.9%)
> 100	8 (12.3%)
Pattern of occurrence	
Daily	47 (72.3%)
Intermittent	
A few per month	9 (13.8%)
A few per year	9 (13.8%)
Premorbid migraine	27 (41.5%)
Previous history of stabbing headaches	14 (21.5%)
Allodynia	24 (36.9%)
Jolt	48 (73.8%)
Bodily jab	8 (12.3%)
Prognosis	
Remission	28 (43.1%)
Persistence	37 (56.9%)
Mode of complete remission	
Spontaneous	17 (45.9%)
By treatment	20 (54.1%)
Treatment	
Indomethacin	8 (12.3%)
Prednisolone	11 (16.9%)
Gabapentin	13 (20.0%)
Tricyclic antidepressants	6 (9.2%)

The data are presented as median (range) or number (%)

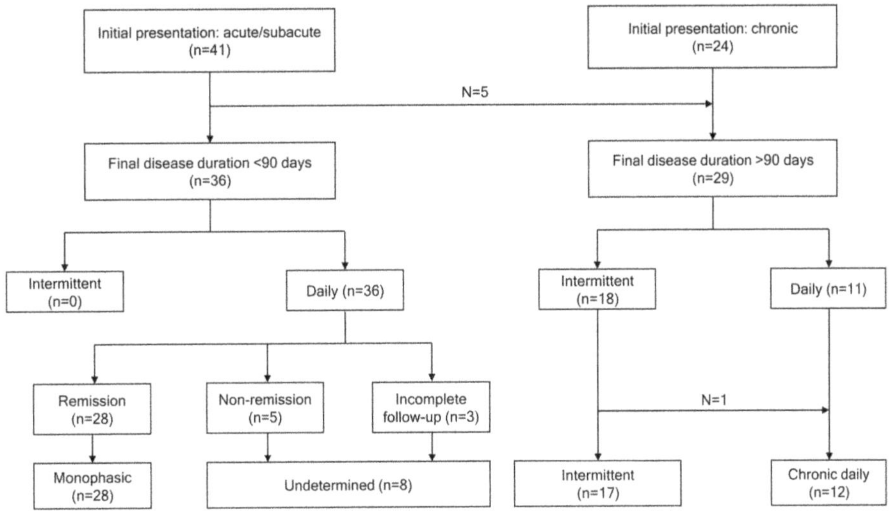

Fig. 2 Algorithm of pattern identification

chronic PSH ($n = 24$) had a female predominance ($p = 0.015$) and a lower frequency of attacks per day ($p = 0.019$). Most patients with acute/subacute PSH had daily stabs (92.5%), while patients with chronic PSH had a more intermittent pattern (p for trend < 0.001). Thirteen (31.7%) patients with acute PSH had a history of PSH ($p = 0.009$) compared to patients with chronic PSH. The prevalence of associated allodynia, jolts, and bodily jabs did not differ between the two groups ($p = 0.672$, >0.999, and 0.149, respectively). Other medical, psychiatric, and social comorbidities did not differ between the groups.

Regarding the clinical course, patients with acute/subacute PSH had a median disease duration of 15 (interquartile range, 6–31) days. They showed a high rate of remission (80.5%), which occurred either spontaneously (51.5%) or as a result of pharmacologic treatment (48.5%). All patients with remission had daily occurrence of stabs at baseline. Five patients with initial acute/subacute presentation progressed to chronic PSH ($n = 3$ with daily stabs, $n = 2$ with a few stabs per month; Fig. 2). All the five patients already had more than 2 months of disease duration at the first visit. Patients with chronic PSH had a low rate of remission (16.7%) and longer disease duration (median, 1,139 days; interquartile range, 275–1,950). Although the number of patients in each group was very small, the steroid response was more prominent in patients with acute/subacute PSH ($p = 0.015$). Patients with chronic PSH showed a high response rate (80.0%) to indomethacin.

Clinical patterns of PSH

The algorithm of pattern identification is shown in Fig. 2. The typical patterns are illustrated in Fig. 3. Twenty-eight patients exhibited the monophasic pattern (Fig. 3a–b). In the monophasic group, 10 patients (35.7%) recalled that they had a similar episode of PSH which remitted before the index event (Fig. 3b; monophasic-relapsing). An intermittent pattern was observed in 17 patients (Fig. 3c–d). Among them, 10 patients showed a clustering of stabs (Fig. 3c), while 7 reported only sporadic stabs (Fig. 3d). Among the 12 patients with chronic daily PSH (Fig. 3e–f), a progressive pattern was identified in six patients (Fig. 3f).

The characteristics of the patients with different clinical courses are summarised in Table 3. The median disease durations were 13 days for monophasic PSH, 9 months for chronic daily PSH, and 2 years for intermittent PSH. The features related to monophasic PSH were greater severity ($p = 0.033$ vs. intermittent PSH), single and side-locked locations ($p = 0.010$ and 0.010, respectively; vs. chronic daily PSH), more frequent attacks per day ($p = 0.001$ vs. intermittent PSH), daily occurrence ($p < 0.001$ vs. intermittent PSH), and good response to treatment. Chronic daily PSH was associated with longer-lasting stabs ($p = 0.071$ vs. monophasic PSH and $p = 0.064$ vs intermittent PSH), and multiple or migrating locations ($p = 0.010$ and 0.017, respectively; vs. monophasic PSH) on bilateral or alternating sides ($p = 0.010$ vs. monophasic PSH). Although statistically not significant, allodynia and bodily jabs were most frequently reported in patients with chronic daily PSH, while jolts were observed less than the other patterns. The characteristics of intermittent PSH included female predominance and sporadic stabs with less intensities, while the other features were similar to or between the patients with monophasic and chronic daily PSH.

Discussion

In this prospective study, we focused on the patterns and clinical courses of PSH. The key findings were the

Table 2 Patient demographics and characteristics according to chronicity at the initial visit

	Acute/subacute ($n = 41$)	Chronic ($n = 24$)	p
Age (y)	54 (48–61)	55 (44–62)	0.822
Female sex	24 (58.5%)	21 (87.5%)	0.015
Severity (Numeric Rating Scale)	8 (7 – 9)	7 (5 – 8)	0.012
Duration (s)	1 (1 – 3)	1 (1 – 3)	0.348
Affected territory (not exclusive)			
Occipital	37 (90.2%)	18 (75.0%)	0.154
V1	4 (9.8%)	4 (16.7%)	0.454
Multiple	7 (17.1%)	9 (37.5%)	0.065
Side			0.044
Side-locked	32 (78.0%)	13 (54.2%)	
Bilateral or alternating	9 (22.0%)	11 (45.8%)	
Migrating location	7 (17.1%)	8 (33.3%)	0.133
Stab frequency per day			0.019*
1 (sporadic stab)	4 (9.8%)	6 (25.0%)	
2 – 10	15 (36.6%)	11 (45.8%)	
10 – 30	6 (14.6%)	4 (16.7%)	
30 – 100	9 (22.0%)	2 (8.3%)	
> 100	7 (17.1%)	1 (4.2%)	
Pattern of occurrence (either single or series of stabs)			<0.001*
Daily	39 (95.1%)	8 (33.3%)	
A few per month	2 (4.9%)	7 (29.2%)	
A few per year	0 (0.0%)	9 (37.5%)	
Disease duration prior to visit (d)	10 (7 – 30)	1,095 (195 – 2,920)	0.000
Follow-up (d)	34 (14 – 64)	49 (29 – 98)	0.086
Total disease duration (d)	15 (6 – 30)	987 (274 – 2,291)	0.000
Complete remission	33 (80.5%)	4 (16.7%)	<0.001
Mode of remission			0.109
Spontaneous	17 (51.5%)	0 (0.0%)	
By treatment	16 (48.5%)	4 (100.0%)	
Treatment response[a]			
Indomethacin	1/3 (33.3%)	4/5 (80.0%)	0.464
Prednisolone	6/7 (85.7%)	0/4 (0.0%)	0.015
Gabapentin	6/9 (66.7%)	1/4 (25.0%)	0.266
Tricyclic antidepressants	1/3 (33.3%)	0/3 (0.0%)	>0.999

The data are presented as median (interquartile range) or number (%)
*p for trend; [a]Only in patients treated by medications (numbers shown in the table)

following: 1) PSH presented with either an acute or chronic course, 2) patients with acute/subacute and chronic PSH had different demographics and headache characteristics, thus implicating different pathophysiologies, and 3) clinical patterns of PSH are either monophasic, intermittent, or chronic daily patterns.

Previous descriptive studies of PSH have reported that both population-based and clinic-based subjects showed a wide range of disease durations, which ranged from days to several years [4, 5]. The results of our study were in line with the results of the previous studies, showing diverse disease durations that ranged from 1 day to 18 years. We found that the distribution of the disease durations had two peaks (<2 weeks and > 1 year), which suggested the presence of two distinctive clinical courses: acute/subacute and chronic. To date, chronic PSH has not been classified as an independent entity in the ICHD-3 beta. However, our study results showed that chronic PSH was not uncommon.

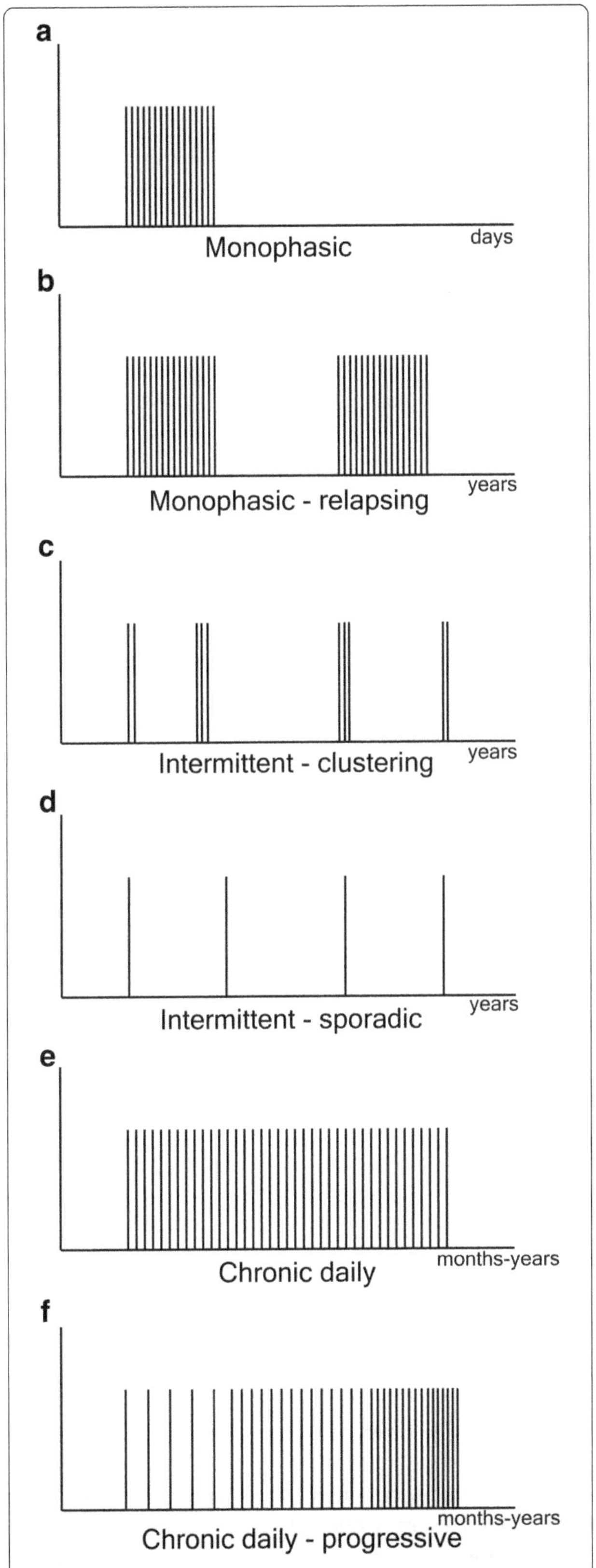

Fig. 3 Clinical patterns of primary stabbing headache. **a-b** Monophasic pattern ($n = 28$). In the monophasic group, a relapse was reported in 10 patients (35.7%). **c-d** Intermittent pattern ($n = 17$). Stabs occur in cluster (**c**) or sporadically (**d**). **e-f** Chronic daily PSH ($n = 12$). Six patients reported a progressive course (**f**)

Previous studies have reported different demographics and characteristics [4, 7, 12, 17, 18]. Our results showed that different characteristics were involved in the chronicity. The characteristics of patients with acute/subacute PSH included more localised locations, greater intensity, more stabs per day, and daily occurrence. Moreover, a history of PSH was more common in the patients with acute/subacute PSH, which suggested a high relapse rate in these patients. In contrast, chronic PSH was associated with female predominance, multifocal and bilateral locations, and both daily and intermittent patterns of occurrence.

Based on these findings, distinct clinical patterns were identified in PSH. The most common pattern was monophasic, which was characterised by the daily occurrence of a series of stabs that lasted days to weeks and a high rate of complete remission. In contrast, the intermittent pattern was defined as a few attacks of sporadic or clustering stabs over a month or year. The stab occurrences did not exceed one day. In this subgroup, pharmacologic treatment was not routinely performed because of its low frequency and negligible impact on routine life. Finally, chronic daily PSH was another extreme of this disorder. Although the frequencies of stabs per day varied among the patients, they had daily or near daily attacks. Some patients reported an evolution from intermittent to daily patterns, which suggested disease progression.

Different disease patterns may have pathophysiological implications, such as different origins of pain or mechanisms of chronification. The monophasic disease might be explained by acute irritation of the peripheral branches of the trigeminal or occipital nerves [5, 19], which resembles a zoster sine herpete that presents with acute-onset neuralgia in the absence of an antecedent rash [20, 21]. Due to assumptions of an inflammatory etiology, we tried steroid treatments for the patients suffering from high-frequency and severe-intensity stabs, and this treatment resulted in an excellent response. Based on these uncontrolled treatment experiences of selected patients, the steroid treatments had the most immediate effects compared with the other therapeutic agents. These results suggest that further investigations of a viral etiology are worthwhile for revealing the mechanisms and optimal treatments of monophasic PSH. The chronic daily pattern was associated with multiple or migrating locations, slightly longer-lasting stabs, frequent allodynia, and bodily jabs, which suggested central sensitisation of the second-order

Table 3 Patient characteristics for different clinical courses

	Monophasic (M; n = 28)	Intermittent (I; n = 17)	Chronic daily (C; n = 12)	P^*	Post-hoc		
					M vs. C	M vs. I	C vs. I
Age (y)	54 (48–61)	57 (48–63)	56 (39–62)	0.970	0.871	0.879	0.825
Female sex	17 (60.7%)	15 (88.2%)	9 (75.0%)	0.203	0.484	0.088	0.622
Chronicity at presentation	0 (0.0%)	16 (94.1%)	8 (66.7%)	<0.001	<0.001	<0.001	0.130
Follow-up (d)	34 (20–63)	43 (22–81)	72 (51–112)	0.020	0.006	0.560	0.048
Total disease duration (d)	13 (5–22)	1,460 (574–3,684)	269(155–398)	<0.001	<0.001	<0.001	0.001
Severity (Numeric Rating Scale)	8 (6–10)	7 (5–8)	7 (5–9)	0.114	0.226	0.046	0.575
Duration (s)	1 (1–3)	1 (1–3)	3 (1–9)	0.163	0.128	0.629	0.064
Affected territory (not exclusive)							
Occipital	25 (89.3%)	14 (82.4%)	9 (75.0%)	0.262	0.341	0.658	0.669
V1	2 (7.1%)	2 (11.8%)	3 (25.0%)	0.205	0.149	0.626	0.622
Multiple	4 (14.3%)	4 (23.5%)	7 (58.3%)	0.008	0.008	0.452	0.119
Side				0.015	0.021	0.284	0.274
Side-locked	23 (82.1%)	11 (64.7%)	5 (41.7%)				
Bilateral or alternating	5 (17.9%)	6 (35.3%)	7 (58.3%)				
Migrating location	4 (14.3%)	4 (23.5%)	6 (50.0%)	0.031	0.041	0.452	0.236
Stab frequency per day				0.118	0.476	0.001	0.018*
1 (sporadic stab)	2 (7.1%)	7 (41.2%)	0 (0.0%)				
2–10	9 (32.1%)	7 (41.2%)	7 (58.3%)				
10–30	6 (21.4%)	2 (11.8%)	2 (16.7%)				
30–100	6 (21.4%)	1 (5.9%)	2 (16.7%)				
>100	5 (17.9%)	0 (0.0%)	1 (8.3%)				
Pattern of occurrence				0.060	0.300	<0.001	<0.001
Daily	28 (100.0%)	0 (0.0%)	11 (91.7%)				
A few per month	0 (0.0%)	8 (47.1%)	1 (8.3%)				
A few per year	0 (0.0%)	9 (52.9%)	0 (0.0%)				
Migraine history	14 (50.0%)	6 (35.3%)	4 (33.3%)	0.314	0.491	0.372	>0.999
Allodynia	10 (35.7%)	4 (23.5%)	6 (50.0%)	0.605	0.490	0.513	0.236
Jolts	22 (78.6%)	14 (82.4%)	6 (50.0%)	0.131	0.130	>0.999	0.106
Bodily jabs	4 (14.3%)	1 (5.9%)	3 (25.0%)	0.636	0.410	0.635	0.279
Depression	4 (14.3%)	0 (0.0%)	0 (0.0%)	0.101	0.297	0.281	>0.999
Anxiety	3 (10.7%)	0 (0.0%)	0 (0.0%)	0.158	0.541	0.279	>0.999
Panic disorder	1 (3.6%)	0 (0.0%)	0 (0.0%)	0.702	>0.999	>0.999	>0.999
Caffeine consumption	22 (78.6%)	13 (76.5%)	8 (66.7%)	0.564	0.451	>0.999	0.683
Smoking	4 (14.3%)	1 (5.9%)	3 (25.0%)	0.636	0.410	0.635	0.279
Insomnia	7 (25.0%)	5 (29.4%)	5 (41.7%)	0.365	0.453	0.743	0.694
Stress scale	60 (30–71)	50 (30–60)	65 (35–80)	0.358	0.412	0.382	0.161

The data are presented as median (interquartile range) or number (%)

*Kruskal-Wallis tests were performed on continuous variables, and linear-by-linear association tests were performed on categorical variables

nociceptive neurons [22, 23]. The mechanism of central sensitisation in PSH might be different from that of migraine because the presence of migraine or factors related to migraine chronification were not associated with chronic daily PSH. It remains to be investigated whether the early treatment of monophasic or intermittent PSHs can reduce the development of chronic daily PSH. The intermittent pattern had features that were similar to or in between monophasic and chronic daily PSH. Future studies need to investigate whether intermittent PSH is an independent entity or a milder form of monophasic or chronic daily PSH.

Although a controversy exist, brain imaging is recommended by some experts to exclude secondary causes of PSH [24]. Investigation of underlying secondary causes may be more important in emergency rooms and tertiary headache clinics [25–27]. Pattern recognition might be helpful for identifying PSHs as a primary headache disorder. In our data, unremitted daily PSHs of recent onset is not common in patients with PSH, warranting an appropriate evaluation for secondary causes. Prevalence of secondary causes in each clinical pattern should be investigated in future studies.

This study has several strengths. This is the first study to focus on the clinical course of PSH. The prospective study setting and homogenous disease-specific evaluation are the main strengths of this study. However, some limitations are also present. The subjects in this study might not represent the general population because they were sampled from a specialised headache clinic in a university hospital. Thus, the prevalence of the acute or chronic PSH cannot be generalized. In order to reduce the selection bias, we recruited patients with a broad spectrum of disease by screening patients whose main complaints were not a stabbing headache. Another limitation is that the treatments were not controlled in this observational study. Therefore, the response rates among drugs could not be directly compared. Finally, headache frequencies were not defined by prospective headache diary.

In conclusion, distinct clinical patterns, such as monophasic, intermittent, and chronic daily patterns, are associated with different clinical characteristics. Different pathophysiologic mechanisms may be present, thus warranting future prospective studies to reveal the etiologies of the different PSH patterns and optimal treatment strategies.

Acknowledgment
We thank Ms. Miran Jung for data management.

Funding
This study was partly supported by Dong-A ST in data management.

Authors' contributions
DYK participated in the design of the study, performed the statistical analysis and drafted the manuscript. MJL conceived of the study, designed and coordinated the study, and drafted the manuscript. HAC and HC participated in data collection and analysis. C-SC conceived of the study and revised the manuscript. All authors read and approved the final manuscript.

Competing interests
The authors declare that they have no competing interests.

Author details
[1]Department of Neurology, Samsung Medical Center, Sungkyunkwan University School of Medicine, Seoul, Korea. [2]Department of Neurology, Eulji University Hospital, Eulji University School of Medicine, Daejeon, Korea.

References

1. Headache Classification Committee of the International Headache S (2013) The International classification of headache disorders, 3rd edition (beta version). Cephalalgia 33(9):629–808. doi:10.1177/0333102413485658
2. Headache Classification Subcommittee of the International Headache S (2004) The International classification of headache disorders: 2nd edition. Cephalalgia 24(Suppl 1):9–160
3. Olesen J (2014) Problem areas in the International classification of headache disorders, 3rd edition (beta). Cephalalgia 34(14):1193–1199. doi:10.1177/0333102414534327
4. Sjaastad O, Pettersen H, Bakketeig LS (2001) The Vaga study; epidemiology of headache I: the prevalence of ultrashort paroxysms. Cephalalgia 21(3):207–215
5. Fuh JL, Kuo KH, Wang SJ (2007) Primary stabbing headache in a headache clinic. Cephalalgia 27(9):1005–1009. doi:10.1111/j.1468-2982.2007.01365.x
6. Mukharesh LO, Jan MM (2011) Primary stabbing "ice-pick" headache. Pediatr Neurol 45(4):268–270. doi:10.1016/j.pediatrneurol.2011.06.017
7. Lee M, Chu MK, Lee J, Yoo J, Song HK (2016) Field testing primary stabbing headache criteria according to the 3rd beta edition of International classification of headache disorders: a clinic-based study. J Headache Pain 17:21. doi:10.1186/s10194-016-0615-z
8. Wang SJ, Fuh JL (2010) The "other" headaches: primary cough, exertion, sex, and primary stabbing headaches. Curr Pain Headache Rep 14(1):41–46. doi:10.1007/s11916-009-0083-0
9. Levy MJ, Matharu MS, Meeran K, Powell M, Goadsby PJ (2005) The clinical characteristics of headache in patients with pituitary tumours. Brain 128 (Pt 8):1921–1930. doi:10.1093/brain/awh525
10. Mascellino AM, Lay CL, Newman LC (2001) Stabbing headache as the presenting manifestation of intracranial meningioma: a report of two patients. Headache 41(6):599–601
11. Guerrero AL, Herrero S, Penas ML, Cortijo E, Rojo E, Mulero P, Fernandez R (2011) Incidence and influence on referral of primary stabbing headache in an outpatient headache clinic. J Headache Pain 12(3):311–313. doi:10.1007/s10194-010-0283-3
12. Pareja JA, Ruiz J, de Isla C, al-Sabbah H, Espejo J (1996) Idiopathic stabbing headache (jabs and jolts syndrome). Cephalalgia 16(2):93–96
13. Sheftell FD, Tepper SJ (2002) New paradigms in the recognition and acute treatment of migraine. Headache 42(1):58–69
14. Heneghan C, Glasziou P, Thompson M, Rose P, Balla J, Lasserson D, Scott C, Perera R (2009) Diagnostic strategies used in primary care. BMJ 338:b946. doi:10.1136/bmj.b946
15. Lipton RB, Dodick D, Sadovsky R, Kolodner K, Endicott J, Hettiarachchi J, Harrison W, study IDMv (2003) A self-administered screener for migraine in primary care: the ID migraine validation study. Neurology 61(3):375–382
16. Schramm SH, Moebus S, Lehmann N, Galli U, Obermann M, Bock E, Yoon MS, Diener HC, Katsarava Z (2015) The association between stress and headache: a longitudinal population-based study. Cephalalgia 35(10): 853–863. doi:10.1177/0333102414563087
17. Sjaastad O, Pettersen H, Bakketeig LS (2005) Long-lasting cephalic jabs (?) The Vaga study of headache epidemiology. Cephalalgia 25(8):581–592. doi:10.1111/j.1468-2982.2005.00927.x
18. Shin JH, Song HK, Lee JH, Kim WK, Chu MK (2007) Paroxysmal stabbing headache in the multiple dermatomes of the head and neck: a variant of primary stabbing headache or occipital neuralgia? Cephalalgia 27(10): 1101–1108. doi:10.1111/j.1468-2982.2007.01395.x
19. Selekler HM, Budak F (2004) Idiopathic stabbing headache and experimental ice cream headache (short-lived headaches). Eur Neurol 51(1):6–9. doi:10.1159/000074910
20. Easton HG (1970) Zoster sine herpete causing acute trigeminal neuralgia. Lancet 2(7682):1065–1066
21. Blumenthal DT, Shacham-Shmueli E, Bokstein F, Schmid DS, Cohrs RJ, Nagel MA, Mahalingam R, Gilden D (2011) Zoster sine herpete: virologic

verification by detection of anti-VZV IgG antibody in CSF. Neurology 76(5): 484–485. doi:10.1212/WNL.0b013e31820a0d28

22. Woolf CJ (2011) Central sensitization: implications for the diagnosis and treatment of pain. Pain 152(3 Suppl):S2–S15. doi:10.1016/j.pain.2010.09.030
23. Milligan ED, Watkins LR (2009) Pathological and protective roles of glia in chronic pain. Nat Rev Neurosci 10(1):23–36. doi:10.1038/nrn2533
24. Mitsikostas DD, Ashina M, Craven A, Diener HC, Goadsby PJ, Ferrari MD, Lampl C, Paemeleire K, Pascual J, Siva A, Olesen J, Osipova V, Martelletti P, committee EHF (2015) European headache federation consensus on technical investigation for primary headache disorders. J Headache Pain 17:5. doi:10.1186/s10194-016-0596-y
25. Tabatabai RR, Swadron SP (2016) Headache in the emergency department: avoiding misdiagnosis of dangerous secondary causes. Emerg Med Clin North Am 34(4):695–716. doi:10.1016/j.emc.2016.06.003
26. Carolei A, Ripa P (2015) Secondary headache in emergency. J Headache Pain 16(Suppl 1):A27. doi:10.1186/1129-2377-16-S1-A27
27. Kim NH, Yang SY, Koo JB, Jeong SW. Occipital neuralgia as the only presenting symptom of foramen magnum meningioma. J Clin Neurol. 2009; 5(4):198–200. doi:10.3988/jcn.2009.5.4.198.

13

Identification of subgroups of patients with tension type headache with higher widespread pressure pain hyperalgesia

César Fernández-de-las-Peñas[1,2,5*], Elena Benito-González[1], María Palacios-Ceña[1,2], Kelun Wang[2], Matteo Castaldo[2,3,4] and Lars Arendt-Nielsen[2]

Abstract

Background: Identification of subgroups of patients with different levels of sensitization and clinical features can help to identify groups at risk and the development of better therapeutic strategies. The aim of this study was to identify subgroups of patients with tension type headache (TTH) with different levels of sensitization, clinical pain features, and psychological outcomes.

Methods: A total of 197 individuals with TTH participated. Headache intensity, frequency, and duration and medication intake were collected with a 4-weeks diary. Pressure pain thresholds were assessed bilaterally over the temporalis muscle, C5-C6 joint, second metacarpal and tibialis anterior muscle to determine widespread pressure pain hyperalgesia. The Hospital Anxiety and Depression Scale assessed anxiety and depression. The State-Trait Anxiety Inventory evaluated the state and trait levels of anxiety. The Headache Disability Inventory evaluated the burden of headache. Health-related quality of life was determined with the SF-36 questionnaire. Groups were considered as positive (three or more criteria) or negative (less than three criteria) on a clinical prediction rule: headache duration <8.5 h/day; headache frequency <5.5 days/week; bodily pain <47 and vitality <47.5.

Results: The ANCOVA revealed that subjects in group 1 (positive rule, $n = 89$) exhibited longer headache history, shorter headache duration, lower headache frequency, higher widespread pressure hyperalgesia, higher anxiety trait levels, and lower quality of life (all, $P < 0.01$) than those subjects within group 2 (negative rule, $n = 108$). Differences were similar between men and women.

Conclusions: This study identified a subgroup of patients with TTH with higher sensitization, higher chronicity of headaches and worse quality of life but lower frequency and duration of headache episodes. This subgroup of individuals with TTH may need particular attention and specific therapeutic programs for avoiding potential chronification.

Keywords: Tension type headache, Pain, Groups, Sensitization

Background

Tension-type headache (TTH) affects up to 80% of the general population at sometime during their life and shows a global prevalence in adults of 42% [1]. The general health costs for headaches in Europe were €13.8 billion, most related to migraine and TTH [2]. In fact, TTH has been found to be the second most prevalent disorder in the world [3]; although it has received far less attention than migraine.

Although the mechanisms underlying the transition from episodic to chronic TTH are not fully understood, the existing literature supports that sensitization mechanisms play an important role [4, 5]. In fact, the most accepted theory is that frequent episodic TTH is peripheral dominant whereas chronic TTH involves more central components [6]. This hypothesis is based on several studies supporting the presence of pressure pain hyperalgesia in

* Correspondence: cesar.fernandez@urjc.es
[1]Department of Physical Therapy, Occupational Therapy, Physical Medicine and Rehabilitation, Universidad Rey Juan Carlos, Alcorcón, Spain
[2]Center for Sensory-Motor Interaction (SMI), Department of Health Science and Technology, Faculty of Medicine, Aalborg University, Aalborg, Denmark
Full list of author information is available at the end of the article

the trigemino-cervical area as a manifestation of altered nociceptive pain processing in TTH [7]. Nevertheless, pressure pain hypersensitivity within the trigeminal area may reflect both peripheral and central sensitization processes. The presence of widespread pressure pain hypersensitivity in distant pain-free areas in TTH supports the role of central sensitization [8, 9].

Identification of subgroups of patients with different levels of sensitization can help to better understanding of chronic and complex pain conditions, such as TTH, and to identify better therapeutic strategies. For instance, a subgroup of individuals with knee osteoarthritis (those with higher pain intensity but minimal radiographic change in the knee) exhibiting strong sensitization has been identified [10]. In individuals with chronic whiplash associated disorders higher widespread pressure sensitivity and cold sensitivity have been associated with higher disability levels [11]. There is a lack of studies investigating sub-classification in individuals with TTH. A clinical prediction rule to identify women with TTH who will be likely to respond favorably to a particular manual therapy approach was identified, but not validated [12]. The results identified 4 variables that were predictive of a positive outcome: headache duration <8.5 h/day, headache frequency < 5.5 days/week, bodily pain <47 points and vitality <47.5 points. If a patient presented with 3 of these 4 variables, the positive likelihood ratio was 3.4 (95%CI 1.4, 8.0) with a posttest probability of success of 80% [12]. It is possible that these variables can be also able to identify groups of patients with TTH with different levels of sensitization or clinical features. In fact, a similar procedure was recently observed in women with carpal tunnel syndrome where those positive on a clinical prediction rule for physical therapy exhibited higher pressure and thermal pain hyperalgesia and higher depressive levels than those negative on the rule [13]. Therefore, the aim of the current study was to characterize groups of patients with TTH by determining if those variables previously associated with a positive outcome for manual therapy are also able to identify patients with TTH with more central sensitization and worse clinical features.

Methods

Participants

A cross-sectional study was conducted. Individuals with headache were recruited from different university-based hospitals between January 2015 and December 2016. All diagnoses were performed following the criteria of the International Classification of Headache Disorders (ICHD-III beta, 2013) by neurologists, expert in headaches [14]. To be included subjects had to exhibit all pain features of TTH; report no more than one among photophobia, phonophobia or mild nausea, and no moderate/severe nausea or vomiting as requested by the ICHD-III diagnostic criteria [14]. A 4-weeks headache diary was used to substantiate the diagnosis and to obtain the headache features [15]. On the headache diary, participants registered the number of days with headache (days/week), the duration of headache episodes (hours/day), and the intensity of pain of each episode on an 11-points numerical pain rate scale (NPRS; 0: no pain; 10: the worst unimaginable pain) [16]. Further, the use of symptomatic and preventive medication intake was also recorded in the diary.

Participants were excluded if presented any of the following criteria: 1, any other primary or secondary headache including medication overuse headache as defined by the ICHD-III; 2, previous cervical or head trauma; 3, cervical herniated disk or cervical osteoarthritis on medical records; 4, systemic medical disease; 5, fibromyalgia syndrome; 6, had received physical therapy or anesthetic blocks in the head/neck within the previous 6 months; or, 7, pregnancy. All subjects read and signed a written consent form prior to their participation in the study. The study design was approved by the local Ethics Committees (URJC 23/2014, HRJ 07/14, Aalborg N20140063, CESU 5/2015) and was conducted following the Helsinki declaration.

Evaluations were conducted when patients were headache-free or, in those with a high frequency of headaches, when the intensity of pain was ≤3 points on the NPRS. They were asked to avoid any analgesic or muscle relaxant 24 h prior to examination. No change was made on their regular pharmacological treatment.

Pressure pain thresholds

An electronic pressure algometer (Somedic® Algometer, Sollentuna, Sweden) was used to measure pressure pain thresholds (PPT) over the temporalis muscle, C5-C6 zygapophyseal joint, second metacarpal and tibialis anterior muscle. PPT is defined as the minimal amount of pressure where a sense of pressure first changes to pain. Participants were instructed to press the "stop-button" of the algometer as soon as the pressure resulted in a first sensation of pressure and pain. Pressure was increased at a rate of approximately 30 kPa/s. The mean of 3 trials on each point, with a 30 s resting period for avoiding temporal summation of pain [17], was calculated and used for the main analyses. The order of assessment was randomized between participants and the assessor was blinded to any other outcome. Participants practiced first on the wrist extensors of the right forearm. The reliability of pressure algometry has been found to be high [18, 19].

Headache Disability Inventory (HDI)

The HDI assesses the burden of headache using 25 items that inquire about the impact of headache on emotional functioning and daily activities [20]. Possible answers for each item include YES (4 points), SOMETIMES (2 point) or NO (0 points). Thirteen items evaluate the emotional burden of the headache (HDI-E, maximum score: 52), and the remaining 12 items the physical burden (HDI-P, maximum score: 48). A greater score suggests a greater burden of the headache. The HDI has exhibited good stability at short and long-terms [21].

State-Trait Anxiety Inventory (STAI)

The STAI is a 40-items scale assessing the state (items l-20, STAI-S) and trait (items 21–40, STAI-T) levels of anxiety [22, 23]. The STAI-S evaluates relatively enduring symptoms of anxiety where subjects use a 4-points response scale ranging from "not at all" to "very much", to indicate the extent to which they experience each emotion. The STAI-T scale measures stable propensity to experience anxiety and tendencies to perceive stressful situations as threatening. It consists of 20 statements requiring individuals to rate how they generally feel on a 4-points scale. Higher scores indicate greater state and/or trait anxiety levels. Both scales have good internal consistency and excellent test-retest reliability [24].

Health-related quality of life

The Short-Form Health Survey 36 (SF-36) was used to assess health-related quality of life. The SF-36 is a self-administered, 36-items questionnaire that measures health-related functions on eight domains: physical function, physical role, bodily pain, general health, vitality, social function, role-emotional, and mental health [25]. After summing Likert-scaled items, each domain is standardized ranging from 0 to 100 points according to established international guidelines where higher scores represent better quality of life [26].

Sub-grouping

Patients were grouped according if they were positive or negative in the rule using identical criteria to those previously reported [12]: headache duration <8.5 h/day; headache frequency <5.5 days per week; bodily pain <47 points and vitality <47.5 points in the domains of the SF-36 questionnaire. Patients who met at least three of the four criteria were classified as positive on the rule (Group 1), whereas patients meeting two or fewer criteria were classified as negative on the rule (Group 2).

Data analysis

Statistical analysis was performed using SPSS software version 20.0 (Chicago, IL, USA). Patients were grouped according to the rule [12]. Differences between groups in clinical features, burden of headache (HDI-E, HDI-P), depression (HADS-D), anxiety (HADS-A, STAI-T, STAI-S) and each domain of SF-36 questionnaire were compared using one-way analysis of covariance (ANCOVA) with gender as covariate, and $\chi 2$ test of independence for categorical data. A two-way ANCOVA was used to evaluate differences in PPTs with side (right/left) as within-subjects factor, group (positive or negative rule) as the between-subjects factor and gender as covariate. The normality and homogeneity criteria were checked for dependent variables with Kurtosis and Skewness for the normality and Levene's test for the homogeneity criteria. Separate ANOVAs were performed for each variable. As multiple comparisons were conducted in the main analysis, a Bonferroni-corrected alpha level of 0.025 (2 independent-samples t tests) was required to support the validity of the sub-groups.

Results

Two hundred and twenty-five ($n = 225$) subjects with headache were screened for possible eligibility criteria. Of these, 197 patients (72% women) satisfied all the eligibility criteria, agreed to participate and signed the written informed consent. The reasons for exclusion were co-morbid migraine ($n = 15$), fibromyalgia ($n = 5$), medication overuse headache ($n = 4$), or previous whiplash ($n = 4$). One hundred and nine ($n = 109$, 56.5%) were classified as frequent episodic tension type headache (FETTH), and 88 (44.5%) were classified as chronic tension type headache (CTTH) accordingly to the ICHD-III diagnostic criteria. Fifty-five (28%) were taking prophylactic intake, i.e., amitriptyline, on a regular basis, and 136 (69%) took symptomatic medication, i.e., NSAIDs, during the headache episodes. Eighty-nine individuals (45%) were classified as group 1 (positive rule) whereas 108 (55%) were classified as group 2 (negative rule).

Headache clinical features and medication intake

Table 1 summarizes demographic and clinical data of each group in the total sample. The ANCOVA revealed significant differences between groups for years with headache ($F = 5.748$; $P = 0.02$), headache duration ($F = 7.836$; $P < 0.001$) and headache frequency ($F = 17.148$; $P < 0.001$), but not for age ($F = 0.813$; $P = 0.488$) or headache intensity ($F = 0.904$; $P = 0.333$): patients in group 1 showed longer history of headache, shorter headache duration, and lower frequency of episodes than those patients within group 2. No interaction of gender was observed for either outcome (age: $F = 0.367$, $P = 0.545$; years with headache: $F = 0.573$, $P = 0.450$; headache intensity: $F = 0.919$, $P = 0.433$; headache duration: $F = 0.182$, $P = 0.670$; headache frequency: $F = 0.187$, $P = 0.666$). A significant ($\chi 2 = 11.594$; $P < 0.001$) greater proportion of FETTH subjects were included in group 1.

Finally, no significant differences in the distribution of gender ($\chi 2 = 0.826$; $P = 0.363$) or medication intake

Table 1 Clinical features, medication intake, psychological and related-disability outcomes in patients with tension-type headache by group

	Group 1 (Rule positive, $n = 89$)	Group 2 (Rule negative, $n = 108$)
Clinical Pain Features		
Gender (male/female) n (%)	22 (25%)/67 (75%)	33 (30%)/75 (70%)
Age (years)	44.8 (41.5, 48.1)	45.8 (42.8, 48.8)
Headache history (years)*	12.9 (10.0, 15.8)	8.8 (6.9, 10.8)
Headache intensity (0-10)	5.3 (4.6, 6.0)	5.1 (4.7, 5.5)
Headache frequency (days/)*	3.7 (3.2, 4.2)	6.0 (5.5, 6.5)
Headache duration (hours per attack)*	5.7 (5.0, 6.4)	8.1 (7.3, 8.9)
FETTH/CTTH n (%)*	60 (67.5%)/29 (32.5%)	49 (45.5%)/59 (55.5%)
Preventive medication (yes/no) n (%)	24 (27%)/65 (73%)	31 (28.5%)/77 (71.5%)
Symptomatic medication (yes/no) n (%)	61 (68.5%)/28 (32.5%)	75 (69.5%)/33 (31.5%)
Psychological and disability-related outcomes		
HADS-D (0–21)	7.8 (6.8, 8.7)	7.8 (6.8, 8.8)
HADS-A (0–21)	9.6 (8.7, 10.6)	10.0 (8.9, 11.1)
HDI-P (0–48)	24.9 (22.2, 27.6)	23.1 (20.5, 25.7)
HDI-E (0–52)	19.7 (16.6, 22.9)	18.3 (15.5, 21.1)
STAI-T (0–60)*	25.8 (23.8, 27.8)	22.1 (20.7, 23.5)
STAI-S (0–60)	21.3 (19.7, 22.9)	21.8 (20.6, 23.0)

HADS Hospital Anxiety and Depression Scale (*D* Depression; *A* Anxiety), *HDI* Headache Disability Inventory (*P* Physical; *E* Emotional), *STAI* State-Trait Anxiety Inventory (*T* Trait; *S* State)
Values are expressed as means (95% confidence interval); *Significant differences between groups (ANOVA, $P < 0.01$)

(preventive drug: $\chi2 = 0.441$, $P = 0.507$; symptomatic drug: $\chi2 = 0.056$, $P = 0.813$) were found between groups.

Burden of headache and mood disorders

Patients in group 1 exhibited higher anxiety trait levels (STAI-T) than those within group 2 ($F = 7.090$; $P = 0.009$). No significant differences in the burden of headache (HDI-P: $F = 1.240$, $P = 0.297$; HDI-E: $F = 0.499$, $P = 0.481$), depression (HADS-D: $F = 0.010$, $P = 0.982$), or anxiety levels (HADS-A: $F = 1.024$, $P = 0.384$; STAI-S: $F = 0.279$, $P = 0.599$) were found (Table 1). Gender did not influence the results (HDI-E: $F = 0.438$, $P = 0.509$; HDI-P: $F = 0.144$, $P = 0.705$; HADS-D: $F = 0.489$, $P = 0.485$; HADS-A: $F = 0.013$, $P = 0.909$; STAI-S: $F = 0.038$, $P = 0.847$; STAI-T: $F = 1.899$, $P = 0.171$).

Widespread pressure pain sensitivity

The two-way ANCOVA revealed significant differences between groups, but not between sides, for PPTs over all the points: temporalis muscle (group: $F = 9.576$, $P = 0.002$; side: $F = 1.249$, $P = 0.304$), C5-C6 joint (group: $F = 12.739$, $P < 0.001$; side: $F = 0.819$, $P = 0.366$), second metacarpal (group: $F = 14.849$, $P < 0.001$; side: $F = 1.026$, $P = 0.312$), tibialis anterior muscle (group: $F = 10.626$, $P < 0.001$; side: $F = 0.346$, $P = 0.557$). No significant side * group interactions were found. Patients within group 1 exhibited bilateral lower widespread PPT than those within group 2 (Fig. 1). A significant effect of gender was also found: temporalis muscle ($F = 13.15$, $P < 0.001$), C5-C6 joint ($F = 12.46$, $P < 0.001$), second metacarpal ($F = 16.317$, $P < 0.001$), tibialis anterior muscle ($F = 11.435$, $P < 0.001$). No group * gender interaction was either observed. PPTs were significantly lower in women than in men in both groups. Table 2 summarizes PPTs in all the assessed points within each group.

Health-related quality of life

The ANCOVA revealed significant differences in all domains of the SF-36 questionnaire (physical function: $F = 6.600$, $P = 0.011$; physical role: $F = 4.428$, $P = 0.014$; bodily pain: $F = 7.654$, $P < 0.001$; general health: $F = 4.715$, $P = 0.018$; vitality: $F = 8.805$, $P < 0.001$; social function: $F = 8.076$ $P < 0.001$; role-emotional: $F = 7.099$, $P = 0.001$) except mental health ($F = 1.503$, $P = 0.195$). Patients from group 1 exhibited lower quality of life than those patients from group 2 (Table 3). No effect of gender was observed for any SF-36 domain (physical function: $F = 0.045$, $P = 0.833$; physical role: $F = 0.1704$, $P = 0.747$; bodily pain: $F = 0.108$, $P = 0.743$; general health: $F = 0.096$, $P = 1.482$; vitality: $F = 0.661$, $P = 0.417$; social function: $F = 0.890$, $P = 0.347$; role-emotional: $F = 0.652$, $P = 0.761$) mental health: $F = 0.659$, $P = 0.418$).

Discussion

The current study has identified a subgroup of patients with TTH with higher widespread pressure pain

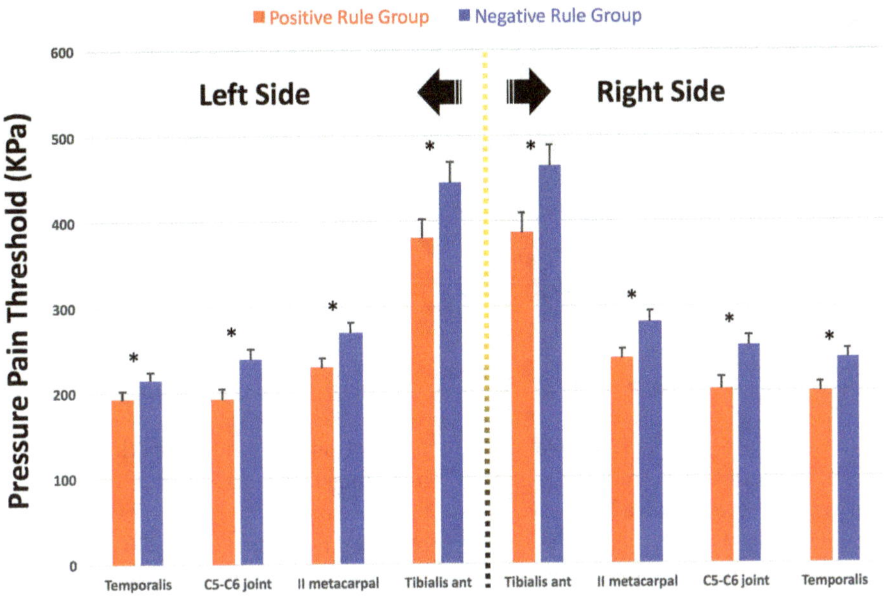

Fig. 1 Differences in widespread pressure pain thresholds (kPa) between patients positive (group 1) or negative (group 2) in the rule. Data are expressed as means and standard error (SE). * Significant differences between groups ($P < 0.01$)

hyperalgesia, longer headache history and lower health-related quality of life but lower frequency and shorter duration of headache episodes. This classification was conducted accordingly to a clinical prediction rule originally developed for identifying women with TTH who were likely to respond favorably to a manual therapy targeting muscle tissues [12].

The group of patients with TTH exhibiting higher pressure hyperalgesia and worse quality of life was identified by applying a simple classification rule [12]. This classification system could potentially help to identify patients with TTH at a higher risk for developing more severe TTH (e.g., transition from episodic to chronic). In fact, it is also possible that this subgroup of patients with higher levels of sensitization would be more susceptible for developing widespread symptoms representing the 35–44% of sufferers with TTH presenting co-morbid fibromyalgia syndrome [27]. This hypothesis would be also supported by the worse health-related quality of life experienced by this subgroup of patients albeit they exhibited lower frequency and shorter duration of headache episodes since patients with TTH and co-morbid widespread symptoms experience worse health-related quality of life [28]. This maybe particularly relevant for the lower scores in one of the domains of the rule, bodily pain, which represents the experience of body pain symptoms by the patient. Nevertheless, the presence of higher sensitization in patients with lower frequency of headaches is contrary to what is observed in patients with migraine and co-morbid fibromyalgia syndrome since a higher frequency of migraine attacks enhances both hyperalgesia and widespread pain symptoms [29]. We do not currently know if the presence of widespread hypersensitivity appears before or after the increase of the frequency of headaches, or both processes are interconnected and therefore one promotes the other.

The presence of higher widespread pain sensitization may suggest different underlying mechanisms in this

Table 2 Differences in pressure pain thresholds (PPT, kPa) between individuals with tension-type headache by group

	Temporalis muscle*	C5-C6 zygapophyseal joint*	Second metacarpal*	Tibialis anterior muscle*
Group 1 (Rule positive, $n = 89$)				
Right side	200.0 (179.6, 220.3)	220.4 (174.5, 230.2)	238.7 (216.6, 261.0)	386.0 (341.2, 430.9)
Left side	192.0 (171.6, 212.3)	192.4 (164.6, 220.2)	229.2 (207.1, 251.5)	379.7 (334.9, 424.6)
Group 2 (Rule negative, $n = 108$)				
Right side	238.7 (220.1, 257.4)	253.0 (227.6, 278.5)	281.8 (261.6, 302.0)	464.1 (423.0, 505.2)
Left side	214.5 (195.8, 233.1)	238.5 (213.0, 263.9)	269.4 (248.9, 289.8)	444.6 (403.1, 486.1)

Values are expressed as means (95% confidence interval)

*Significant differences between both groups (2-two way ANOVA test, $P < 0.001$)

Table 3 Differences in health-related quality of life in individuals with tension-type headache by group

	Group 1 (Rule positive, $n = 89$)	Group 2 (Rule negative, $n = 108$)
Physical Function (0–100)*	72.9 (67.6, 78.2)	83.7 (79.4, 87.8)
Physical Role (0–100)*	44.9 (36.7, 53.1)	58.7 (51.0, 66.4)
Bodily pain (0–100)*	39.4 (35.6, 43.2)	61.1 (57.0, 65.2)
General Health (0–100)*	52.9 (48.2, 57.6)	60.3 (56.3, 64.3)
Vitality (0–100)*	40.8 (37.1, 44.6)	59.1 (54.7, 63.5)
Social Function (0–100)*	58.0 (53.0, 63.0)	72.3 (68.5, 78.0)
Role Emotional (0–100)*	52.3 (43.4, 61.2)	51.1 (63.8, 78.3)
Mental Health (0–100)	55.4 (50.9, 59.9)	59.7 (55.5, 64.0)

Values are expressed as means (95% confidence interval)
*Significant differences between groups (ANOVA, $P < 0.02$)

group of patients. It is accepted that prolonged nociception from peripheral tissues, i.e., muscles, is the main responsible for triggering centralized sensitization mechanisms and the evolution from the episodic to the chronic form [6, 30]. In the chronification process, the frequency of the headache episodes is found to play an important role [31]. However, our study found that the subgroup of patients exhibiting higher widespread pressure pain hypersensitivity reported lower frequency of headaches. This is supported by the fact that there was a greater distribution of patients with FETTH within group 1. Other possibility is that higher chronicity (history with pain symptoms) of headache can also explain higher sensitization levels [32]. We also observed that the group of patients with TTH with higher sensitization levels also exhibited a longer history of headache, supporting this hypothesis. This finding would suggest that, not only the frequency of headaches as previously reported, but also the chronicity of symptoms, may be also relevant for the development of central sensitization. Therefore, early therapeutic interventions for preventing development of central sensitization should be encouraged in this subgroup. An interesting finding was that the identified subgroup of patients with TTH with higher levels of sensitization also exhibited higher trait anxiety. Since stress is one of the most common trigger and aggravating factors of TTH [33, 34], it is possible that this subgroup of subjects would be more susceptible to stressful situations and therefore promoting development of central sensitization. Therefore, psychological approaches targeting anxiety trait levels should be also implemented in this subgroup of patients. Finally, it is also possible that this subgroup of patients with TTH exhibits different neurotransmitter concentrations or differences in brainstem processing [35] explaining the altered nociceptive processing; although this hypothesis should be investigated in future studies.

Although this is the first study investigating a classification system in patients with TTH, we should recognize some potential limitations. First, we recruited our patients from tertiary care hospitals; therefore, multi-center studies including individuals from the general population would help to extrapolate the results. Second, we only tested the response to pressure stimulation as it has been previously found that pressure pain sensitivity is a clear feature of TTH [6, 7]. It would be interesting to investigate other outcomes of central sensitization, e.g., thermal pain thresholds, conditioning pain modulation (CPM) or nociception flexor reflex (NFR) in these subgroups of patients with TTH.

Conclusions

Patients with TTH who meet a clinical prediction for group 1 (at least 3 of the criteria) tended to exhibit higher widespread pressure hyperalgesia, longer headache history, higher trait anxiety levels, and worse quality of life but lower frequency and shorter duration of headache episodes than those within group 2 (met two or fewer criteria).

Abbreviations

ANOVA: Analysis of variance; CI: Confidence interval; CTT: Chronic tension type headache; FETTH: Frequent episodic tension type headache; HADS: Hospital Anxiety and Depression Scale; HDI: Headache Disability Inventory; ICHD3: International Classification of Headache Disorders, third edition; NPRS: Numerical pain rate scale; PPT: Pressure pain thresholds; SF-36: Short-Form Health Survey 36; STAI: State-Trait Anxiety Inventory; TTH: Tension-type headache

Authors' contributions

All authors contributed to the study concept and design. CFdlP and EBG did the statistical analysis. MPC, KW and MC contributed to analysis and interpretation of data. CFdlP and LAN contributed to drafting the paper. LAN obtained funding, provided administrative, technical, and material support. KW, MC and LAN supervised the study. All authors revised the text for intellectual content and have read and approved the final version of the manuscript.

Competing interests

The authors declare that they have no competing interests.

Disclosures

Financial disclosure statements have been obtained. No conflicts of interest have been reported by the authors or by any individuals in control of the content of this article.

Author details

[1]Department of Physical Therapy, Occupational Therapy, Physical Medicine and Rehabilitation, Universidad Rey Juan Carlos, Alcorcón, Spain. [2]Center for Sensory-Motor Interaction (SMI), Department of Health Science and Technology, Faculty of Medicine, Aalborg University, Aalborg, Denmark. [3]Department of Physical Therapy, University of Siena, Siena, Italy. [4]Poliambulatorio Fisiocenter, Collecchio, Parma, Italy. [5]Facultad de Ciencias de la Salud, Universidad Rey Juan Carlos, Avenida de Atenas s/n, 28922 Alcorcón, Madrid, Spain.

References

1. Ferrante T, Manzoni GC, Russo M, Camarda C, Taga A, Veronesi L, Pasquarella C, Sansebastiano G, Torelli P (2013) Prevalence of tension-type headache in adult general population: the PACE study and review of the literature. Neurol Sci 34:S137–8
2. Raggi A, Leonardi M (2015) Burden and cost of neurological diseases: a European North-South comparison. Acta Neurol Scand 132:16–22
3. Global Burden of Disease Study 2013 Collaborators (2015) Global, regional, and national incidence, prevalence, and years lived with disability for 301 acute and chronic diseases and injuries in 188 countries, 1990-2013: a systematic analysis for the Global Burden of Disease Study 2013. Lancet 386:743–800
4. Yu S, Han X (2015) Update of chronic tension-type headache. Curr Pain Headache Rep 19:469
5. Bezov D, Ashina S, Jensen R, Bendtsen L (2011) Pain perception studies in tension-type headache. Headache 51:262–71
6. de Tommaso M, Fernández-de-las-Peñas C (2016) Tension type headache. Curr Rheumatol Rev 12:127–39
7. Andersen S, Petersen MW, Svendsen AS, Gazerani P (2015) Pressure pain thresholds assessed over temporalis, masseter, and frontalis muscles in healthy individuals, patients with tension-type headache, and those with migraine: a systematic review. Pain 156:1409–23
8. Ashina S, Bendtsen L, Ashina M, Magerl W, Jensen R (2006) Generalized hyperalgesia in patients with chronic tension type headache. Cephalalgia 26:940–8
9. Palacios-Ceña M, Castaldo M, Wang K, Torelli P, Pillastrini P, Fernández-de-las-Peñas C, Arendt-Nielsen L (2017) Widespread pressure pain hypersensitivity is similar in women with frequent episodic and chronic tension-type headache: a blinded case-control study. Headache 57:217–225
10. Arendt-Nielsen L, Egsgaard LL, Petersen KK, Eskehave TN, Graven-Nielsen T, Hoeck HC, Simonsen O (2015) A mechanism-based pain sensitivity index to characterize knee osteoarthritis patients with differentdisease stages and pain levels. Eur J Pain 19:1406–17
11. Pedler A, Sterling M (2013) Patients with chronic whiplash can be subgrouped on the basis of symptoms of sensory hypersensitivity and posttraumatic stress. Pain 154:1640–8
12. Fernández-de-las-Peñas C, Cleland JA, Cuadrado ML, Pareja JA (2008) Predictor variables for identifying patients with chronic tension type headache who are likely to achieve short-term success with muscle trigger point therapy. Cephalalgia 28:264–75
13. Fernández-de-las-Peñas C, Fernández-Muñoz JJ, Navarro-Pardo E, Da-Silva-Pocinho RF, Ambite-Quesada S, Pareja J (2016) Identification of subgroups of women with carpal tunnel syndrome with central sensitization. Pain Med 17:1749–1756
14. ICHD-III International Classification of Headache Disorders (2013) Headache classification subcommittee of the International Headache Society, 3nd edition. Cephalalgia 33:629–808
15. Phillip D, Lyngberg AC, Jensen R (2007) Assessment of headache diagnosis: a comparative population study of a clinical interview with a diagnostic headache diary. Cephalalgia 27:1–8
16. Jensen MP, Turner JA, Romano JM, Fisher L (1999) Comparative reliability and validity of chronic pain intensity measures. Pain 83:157–162
17. Nie H, Arendt-Nielsen L, Andersen H, Graven-Nielsen T (2005) Temporal summation of pain evoked by mechanical stimulation in deep and superficial tissue. J Pain 6:348–355
18. Walton DM, Macdermid JC, Nielson W, Teasell RW, Chiasson M, Brown L (2011) Reliability, standard error, and minimum detectable change of clinical pressure pain threshold testing in people with and without acute neck pain. J Orthop Sports Phys Ther 41:644–50
19. Chesterson LS, Sim J, Wright CC, Foster NE (2007) Inter-rater reliability of algometry in measuring pressure pain thresholds in healthy humans, using multiple raters. Clin J Pain 23:760–6
20. Jacobson GP, Ramadan NM, Norris L, Newman CW (1994) The Henry Ford Hospital headache disability inventory. Neurology 44:837–42
21. Jacobson GP, Ramadan NM, Norris L, Newman CW (1995) Headache disability inventory (HDI): short-term test-retest reliability and spouse perceptions. Headache 35:534–9
22. Spielberger CD (1983) Manual for the State-Trait Anxiety Inventory STAI (Form Y). Mind Garden, Palo Alto, CA
23. Spielberger CD (1989) State-Trait Anxiety Inventory: a comprehensive bibliography. Consulting Psychologists Press, Palo Alto, CA
24. Barnes LLB, Harp D, Jung WS (2002) Reliability generalization of scores on the Spielberger State-Trait Anxiety Inventory. Educ Psychol Meas 62:603–618
25. Ware JE Jr, Sherbourne CD (1992) The MOS 36-item short-form health survey (SF-36). I. Conceptual framework and item selection. Med Care 30:473–483
26. Ware JE, Snow KK, Kosinski M, Gandek B (1993) SF-36 Health Survey: manual and interpretation guide. New England Medical Center, The Health Institute, Boston, MA
27. de Tommaso M, Sardaro M, Serpino C, Costantini F, Vecchio E, Prudenzano MP, Lamberti P, Livrea P (2009) Fibromyalgia comorbidity in primary headaches. Cephalalgia 29:453–64
28. de Tommaso M, Federici A, Serpino C, Vecchio E, Franco G, Sardaro M, Delussi M, Livrea P (2011) Clinical features of headache patients with fibromyalgia comorbidity. J Headache Pain 12:629–38
29. Giamberardino MA, Affaitati G, Martelletti P, Tana C, Negro A, Lapenna D, Curto M, Schiavone C, Stellin L, Cipollone F, Costantini R (2015) Impact of migraine on fibromyalgia symptoms. J Headache Pain 17:28
30. Bendtsen L, Ashina S, Moore A, Steiner TJ (2016) Muscles and their role in episodic tension-type headache: implications for treatment. Eur J Pain 20:166–75
31. Buchgreitz L, Lyngberg AC, Bendtsen L, Jensen R (2006) Frequency of headache is related to sensitization: a population study. Pain 123:19–27
32. Woolf CJ (2011) Central sensitization: implications for the diagnosis and treatment of pain. Pain 152:S2–15
33. Cathcart S, Petkov J, Winefield AH, Lushington K, Rolan P (2010) Central mechanisms of stress-induced headache. Cephalalgia 30:285–95
34. Cathcart S, Winefield A, Lushington K, Rolan P (2010) Stress and tension-type headache mechanisms. Cephalalgia 30:1250–67
35. Wang P, Du H, Chen N, Guo J, Gong Q, Zhang J, He L (2014) Regional homogeneity abnormalities in patients with tension-type headache: a resting-state fMRI study. Neurosci Bull 30:949–55

14

Restless legs syndrome and tension-type headache

Pil-Wook Chung[1], Soo-Jin Cho[2], Won-Joo Kim[3], Kwang Ik Yang[4], Chang-Ho Yun[5] and Min Kyung Chu[6*]

Abstract

Background: Recent studies have shown a significant association between restless legs syndrome (RLS) and primary headache disorders. Nevertheless, information regarding the association between tension-type headache (TTH) and RLS is limited. This study aimed to investigate the association between RLS and TTH in a population-based sample.

Methods: We selected a stratified random population sample of Koreans aged 19–69 years and assessed them using a semi-structured interview designed to identify RLS, headache type, and clinical characteristics of TTH. We determined the prevalence and clinical impact of RLS in participants with TTH.

Results: Of the 2695 participants, 570 (21.2%) and 142 (5.3%) were classified as having TTH and RLS, respectively. Among the 570 individuals with TTH, 113 (19.8%) also met the criteria for probable migraine (PM). The prevalence of RLS was significantly higher among individuals with TTH than among those with non-headache (6.0% vs 3.6%, $p = 0.018$). The prevalence of RLS was significantly higher in subjects with TTH who fulfilled PM criteria than in those with non-headache participants (8.0% vs. 3.6%, $p = 0.018$). However, RLS prevalence in individuals with TTH who did not fulfil PM criteria did not differ from that of participants with non-headache (5.5% vs. 3.6%, $p = 0.063$). TTH participants with RLS had higher visual analogue scale scores for headache intensity (5.1 ± 2.0 vs. 4.3 ± 1.8, $p = 0.038$), and higher prevalence of anxiety (20.6% vs. 8.8%, $p = 0.022$) and depression (14.7% vs. 3.5%, $p = 0.002$) than TTH participants without RLS. Multivariable analyses revealed that headache aggravation by movement (odds ratio [OR] = 2.4, 95% confidence interval [CI] = 1.1–5.2) and depression (OR = 3.5, 95% CI = 1.1–11.4) were significant indicators of RLS among individuals with TTH.

Conclusions: The prevalence of RLS was higher among individuals with TTH than among those with non-headache. Some clinical presentations varied in accordance with the presence of RLS among participants with TTH.

Keywords: Restless legs syndrome, Tension-type headache, Anxiety, Depression

Background

Tension-type headache (TTH) is the most common type of primary headache disorder and is the third most common disease in the world [1]. TTH has been considered a non-serious disorder compared to migraine. However, it is a major health problem and leads to a severe socioeconomic burden owing to its high prevalence and comorbidities such as anxiety, depression, temporo-mandibular disorders, fibromyalgia, and obstructive sleep apnoea [2–6]. Patients with TTH with comorbidities have more severe symptoms than those without comorbidities [2]. Therefore, identification of the associated comorbidities of TTH is important for better management of TTH and may reduce the burden of the disease.

Restless legs syndrome (RLS) is a sleep-related sensory-motor disorder characterized by unpleasant feelings in the legs, especially during rest or at bedtime. The unpleasant feelings are relieved by voluntary leg movement [7]. Previous population-based and clinic-based studies have consistently reported a significant association between RLS and migraine [8–14].

The mechanism for the association between migraine and RLS is still uncertain. Dopamine and iron

* Correspondence: chumk@hallym.ac.kr
[6]Department of Neurology, Kangnam Sacred Heart Hospital, Hallym University College of Medicine, 1 Singil-ro, Yeongdeungpo-gu, Seoul 07441, Republic of Korea

dysregulation have been proposed to be mechanism both for migraine and RLS [7, 15–17]. Therefore, they were considered as mechanisms for the comorbidity of two disorders. Furthermore, genetic associations between RLS and migraine have been suggested [18]. Although numerous reports have suggested a close association between migraine and RLS, population-based information regarding the association between RLS and TTH, which is the most common type of headache, is limited. Nevertheless, a few studies have suggested the presence of significant associations between RLS and TTH. A population-based report indicates that RLS has a significant association with non-migraine headache [14]. A health-insurance database study in Taiwan revealed that individuals with TTH have an increased risk for developing RLS [19].

We hypothesized that RLS and TTH would have a significant association in a general population-based sample. The Korean Headache-Sleep Study (KHSS) is a cross-sectional nationwide population-based survey on sleep and headache in Korean adults aged 19–69 years and may provide an opportunity for us to assess the association between RLS and TTH. Therefore, we estimated the prevalence of TTH and RLS in a Korean general population-based sample, compared the association between TTH and RLS in comparison with individuals with non-headache, and assessed the clinical impact of RLS in individuals with TTH using data from the KHSS.

Methods

Survey

The KHSS, used in this study, was approved by the institutional review board and ethics committee of Hallym University Sacred Heart Hospital and written informed consent was obtained from all participants. Details of the KHSS have previously been described [14, 20]. Briefly, we used a 2-stage clustered random sampling method to obtain a sample proportional to the population distribution of Korea, with the exception of Jeju Island. Participants were stratified by age, sex, and occupation. We informed candidates that the survey topic was general health rather than headache and sleep to avoid interest bias. All interviewers were employees of Gallup Korea. The survey was conducted between November 2011 and January 2012 via personal visits and interviews, using a questionnaire that was designed to identify headache type, anxiety, depression, and RLS.

Diagnosis of TTH

Diagnosis of TTH was based on the criteria for infrequent TTH (code 2.1) of the third edition beta version of the International Classification of Headache Disorders (ICDH-3 beta) [21]. Participants were considered to have TTH if they met criteria B through E (B: lasting from 30 min to 7 days; C: at least two of the four typical headache characteristics [i.e. bilateral pain, non-pulsating quality, mild-to-moderate pain intensity, and no aggravation by routine physical activity]; D: attacks associated with both of the following: no nausea or vomiting, not having both photophobia and phonophobia, and E: not better accounted for by another ICHD-3 diagnosis). The questionnaire used in the present study had 75.0% sensitivity and 88.2% specificity when compared to physicians' diagnoses [22]. We did not apply the frequency criterion (criterion A) in the diagnosis of TTH. Thus, patients with TTH evaluated in this study included those with infrequent TTH (code 2.1), frequent TTH (code 2.2), and chronic TTH (code 2.3). According to ICHD-3 beta, if a participant's headache met the criteria for both TTH and probable migraine (PM), he or she was considered to have TTH [21].

Diagnosis of RLS

Diagnosis of RLS was based on the Korean version paradigm of questions for the epidemiology studies of RLS [7, 23]. The paradigm for question for the epidemiology studies for RLS was based on the International Restless Legs Syndrome Study Group criteria published in 2003 [7]. The Korean version paradigm of question for the epidemiology studies of RLS was composed of 3 questions: (1) 'Do you have unpleasant sensations in your legs combined with an urge or need to move your legs?' (2) 'Do these feelings occur mainly or only at rest and do they improve with movement?' (3) 'Are these feelings worse in the evening or night than in the morning?'. The Korean version paradigm of question for the epidemiology studies for RLS was validated with 85.3% sensitivity and 89.5% specificity by comparing doctors' diagnosis of RLS [23].

Assessment of anxiety and depression

Anxiety was measured using the Goldberg Anxiety Scale (GAS) [24]. The Korean version of GAS has 82.0% sensitivity and 94.4% specificity for the diagnosis of anxiety and has previously been validated [25]. To diagnose depression, the Patient Health Questionnaire-9 was used [26]. Participants with scores of 10 or higher on this measure were considered to have depression. The Korean version of the Patient Health Questionnaire-9 has 81.1% sensitivity and 89.9% specificity [27]. To assess headache intensity and the impact of the headache, we used the Visual Analogue Scale (VAS) and the Headache Impact Test-6, respectively.

Statistical Analyses

The Kolmogorov-Smirnov test was used to confirm the normality of the distributions. Following confirmation of a normal distribution, we used Student's t-tests or Analysis of Variance to compare continuous variables. In cases of non-normal distribution, we used Mann–Whitney U tests or Kruskal-Wallis tests. Categorical variables were compared using Chi-square tests.

We investigated factors contributing to RLS among individuals with TTH using univariable and multivariable analyses. To perform univariable analyses, we considered factors with significant differences between TTH participants with RLS and those without RLS. To perform multivariable analyses, we developed 4 models for the association between RLS and TTH. Model 1 included sociodemographic variables (age, sex, size of residential area, and education level) and headache aggravation by movement. Model 2 added anxiety as a variable to Model 1. In Model 3, we added depression to Model 1. The final model, Model 4, incorporated sociodemographic variables, aggravation by movement, and anxiety and depression. A significance level of $p < 0.05$ was used for all analyses. Analyses were conducted using the Statistical Package for the Social Sciences 22.0 (SPSS 22.0; IBM, Armonk, NY).

Similar to most survey sampling designs, there were missing data (resulting from non-response) for several variables. All of the reported results are based on the available data. As such, the total numbers for some variables diverge from 2695 because of missing data for that particular variable. Imputation techniques were not used because we wanted to minimize non-response effects [28].

Results

Survey

Interviewers approached 7430 individuals. Of the 7430 individuals, 3114 agreed to participate in this survey (rejection rate, 58.1%). Of these participants, 2695 completed the survey (cooperation rate, 36.3%; Fig. 1). Distributions of age, sex, size of residential area, and education level were not significantly different between our survey participants and the general population of Korea (Additional file 1: Table S1).

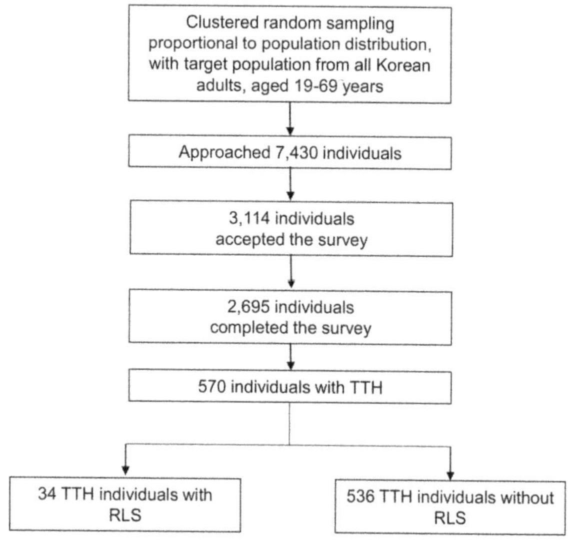

Fig. 1 Flowchart depicting the participation of subjects in the Korean Headache-Sleep Study. *RLS*, restless legs syndrome; *TTH*, tension-type headache

Prevalence of TTH and RLS

Of the 2695 participants, 570 (21.2%) were considered to have TTH and 1422 (52.8%) were classified as non-headache participants. Of the 570 participants who were classified as TTH, 14 participants (2.5%) were classified as chronic TTH (code 2.3), 229 (40.2%) as infrequent episodic TTH (code 2.1), and 327(57.3%) as frequent episodic TTH (code 2.2). Among the individuals with TTH, 113 (19.8%) also met the criteria for PM. The prevalence of TTH was not significantly affected by age, sex, or educational level. The prevalence of TTH was higher in rural areas compared to large cities and small-to-medium cities (Table 1). One hundred and forty-two (5.3%) participants were classified as having RLS. Restless legs syndrome was more prevalent in women and participants with lower educational level (middle school or less) than among men and those with higher educational level. The prevalence of RLS had a trend toward an increase with increasing age (Additional file 1: Table S1). Sociodemographic characteristics of individuals with TTH and non-headache are summarized in Table 1. Women and participants living in rural areas were more common among individuals with TTH than among those with non-headache. However, distributions of age and educational level were not significantly different between the two groups.

Prevalence of anxiety and depression

Two-hundred and sixty-eight (9.9%) and 116 (4.3%) participants were classified as having anxiety and depression, respectively. The prevalence of anxiety (9.5% vs. 5.3%, $p = 0.001$) and depression (4.2% vs. 1.8%, $p = 0.001$) were significantly higher among individuals with TTH than among those with non-headache.

Prevalence of RLS in participants with TTH

Among the 570 individuals with TTH, 34 (6.0%) were classified as having RLS. The prevalence of RLS was significantly higher among individuals with TTH than among individuals with non-headache (6.0% vs 3.6%, $p = 0.018$). Among the 113 participants with TTH who fulfilled PM criteria, 9 participants (8.0%) were classified as having RLS. The prevalence of RLS among participants with TTH who also fulfilled PM

Table 1 Sociodemographic characteristics and RLS status in participants with TTH and participants with non-headache

	All participants, N	Participants with TTH, N (%)	Participants with non-headache, N (%)	P^a
Sex				<0.001
Male	1345	268 (19.9)	838 (62.3)	
Female	1350	302 (22.3)	584 (43.3)	
Age				0.405
19–29	542	119 (22.0)	286 (52.8)	
30–39	604	127 (21.0)	293 (48.5)	
40–49	611	131 (21.4)	295 (48.3)	
50–59	529	107 (20.2)	303 (57.3)	
60–69	409	86 (21.0)	245 (59.9)	
Size of the residential area				0.009
Large city	1248	251 (20.1)	647 (51.8)	
Small-to-medium city	1186	243 (20.5)	650 (54.8)	
Rural area	261	76 (29.1)	125 (47.9)	
Education level				0.345
Middle school or lower	393	96 (24.5)	208 (52.4)	
High school	1208	247 (20.5)	646 (53.5)	
College or higher	1068	223 (20.9)	551 (51.6)	
No response	26	4 (15.4)	19 (73.1)	
RLS	142	34 (6.0)	51 (3.6)	0.018

[a]Comparison between participants with tension-type headache and those without headache. *TTH* Tension-type headache, *RLS* Restless legs syndrome

criteria was not significantly different from that among those with TTH not fulfilling PM criteria (8.0% vs. 5.5%, $p = 0.318$). The prevalence of RLS in participants with TTH not fulfilling PM criteria did not differ from that of individuals with non-headache (5.5% vs. 3.6%, $p = 0.063$). Nevertheless, the prevalence of RLS among individuals with TTH fulfilling PM criteria was significantly higher than that among those with non-headache (8.0% vs. 3.6%, $p = 0.018$; Fig. 2). Prevalence of RLS was analysed according to headache frequency. Prevalence of RLS in participants with TTH with 1-10 attacks per month (5.9%, $p = 0.861$) and participants with TTH with >10 attacks per month (13.6%, $p = 0.116$) was numerically higher compared to that of those with <1 attack per month (5.5%). However, it did not reach statistical significance.

We also investigated the prevalence of RLS in individuals with TTH grouped on the basis of anxiety and depression status (Table 2). The prevalence of RLS was significantly higher among TTH participants with anxiety than among those without anxiety (13.0% vs. 5.2%, $p = 0.022$). The prevalence of RLS was significantly higher among TTH subjects with depression than among those without depression (20.8% vs. 5.3%, $p = 0.002$).

Demographics and clinical presentations of participants with TTH according to RLS status

The demographics and clinical presentations of participants with TTH according to the presence of RLS are summarized in Table 2. Demographic variables, headache characteristics (except for non-aggravation by

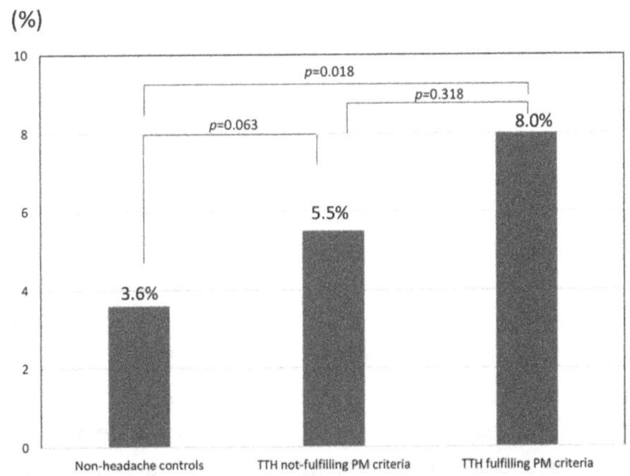

Fig. 2 Prevalence of RLS among individuals with non-headache, those with TTH fulfilling PM criteria, and those with TTH not fulfilling PM criteria. *PM*, probable migraine; *RLS*, restless legs syndrome; *TTH*, tension-type headache

Table 2 Demographics, headache characteristics, and associated symptoms in subjects with TTH according to the presence of RLS

	TTH subjects with RLS N = 34	TTH subjects without RLS N = 536	P
Demographics			
Mean age ± SD (years)	46.4 ± 13.3	42.5 ± 13.7	0.108
Women, N (%)	20 (58.8)	282 (52.6)	0.482
Headache characteristics			
Bilateral pain, N (%)	23 (67.6)	351 (65.5)	0.797
Non-pulsating quality, N (%)	16 (47.1)	211 (39.4)	0.374
Mild-to-moderate severity, N (%)	34 (100.0)	526 (98.1)	0.422
Non-aggravation by movement, N (%)	22 (64.7)	429 (80.0)	0.033
Associated symptoms			
Photophobia, N (%)	5 (14.7)	41 (7.6)	0.143
Phonophobia, N (%)	9 (26.5)	172 (32.1)	0.495
Osmophobia, N (%)	7 (20.6)	88 (16.4)	0.527
Mood			
Anxiety	7 (20.6)	47 (8.8)	0.022
Depression	5 (14.7)	19 (3.5)	0.002
Headache frequency per month	2.3 ± 3.5	1.9 ± 4.9	0.054
VAS score for headache intensity	5.1 ± 2.0	4.3 ± 1.8	0.038

RLS Restless legs syndrome, *TTH* Tension-type headache, *VAS* Visual Analogue Scale

movement), and accompanying symptoms were not significantly different between TTH subjects with RLS and those without RLS. Visual Analogue Scale scores for headache intensity were significantly higher among TTH subjects with RLS than among those without RLS. Headache frequency was marginally different between the two groups, although this difference was not significant. The prevalence of anxiety and depression were significantly higher among participants with TTH with RLS than in those without RLS.

Factors contributing to RLS among participant with TTH

Univariate analyses revealed that headache aggravation by movement (odds ratio [OR] = 2.2, 95% confidence interval [CI] = 1.1–4.6), anxiety (OR = 2.7, 95% CI = 1.2–6.5), and depression (OR = 4.7, 95% CI = 1.6–13.5) are associated with an increased risk for RLS. Multivariable analyses including sociodemographic variables and aggravation by movement (Model 1) indicated that aggravation by movement leads to an increased OR for RLS (OR = 2.3, 95% CI = 1.1–4.8). In Model 2 (including sociodemographic variables, aggravation by movement, and anxiety), aggravation by movement (OR = 2.3, 95% CI = 1.1–4.9) and anxiety (OR = 3.4, 95% CI = 1.3–8.8) had significant effects on RLS status. In Model 3 (including sociodemographic variables, aggravation by movement, and depression), aggravation by movement (OR = 2.4, 95% CI = 1.1–5.2) and depression (OR = 4.9, 95% CI = 1.6–15.0) led to increased ORs for RLS. Model 4 (including sociodemographic variables, aggravation by movement, anxiety, and depression) revealed that aggravation by movement (OR = 2.4, 95% CI = 1.1–5.2) and depression (OR = 3.5, 95% CI = 1.1–11.4) have significant effects on RLS status (Table 3).

Discussion

The main findings of the present study are as follows: 1) The prevalence of TTH and RLS are 21.1% and 5.3%, respectively, in the Korean general population sample used; 2) The prevalence of RLS among subjects with TTH was significantly higher than among participants with non-headache; and 3) TTH participants with RLS had more severe headache intensity and higher prevalence of anxiety and depression than those without RLS.

While a significant association between RLS and migraine has been consistently reported, information regarding the association between RLS and TTH, which is another common primary headache, is limited. Recently, a retrospective cohort study using a health insurance database suggested that patients with TTH had an increased risk of developing RLS [19]. Nevertheless, the study did not provide cross-sectional evidence for an association between RLS and TTH, identified TTH and RLS cases on the basis of diagnostic codes rather than diagnostic criteria and did not assess the impact of RLS on the clinical presentation of TTH. Here, we identified RLS and TTH cases on the basis of validated criteria and found that RLS was more prevalent among individuals with TTH than among those with non-headache in a general population-based sample. In addition, we found that participants with TTH with RLS had more severe headache intensity than those with TTH without RLS.

In the present study, TTH individuals with anxiety and depression had higher RLS prevalence than those without anxiety and depression. Multivariable regression analyses revealed that depression is an independent predictor of RLS. These findings are concurrent with those of previous studies of the association between RLS and mood symptoms. Individuals with anxiety or depression have been shown to have a higher risk of RLS and vice versa [29–31]. Anxiety and depression are also common comorbid conditions of TTH [3]. Therefore, it is plausible that mood symptoms, such as anxiety and depression, are important factors linking RLS to TTH. Further studies are required among TTH subjects regarding

Table 3 Univariate and multivariable logistic regression analyses of RLS among individuals with tension-type headache ($N = 570$)

	Univariable analyses	Multivariable analyses			
		Model 1[a]	Model 2[b]	Model 3[c]	Model 4[d]
	OR (95% CI)	OR (95% CI)	OR (95% CI)	OR (95% CI)	OR (95% CI)
Aggravation by movement	2.2 (1.1–4.6)	2.3 (1.1–4.8)	2.3 (1.1–4.9)	2.4 (1.1–5.2)	2.4 (1.1–5.2)
Anxiety	2.7 (1.2–6.5)		3.4 (1.3–8.8)		2.6 (0.9–7.0)
Depression	4.7 (1.6–13.5)			4.9 (1.6–15.0)	3.5 (1.1–11.4)

OR odds ratio, *CI* confidence interval
[a]Including sociodemographic variables (age, sex, size of residential area, and educational level) and aggravation by movement
[b]Including sociodemographic variables, aggravation by movement, and anxiety
[c]Including sociodemographic variables, aggravation by movement, and depression
[d]Including sociodemographic variables, aggravation by movement, anxiety, and depression

mood symptoms and RLS to elucidate the associations among RLS, mood symptoms, and TTH.

We classified 113 participants fulfilling both TTH and PM criteria as subjects with TTH in accordance with the general rule of ICHD-3 beta. Although RLS prevalence in participants with TTH fulfilling PM criteria did not significantly differ from that in those with TTH not fulfilling PM criteria, RLS prevalence in participants with TTH fulfilling PM criteria was significantly higher than in those with non-headache. However, RLS prevalence among participants with TTH not fulfilling PM criteria was not different from that in participants with non-headache (Fig. 2). Among migrainous features, aggravation by movement was more frequently found in TTH participants with RLS than in those without RLS (Table 2). Univariable and multivariable analyses indicated that headache aggravation by movement is an independent predictor of RLS among participants with TTH (Table 3). These findings were concurrent with previous findings that the frequency of RLS may increase with an increase in the number of migrainous symptoms among migraineurs [8]. However, other migrainous features, such as unilateral pain, pulsating quality, moderate-to-severe headache intensity, photophobia, and phonophobia were not significantly different between individuals with and those without RLS in the present study. Further studies including various headache populations will validate the association between migrainous features and RLS among headache sufferers.

The 1-year TTH prevalence rate (21.2%) in the present study was somewhat lower than that previously observed in Western countries (20–78%) [32]. The 1-year prevalence of TTH in Asian countries ranges from 10.3 to 33.3% in most studies of Asian populations, which is somewhat lower than those reported in studies of European and North American countries [32, 33]. RLS prevalence (5.3%) in the present study was similar to those reported in previous studies from Korea and other Asian countries, which range from 1.8 to 8.3%. Similar to TTH, the reported RLS prevalence in Asian populations is lower than that observed in Western countries [5, 23, 30, 34]. Therefore, the prevalence of RLS and TTH in the present study is similar to the reported prevalence in Asian countries. The similarities between the prevalence of RLS and TTH in the present study and in previous reports from Asian countries suggest that our study properly evaluated RLS and TTH.

Restless leg syndrome has long been considered to be caused by dopaminergic system dysfunction and disturbed iron metabolism [16, 35]. Unbalanced level of dopaminergic neurotransmitter might also be involved in migraine pathogenesis and dysfunctional iron metabolism in the brain of migraine has been suggested [15, 17, 18]. Therefore, it is plausible that some underlying migraine characteristics may be a substrate for linking TTH and RLS in consideration of more strong association between TTH fulfilling PM criteria and RLS than between TTH not fulfilling PM criteria and RLS in the present study.

In the present study, depression was significant contributing factor for RLS among individuals with TTH in univariable and multivariable analyses. Association of depression and RLS has been documented in population-based studies [34, 36]. Dopaminergic dysfunction was noted in depression [37]. It also has been considered as a key mechanism of RLS as mentioned above [35]. Dopaminergic dysregulation in TTH has been proposed in previous studies [38, 39]. Accordingly, dopaminergic dysfunction could be a mechanism for connecting depression and RLS among individuals with TTH. Further experimental and clinical studies were needed for the association of depression, RLS and TTH.

There are several limitations to the present study. Firstly, we diagnosed RLS by using the Korean version paradigm of questions for the epidemiology studies of RLS based on participant's report [23]. Therefore, some conditions similar to RLS may have been included. Akathisia, meralgia paresthetica, peripheral neuropathy, and nocturnal cramping can mimic RLS. Nevertheless, the Korean version paradigm of questions for the epidemiology studies of RLS showed high sensitivity and specificity for the diagnosis of RLS when comparing doctors' diagnosis of RLS [7, 23]. Secondly, we did not assess the severity of RLS owing to limitations on questionnaire length. An attempt to quantitatively correlate RLS and headache may add more insight to the association between TTH and RLS. Thirdly, although the current study used a population-based sample with low sampling error, its statistical power was limited in terms of examining the subgroups of interest. In other words, the lack of significant findings in the subgroup analyses might be the result of the limited sample size.

Our study has several strengths. Firstly, we used the data of KHSS which was based on clustered random sampling proportional to the Korean population distribution with low sampling error. This condition allowed us to precisely investigate the association between RLS and TTH in a population-base setting. Secondly, we investigated anxiety and depression, which are common comorbidities among individuals of RLS and assessed the effect of anxiety and depression in the association between RLS and TTH. Thirdly, we assessed the prevalence of RLS among individuals with TTH according to migrainous features.

Conclusions

In conclusion, the prevalence of RLS among individuals with TTH was significantly higher than that among those with non-headache in a population-based sample in Korea. TTH participants with RLS had higher VAS scores for headache intensity than those without RLS. Headache aggravation by movement and depression were significant indicators of the presence of RLS among individuals with TTH. Our findings may provide a better understanding of the comorbidity between RLS and TTH.

Abbreviations

CI: Confidence interval; GAS: Goldberg anxiety scale; ICHD: International classification of headache disorders; IRLSSG: International restless legs syndrome study group; KHSS: Korean headache-sleep study; OR: Odds ratio; PM: Probable migraine; RLS: Restless legs syndrome; TTH: Tension-type headache; VAS: Visual analogue scale

Acknowledgements

The authors would like to thank Gallup Korea for providing technical support for the Korean Headache-Sleep study.

Funding

This study was supported by a 2011 grant from the Korean Academy of Medical Sciences.

Author's contributions

MKC conceived and designed the study, collected and analyzed data, and wrote the manuscript. PWC conceived and designed the study, and wrote the manuscript. SJC designed the study and analyzed data. WJK conceived the study and collected the data. KIY conceived the study and analyzed data. CHY conceived and designed the study, and collected data. All authors read and approved the final manuscript.

Competing interests

Dr. Pil-Wook Chung declared no conflict of interest.
Dr. Soo-Jin Cho was involved as a site investigator of multicenter trial sponsored by Otsuka Korea, Eli Lilly and Company, Korea BMS, and Eisai Korea, and received research support from Hallym University Research Fund 2016 and received lecture honoraria from Yuyu Pharmaceutical Company.
Dr. Won-Joo Kim declared no conflict of interest.
Dr. Kwang Ik Yang declared no conflict of interest.
Dr. Chang-Ho Yun declared no conflict of interest.
Dr. Min Kyung Chu was as a site investigator for a multicenter trial sponsored by Eli Lilly, worked an advisory member for Teva, and received lecture honoraria from Allergan Korea and Yuyu Pharmaceutical Company.

Author details

[1]Department of Neurology, Kangbuk Samsung Hospital, Sungkyunkwan University School of Medicine, Seoul, Republic of Korea. [2]Department of Neurology, Dongtan Sacred Heart Hospital, Hallym University College of Medicine, Hwaseong, Republic of Korea. [3]Department of Neurology, Gangnam Severance Hospital, Yonsei University, College of Medicine, Seoul, Republic of Korea. [4]Department of Neurology, Soonchunhyang University College of Medicine, Cheonan Hospital, Cheonan, Republic of Korea. [5]Department of Neurology, Bundang Clinical Neuroscience Institute, Seoul National University Bundang Hospital, Seongnam, Republic of Korea. [6]Department of Neurology, Kangnam Sacred Heart Hospital, Hallym University College of Medicine, 1 Singil-ro, Yeongdeungpo-gu, Seoul 07441, Republic of Korea.

References

1. Global Burden of Disease Study 2013 Collaborators (2015) Global, regional, and national incidence, prevalence, and years lived with disability for 301 acute and chronic diseases and injuries in 188 countries, 1990-2013: a systematic analysis for the Global Burden of Disease Study 2013. Lancet 386(9995):743–800. doi:10.1016/S0140-6736(15)60692-4
2. Puca F, Genco S, Prudenzano MP, Savarese M, Bussone G, D'Amico D et al (1999) Psychiatric comorbidity and psychosocial stress in patients with tension-type headache from headache centers in Italy. The Italian collaborative group for the study of psychopathological factors in primary headaches. Cephalalgia 19(3):159–164
3. Song TJ, Cho SJ, Kim WJ, Yang KI, Yun CH, Chu MK (2016) Anxiety and depression in tension-type headache: a population-based study. PLoS One 11(10):e0165316. doi:10.1371/journal.pone.0165316
4. Freedom T, Evans RW (2013) Headache and sleep. Headache 53(8): 1358–1366. doi:10.1111/head.12178
5. Ohayon MM, O'Hara R, Vitiello MV (2012) Epidemiology of restless legs syndrome: a synthesis of the literature. Sleep Med Rev 16(4):283–295
6. Cho YW, Shin WC, Yun CH, Hong SB, Kim JH, Allen RP, Earley CJ (2008) Epidemiology of restless legs syndrome in Korean adults. Sleep 31(2):219–223
7. Allen RP, Picchietti D, Hening WA, Trenkwalder C, Walters AS, Montplaisi J (2003) Restless legs syndrome: diagnostic criteria, special considerations, and epidemiology. A report from the restless legs syndrome diagnosis and epidemiology workshop at the National Institutes of Health. Sleep Med 4(2): 101–119
8. Chen PK, Fuh JL, Chen SP, Wang SJ (2010) Association between restless legs syndrome and migraine. J Neurol Neurosurg Psychiatry 81(5):524–528. doi: 10.1136/jnnp.2009.191684
9. Suzuki S, Suzuki K, Miyamoto M, Miyamoto T, Watanabe Y, Takashima R et al (2011) Evaluation of contributing factors to restless legs syndrome in migraine patients. J Neurol 258(11):2026–2035. doi:10.1007/s00415-011-6064-3
10. Winter AC, Schurks M, Berger K, Buring JE, Gaziano JM, Kurth T (2013)

Migraine and restless legs syndrome in men. Cephalalgia 33(2):130–135. doi:10.1177/0333102412466965
11. Zanigni S, Giannini G, Melotti R, Pattaro C, Provini F, Cevoli S et al (2014) Association between restless legs syndrome and migraine: a population-based study. Eur J Neurol 21(9):1205–1210. doi:10.1111/ene.12462
12. Schurks M, Winter A, Berger K, Kurth T (2014) Migraine and restless legs syndrome: a systematic review. Cephalalgia 34(10):777–794. doi:10.1177/0333102414537725
13. Yang FC, Lin TY, Chen HJ, Lee JT, Lin CC, Huang WY et al (2016) Increased risk of restless legs syndrome in patients with migraine: a nationwide population-based cohort study. Medicine (Baltimore) 95(5):e2646. doi:10.1097/md.0000000000002646
14. Cho SJ, Chung YK, Kim JM, Chu MK (2015) Migraine and restless legs syndrome are associated in adults under age fifty but not in adults over fifty: a population-based study. J Headache Pain 16:554. doi:10.1186/s10194-015-0554-0
15. D'Andrea G, D'Arrigo A, Dalle Carbonare M, Leon A (2012) Pathogenesis of migraine: role of neuromodulators. Headache 52(7):1155–1163. doi:10.1111/j.1526-4610.2012.02168.x
16. Earley CJ, Connor J, Garcia-Borreguero D, Jenner P, Winkelman J, Zee PC et al (2014) Altered brain iron homeostasis and dopaminergic function in restless legs syndrome (Willis-Ekbom disease). Sleep Med 15(11):1288–1301. doi:10.1016/j.sleep.2014.05.009
17. Kruit MC, Launer LJ, Overbosch J, van Buchem MA, Ferrari MD (2009) Iron accumulation in deep brain nuclei in migraine: a population-based magnetic resonance imaging study. Cephalalgia 29(3):351–359. doi:10.1111/j.1468-2982.2008.01723.x
18. Fuh JL, Chung MY, Yao SC, Chen PK, Liao YC, Hsu CL et al (2015) Susceptible genes of restless legs syndrome in migraine. Cephalalgia. doi:10.1177/0333102415620907
19. Yang FC, Lin TY, Chen HJ, Lee JT, Lin CC, Kao CH (2015) Risk of restless legs syndrome following tension-type headache: a nationwide population-based cohort study. Medicine (Baltimore) 94(46):e2109. doi:10.1097/md.0000000000002109
20. Oh K, Cho SJ, Chung YK, Kim JM, Chu MK (2014) Combination of anxiety and depression is associated with an increased headache frequency in migraineurs: a population-based study. BMC Neurol 14:238. doi:10.1186/s12883-014-0238-4
21. Headache Classification Committee of the International Headache Society (IHS) The International Classification of Headache Disorders, 3rd edition (beta version) (2013). Cephalalgia 33 (9):629-808. doi:10.1177/0333102413485658
22. Kim BK, Chu MK, Lee TG, Kim JM, Chung CS, Lee KS (2012) Prevalence and impact of migraine and tension-type headache in Korea. J Clin Neurol 8(3):204–211. doi:10.3988/jcn.2012.8.3.204
23. Cho YW, Lee MY, Yun CH, Shin WC, Hong SB, Kim JH (2007) The reliability and validity of the Korean version of paradigm of questions for epidemiology studies of restless legs syndrome and the Johns Hopkins telephone diagnostic interview form for the restless legs syndrome. J Kor Nerol Assoc 25(4):494–499
24. Goldberg D, Bridges K, Duncan-Jones P, Grayson D (1988) Detecting anxiety and depression in general medical settings. BMJ 297(6653):897–899
25. Park HS, Lim JY, Lee SH, Cha YS, Sun WS (2001) Reliability and validity of anxiety screening scale. Korean J Fam Med 22(8):1224–1232
26. Pignone MP, Gaynes BN, Rushton JL, Burchell CM, Orleans CT, Mulrow CD et al (2002) Screening for depression in adults: a summary of the evidence for the U.S. Preventive Services Task Force. Ann Intern Med 136(10):765–776
27. Choi HS, Choi JH, Park KH, Joo KJ, Ga H, Ko HJ et al (2007) Standardization of the Korean version of patient health questionnaire-9 as a screening instrument for major depressive disorder. Korean J Fam Med 28(2):114–119
28. Rubin DB, Little RJ (2002) Statistical analysis with missing data. J Wiley & Sons, Hoboken
29. Sevim S, Dogu O, Kaleagasi H, Aral M, Metin O, Camdeviren H (2004) Correlation of anxiety and depression symptoms in patients with restless legs syndrome: a population based survey. J Neurol Neurosurg Psychiatry 75(2):226–230
30. Nomura T, Inoue Y, Kusumi M, Uemura Y, Nakashima K (2008) Prevalence of restless legs syndrome in a rural community in Japan. Mov Disord 23(16):2363–2369. doi:10.1002/mds.22274
31. Becker PM, Sharon D (2014) Mood disorders in restless legs syndrome (Willis-Ekbom disease). J Clin Psychiatry 75(7):e679–694. doi:10.4088/JCP.13r08692
32. Stovner L, Hagen K, Jensen R, Katsarava Z, Lipton R, Scher A et al (2007) The global burden of headache: a documentation of headache prevalence and disability worldwide. Cephalalgia 27(3):193–210
33. Peng KP, Wang SJ (2014) Epidemiology of headache disorders in the Asia-Pacific region. Headache 54(4):610–618
34. Kim WH, Kim BS, Kim SK, Chang SM, Lee DW, Cho MJ et al (2012) Restless legs syndrome in older people: a community-based study on its prevalence and association with major depressive disorder in older Korean adults. Int J Geriatr Psychiatry 27(6):565–572
35. Allen R (2004) Dopamine and iron in the pathophysiology of restless legs syndrome (RLS). Sleep Med 5(4):385–391. doi:10.1016/j.sleep.2004.01.012
36. Lee HB, Hening WA, Allen RP, Kalaydjian AE, Earley CJ, Eaton WW et al (2008) Restless legs syndrome is associated with DSM-IV major depressive disorder and panic disorder in the community. J Neuropsychiatry Clin Neurosci 20(1):101–105
37. Dunlop BW, Nemeroff CB (2007) The role of dopamine in the pathophysiology of depression. rch. Gen Psychiatry 64(3):327–337
38. Castillo J, Martinez F, Leira R, Lema M, Noya M (1994) Plasma monoamines in tension-type headache. Headache 34(9):531–535
39. Friedman BW, Adewunmi V, Campbell C, Solorzano C, Esses D, Bijur PE et al (2013) A randomized trial of intravenous ketorolac versus intravenous metoclopramide plus diphenhydramine for tension-type and all nonmigraine, noncluster recurrent headaches. Annal Emerg Med 62(4):311–318, e314

15

The course of headache in patients with moderate-to-severe headache due to mild traumatic brain injury

Chang-Ki Hong[1,2], Jin-Yang Joo[1], Yu Shik Shim[3], Sook Young Sim[4], Min A Kwon[1], Yong Bae Kim[1] and Joonho Chung[1,2,5*]

Abstract

Background: Little is known about the long-term course of headache in patients with moderate-to-severe headache due to traumatic brain injury (TBI). We evaluated the course of headache in patients with moderate-to-severe headache due to mild TBI.

Methods: Since September 2009, patients with TBI prospectively rated their headache using a numeric rating scale (NRS). From the database containing 935 patients with TBI between September 2009 and December 2013, 259 patients were included according to following criteria: (1) newly onset moderate-to-severe headache (NRS ≥ 4) due to head trauma; (2) age ≥ 15 years; (3) Glasgow Coma Scale ≥ 13; (4) transient loss of consciousness ≤ 30 min; and (5) radiographic evaluation, such as computed tomography or magnetic resonance image. We evaluated initial and follow-up NRS scores to determine the significance of NRS changes and identified risk factors for moderate-to-severe headache at 36-month follow-up.

Results: At 36-month follow-up, 225 patients (86.9%) reported improved headache (NRS ≤ 3) while 34 (13.1%) reported no improvement. The NRS scores were significantly decreased within a month ($P < 0.001$). The follow-up NRS scores at 12-, 24-, and 36-months were lower than those at one month ($P < 0.001$). Multiple logistic regression analysis showed that post-traumatic seizure (odds ratio, 2.162; 95% CI, 1.095–6.542; $P = 0.041$) and traumatic intracranial hemorrhage (odds ratio, 2.854; 95% CI, 1.241–10.372; $P = 0.024$) were independent risk factors for moderate-to-severe headache at 36-month follow-up.

Conclusions: The course of headache in patients with mild TBI continuously improved until 36-month follow-up. However, 13.1% of patients still suffered from moderate-to-severe headache at 36-month follow-up, for whom post-traumatic seizure and traumatic intracranial hemorrhage might be risk factors.

Keywords: Headache, Head injury, Post-traumatic headache, Traumatic brain injury

Background

It has been reported that 18–33% of subjects continue to experience persistent headache after traumatic brain injury (TBI) even beyond one year post-injury. Most headaches after TBI resolves within 6–12 months [1]. Previously, studies that addressed headache in patients with TBI received little attention since achieving a good clinical outcome was of higher importance than headache improvement. However, headache has become one of the most frequently reported symptoms after mild TBI [1–3] and has affected quality of life [4]. Thus, persistent post-traumatic headache, rather than some mild morbidity after mild TBI, has received more attention because of its potential impact on patient quality of life. According to the International Classification of Headache Disorders, 3rd edition (beta version), headache attributed to trauma or

* Correspondence: ns.joonho.chung@gmail.com
[1]Department of Neurosurgery, Gangnam Severance Hospital, Yonsei University College of Medicine, 211, Eonjuro, Gangnam-gu, Seoul 135-720, Republic of Korea
[2]Severance Institute for Vascular and Metabolic Research, Yonsei University, Seoul, Republic of Korea
Full list of author information is available at the end of the article

injury to the head and/or neck are the most common secondary headache disorders [5]. Post-traumatic headache is reported to have developed within 7 days after one of the following: (1) the injury to the head, (2) regaining of consciousness following the injury to the head, or (3) discontinuation of medications that impair ability to sense or report headache following the injury to the head [5]. During the first 3 months from onset, post-traumatic headache is considered acute. Persistent post-traumatic headache was described as headache of greater than 3 months' duration caused by traumatic injury to the head. The term persistent has been adopted in place of chronic [5]. However, little is known about how these headaches change over time and what makes these headaches persistent. Thus, it is important to know about the course of headache after mild TBI. The purpose of this study was to evaluate the courses of headache in patients who had moderate-to-severe headache initially after mild TBI and to identify associated risk factors.

Methods

This retrospective cross-sectional study using prospectively collected data was approved by our institutional review board, and informed consent was waived. Since September 2009, we prospectively rated patient headache using a numeric rating scale (NRS). From the database containing 935 patients with TBI between September 2009 and December 2013, 259 patients were included in the present study according to the following inclusion criteria: (1) newly onset moderate-to-severe headache (NRS ≥ 4) due to head trauma; (2) age ≥ 15 years; (3) Glasgow Coma Scale [GCS] ≥ 13; (4) transient loss of consciousness (LOC) ≤ 30 min; and (5) radiographic evaluation, such as computed tomography (CT) or magnetic resonance image (MRI). The remaining 676 case from the database were excluded for the following reasons: (1) GCS < 13 ($n = 228$); (2) initial or follow-up modified Rankin Scale (mRS) ≥ 3 ($n = 59$); (3) history of neurosurgery (craniotomy due to any cause) ($n = 37$); (4) TBI due to any cerebrovascular disease ($n = 87$); (5) history of previously diagnosed intracranial disease ($n = 45$); (6) post-traumatic amnesia > 24 h ($n = 33$); (7) delayed hemorrhage (>24 h) ($n = 25$); (8) combined spinal cord injury ($n = 93$); (9) incomplete NRS score data ($n = 17$); and (10) loss to follow-up ($n = 52$). Our inclusion/exclusion criteria have contained the definition of mild TBI since mild TBI, in general, is defined as TBI resulting in GCS ≥ 13, LOC ≤ 30 min, and post-traumatic amnesia ≤ 24 h [6, 7]. Most mild TBI are not associated with visible abnormalities on structural neuroimaging. A complicated mild TBI was differentiated from an uncomplicated mild TBI by the presence of (a) a depressed skull fracture and/or (b) a trauma-related intracranial abnormality, such as hemorrhage, contusion, or edema [8]. According to the GCS scoring system, moderate TBI is defined as a GCS of 9 to 12 and severe TBI is defined as a GCS of 3 to 8.

Intensity of headache was assessed with the NRS, an 11-point numeric scale for rating pain intensity. The quantitative scale ranges from 0 to 10, with 0 meaning "no headache at all" and 10 meaning "the worst possible headache." This 11-point scale has been previously applied to headache assessment [9–11]. We defined NRS scores of 1 to 3, 4 to 6, and 7 to 10 as mild, moderate, and severe headaches, respectively. Mild headache was described as nagging, annoying, or interfering little with active daily living. Moderate headache was described as interfering significantly with active daily living. Severe headache was described as disabling or interfering to the point that patients were unable to perform daily activities. Thus, we defined an NRS score ≥ 4 as significant. All included patients visited the emergency department or the outpatient office within 48 h of onset. NRS score was determined every 8 h (three times per day) during a patient's hospitalization or twice during each outpatient visit. Analgesics were prescribed to all included patients. Patient NRS scores were collected and averaged for the onset (within a week from TBI), and at 1-month, 6-month, 12-month, 24-month, and 36-month follow-ups.

Three independent investigators blinded to the data retrospectively reviewed the clinical and radiographic data of the included patients using their medical records. Variables evaluated were age, gender, initial GCS score, cause of TBI, mechanism of TBI, traumatic intracranial hemorrhage, initial symptoms and signs (LOC, vomiting, tinnitus, visual symptoms, confusion, post-traumatic amnesia, and post-traumatic seizure), and previous physician-diagnosed headache (treated with medications). A follow-up NRS score ≤ 3 (mild headache or no headache) was defined as improvement, as NRS scores rated 1 to 3 were regarded as headache interfering minimally with most activities [11]. We evaluated the initial and follow-up NRS scores to determine the significance of NRS changes and identified risk factors for moderate-to-severe headache (NRS ≥ 4) at 36-month follow-up.

Statistical analysis

All statistical analyses were performed in consultation with a biostatistician and performed using R language ver. 3.01 (R Foundation for Statistical Computing, Vienna, Austria). Paired *t*-tests or Wilcoxon signed rank tests were used to evaluate NRS changes between baseline and follow-up scores. For these multiple comparisons, we applied the Bonferroni adjustment to the interpretations; therefore, statistical significance was defined by $P < 0.01$ (0.05/5). Mann-Whitney *U*-tests were used for numeric variables. Chi-square tests or Fisher's exact tests were used for nominal variables. Logistic regression analysis was performed to determine the independent risk factors of moderate-to-severe headache at 36-month follow-up (with regard to NRS score change). Multiple logistic regression analysis was performed on variables with an unadjusted effect and a $P < 0.1$ on simple logistic regression analysis. Statistical significance was defined as $P < 0.05$ with a 95% confidence interval (CI).

Results

Table 1 presents patient clinical characteristics. On admission, the most frequent cause of TBI was motor vehicle accident (142 patients, 54.8%) and the most frequent mechanism was head striking an object (170 patients, 65.6%). LOC was experienced in 144 patients (55.6%), post-traumatic amnesia in 57 patients (22.0%), post-traumatic seizure in 16 patients (6.2%), traumatic intracranial hemorrhage in 42 patients (16.2%), and previously physician-diagnosed headache in 52 patients (20.1%). Forty-two patients with traumatic intracranial hemorrhage had neurologically asymptomatic minimal hemorrhage on their CT or MRI. At 12-month follow-up, 154 patients (59.5%) improved their headache (NRS ≤ 3) and 105 patients (40.5%) still suffered from moderate-to-severe headache. There were no significant differences in characteristics between patients with headache improvement and those without headache improvement.

At the 36-month follow-up, 225 patients (86.9%) reported their headache improved and 34 patients (13.1%) still suffered from moderate-to-severe headache. Four patients of the 154 patients with headache improvement at 12-month follow-up reported aggravated headache (NRS ≥ 4) at 36-month follow-up. Seventy-five patients of the 105 patients without headache improvement at 12-month follow-up became better (NRS ≤ 3) at 36-month follow-up. Post-traumatic seizure ($P = 0.041$) and traumatic intracranial hemorrhage ($P = 0.008$) were significantly different between patients with headache improvement and those without headache improvement.

Mean NRS scores were 8.37, 5.23, 2.94, 2.62, and 2.35 at onset, 1-month, 12-month, 24-month, and 36-month follow-ups, respectively. The NRS scores were significantly decreased within a month ($P < 0.001$). Then, the follow-up NRS scores at 12-, 24-, and 36-months were lower than those at one month ($P < 0.001$). Follow-up NRS scores decreased continuously until the 36-month follow-up (Fig. 1).

Multiple logistic regression analysis showed that post-traumatic seizure (odds ratio, 2.162; 95% CI, 1.095–6.542; $P = 0.041$) and traumatic intracranial hemorrhage (odds ratio, 2.854; 95% CI, 1.241–10.372; $P = 0.024$) were independent risk factors for moderate-to-severe headache at the 36-month follow-up (Table 2). Previously diagnosed headache had a *P*-value of 0.046 in simple logistic regression analysis, but was not statistically significant after adjustment ($P = 0.097$).

Discussion

The course of headache in patients with moderate-to-severe headache due to mild TBI continuously improved until 36-month follow-up. However, persistence of moderate-to-severe headache occurred in 13.1% of the 259 patients throughout the 36-month follow-up. Patients who experienced post-traumatic seizure and those who had traumatic intracranial hemorrhage on their radiographic images might be expected to have persistent moderate-to-severe headache at 36-month follow-up.

The reported prevalence of headache due to TBI ranges between 20 and 89% at baseline, and the cumulative incidence of headache over one year has been reported to be 71–91%. Many studies have reported that more than one-third of patients complained of persistent headache throughout the follow-up period [1, 3, 12–16]. The present study is different from previous reports because we included selective patients who had moderate-to-severe headache due to TBI. Thus, it was difficult to assess the prevalence of new onset post-traumatic headache throughout the follow-up period. It was only possible to determine if headache intensity became better or worse over time. Four of the 154 patients whose headache was better at 12-month follow-up might be considered to have new onset post-traumatic headache or headache unrelated to TBI because their headache became better but was then aggravated again at 36-month follow-up. All included patients had follow-up NRS scores that were continuously decreased until 36-month follow-up, except 34 patients (13.1%) who suffered from moderate-to-severe headache over the entire 36 months after TBI. Among those 34 patients, however, their headaches might not have originated from TBI because we did not evaluate NRS continuously and there were time intervals between the follow-up periods. These headaches might be new onset migraines because the prevalence of migraine with severe headache has been reported in 14.2% of Americans and 8.4% of Japanese annually [17, 18]. The characteristics and pathophysiologic mechanisms are similar between post-traumatic

Table 1 Clinical Characteristics of the patients

	Baseline characteristics (n = 259)	12-month follow-up			36-month follow-up		
		Headache improved (n = 154)	Headache not improved (n = 105)	P value	Headache improved (n = 225)	Headache not improved (n = 34)	P value
Age (mean ± SD)	37.9 ± 10.4	39.4 ± 11.4	38.6 ± 12.1	0.801	40.4 ± 12.5	42.1 ± 12.8	0.545
Female (n, %)	116 (44.8)	72 (46.8)	44 (41.9)	0.685	102 (45.3)	14 (41.2)	0.617
Cause of traumatic brain injury (n, %)				0.651			0.452
Motor vehicle accident	142 (54.8)	93 (60.4)	59 (56.2)		122 (54.2)	20 (58.8)	
Fall from height	61 (23.6)	33 (21.4)	28 (26.7)		57 (25.3)	4 (11.8)	
Direct hit on the head	56 (21.6)	28 (18.2)	28 (26.7)		46 (20.4)	10 (29.4)	
Mechanism of traumatic brain injury (n, %)				0.434			0.885
Whiplash	36 (13.9)	22 (14.3)	14 (13.3)		31 (13.8)	5 (14.7)	
Head being struck	53 (20.5)	33 (21.4)	20 (19.0)		45 (20.0)	8 (23.5)	
Head striking an object	170 (65.6)	99 (64.3)	71 (67.6)		149 (66.2)	21 (61.8)	
Loss of consciousness (n, %)	144 (55.6)	79 (51.3)	65 (61.9)	0.148	123 (54.7)	21 (61.8)	0.264
Vomiting (n, %)	73 (28.2)	41 (26.6)	32 (20.8)	0.353	66 (29.3)	7 (20.6)	0.192
Tinnitus (n, %)	25 (9.7)	16 (10.4)	7 (8.6)	0.638	23 (10.2)	2 (5.9)	0.312
Visual symptoms (n, %)	18 (6.9)	12 (7.8)	6 (5.7)	0.755	16 (7.1)	2 (5.9)	0.863
Confusion (n, %)	50 (19.3)	32 (20.8)	18 (17.1)	0.621	41 (18.2)	9 (26.5)	0.206
Post-traumatic amnesia (n, %)	57 (22.0)	38 (24.7)	19 (18.1)	0.446	47 (20.9)	10 (29.4)	0.127
Post-traumatic seizure (n, %)	16 (6.2)	3 (1.9)	13 (12.4)	0.145	6 (2.7)	10 (29.4)	0.041
Traumatic intracranial hemorrhage (n, %)	42 (16.2)	10 (6.5)	32 (20.8)	0.072	19 (8.4)	23 (67.6)	0.008
Previously diagnosed headache (n, %)	52 (20.1)	25 (16.2)	27 (25.7)	0.096	41 (18.2)	11 (32.4)	0.076
Hypertension (n, %)	110 (42.5)	71 (46.1)	39 (37.1)	0.185	96 (42.7)	14 (41.2)	0.814
Diabetes (n, %)	51 (19.7)	33 (21.4)	18 (17.1)	0.549	44 (19.6)	7 (20.6)	0.905
Dyslipidemia (n, %)	59 (22.8)	41 (26.6)	18 (17.1)	0.177	54 (24.0)	5 (14.7)	0.258
Smoking (n, %)	76 (29.3)	43 (27.9)	33 (31.4)	0.646	65 (28.9)	11 (32.4)	0.649
Alcohol (n, %)	63 (24.3)	42 (27.3)	21 (20.0)	0.225	56 (24.9)	7 (20.6)	0.561
Antiplatelet agent (n, %)	21 (8.1)	15 (9.7)	6 (5.7)	0.376	19 (8.4)	2 (5.9)	0.454
Anticoagulant (n, %)	5 (1.9)	3 (1.9)	2 (1.9)	0.889	5 (2.2)	0 (0.0)	0.623

SD standard deviation

headache and migraine [19–22]. In addition, there are no specific headache features known to distinguish the subtypes of headache attributed to trauma or injury to the head and/or neck from other headache types; most often these resemble tension-type headache or migraine [5].

We included patients with moderate-to-severe headache initially, who did not have neurological disability with GCS ≥ 13 because disability could affect post-traumatic headache. In fact, it was reported that disability related to post-traumatic headache was high with an average NRS ranging from 5.5 at baseline to 5.7 at 60-month follow-up [14]. Moderate-to-severe TBI makes post-traumatic headache worse compared to mild TBI [23]. However, we did not focus on the intensity (mild, moderate, or severe) of TBI, but just on moderate-to-severe headache over time in neurologically asymptomatic patients who have frequently received little attention since their clinical course was mostly good. Additionally, moderate-to-severe headache (NRS ≥ 4) might have more clinical relevance compared to mild headache (NRS ≤ 3), because mild headache was described as interfering little with activities of daily living, while moderate-to-severe headache interfered with or prevented activities of daily living. We, also, excluded patients with spinal cord injury because some patients with mild TBI could have headaches secondary to spinal cord injury. In the same context, 55.6% (144/259) of LOC in the present study, that seemed a bit high for patients with mild TBI, can be understood. The initial impact to the head could be more severe in patients of the

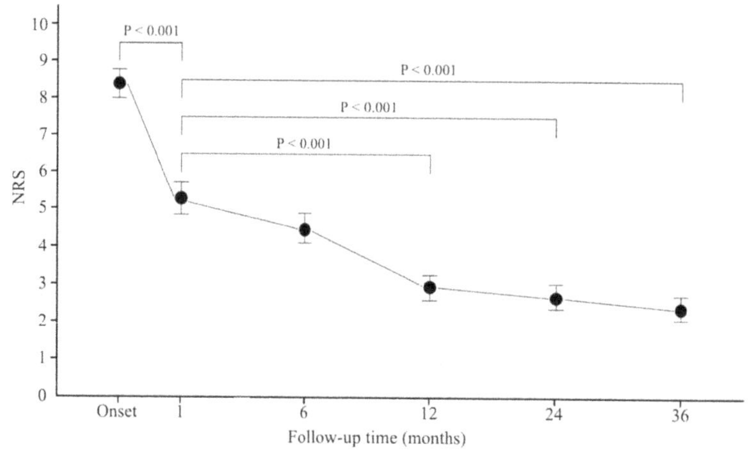

Fig. 1 The course of headache in patients with mild traumatic brain injury is represented by changes in numeric rating scale (NRS) score from onset to 36-month follow-up. Compared with NRS scores at onset, those at 1-month follow-up were significantly decreased. Follow-up NRS scores were significantly lower at 12-, 24-, and 36-month follow-ups compared to 1-month follow-up. The NRS scores decreased continuously until 36-month follow-up. *Dots* indicate mean NRS scores at each time point and *error bars* indicate the 95% confidence intervals

present study than those with mild TBI in general because our patients had moderate-to-severe headache initially as well as visible abnormalities on structural neuroimaging. In addition, Beetar et al. have previously reported that 62.9% (127/202) of their patients with mild TBI had LOC [24].

We identified two risk factors, post-traumatic seizure and traumatic intracranial hemorrhage, that were related to moderate-to-severe headache at 36-month follow-up. Because our data included patients with traumatic intracranial hemorrhage, we did enroll patients with complicated mild TBI. However, we excluded patients with disability (mRS ≥ 3) because we had tried to get rid of probable effects of disability on the course of headache in patients with TBI. Neurological deficits may affect more seriously to patients' daily living or quality of life than post-traumatic headache. Thus, our findings on risk factors for moderate-to-severe headache at 36-month follow-up might be natural for patients with complicated mild TBI because post-traumatic seizure and traumatic intracranial hemorrhage usually occur in patients with complicated mild TBI compared to patients with uncomplicated mild TBI. Up to 3 years after TBI, however, patients could have post-traumatic headache that interfered with or prevented activities of daily living according to our results. These results may allow providers to educate their patients who present with initially alert consciousness and no disability about what they can expect with respect to moderate-to-severe headache after TBI. Additionally, this suggests that management of post-traumatic headache should not be neglected.

There are several limitations to this study. First, it was a retrospective study based on a prospectively collected database and had no true control group. Patients with incomplete NRS data ($n = 17$) and those lost to follow-up ($n = 52$) were excluded from the analyses. Second, we did not distinguish headache characteristics, such as type, intensity, onset, duration, or frequency. In prior studies, the most frequent type of headache reported after TBI was migraine [13, 25]. Up to 49% of post-traumatic headache met the criteria for migraine, followed by tension-type headache (up to 40%) [13]. Although little is known about the natural history of headache after TBI, it has been reported that TBI-attributed headache was persistent over five years or longer after TBI [12, 14, 26, 27]. Some studies reported that new or worse headache prevalence remained consistent with at least 33% of patients [14]. Therefore, our results may have been different if we had evaluated headache characteristics. However, we were only concerned with a subjective measure of headache intensity (NRS), as our focus was on headaches after TBI in general and their potential effects on daily activities. Finally, we did not obtain sufficient information about headache medications. Analgesics were given to all included patients. However, medication may affect headache improvement or may provoke medication-overuse headache [14]. Approximately half of people with headache on 15 or more days per month for more than 3 months have medication-overuse headache [14]. It is very difficult to analyze when or how medications were used. However, we attempted to evaluate the correlation between previously diagnosed headache treated with medication and headache improvement after TBI.

Table 2 Risk factors for moderate-to-severe headache at the 36-month follow-up

	Unadjusted		Adjusted	
	OR (95% CI)	*p* value	OR (95% CI)	*p* value
Age in years				
< 40	1		1	
≥ 40	1.628 (0.636–3.743)	0.708	1.446 (0.423–3.190)	0.845
Gender				
Female	1		1	
Male	0.954 (0.438–2.285)	0.713	0.912 (0.497–2.559)	0.776
Initial GCS				
15	1			
13 and 14	1.898 (0.845–5.562)	0.294		
Cause of traumatic brain injury				
Motor vehicle accident	1			
Fall from height	0.733 (0.433–2.632)	0.535		
Direct hit on the head	1.865 (0.524–3.356)	0.629		
Mechanism of traumatic brain injury				
Whiplash	1			
Head being struck	1.438 (0.754–4.224)	0.472		
Head striking an object	0.872 (0.637–3.325)	0.486		
Loss of conscious				
No	1			
Yes	2.762 (0.805–6.433)	0.154		
Vomiting				
No	1			
Yes	0.949 (0.475–1.768)	0.512		
Tinnitus				
No	1			
Yes	0.886 (0.396–2.267)	0.564		
Visual symptoms				
No	1			
Yes	0.821 (0.358–1.947)	0.607		
Confusion				
No	1			
Yes	1.504 (0.526–3.435)	0.658		
Post-traumatic amnesia				
No	1		1	
Yes	2.083 (0.889–6.219)	0.069	1.921 (0.816–4.945)	0.154
Post-traumatic seizure				
No	1		1	
Yes	2.435 (1.218–6.105)	0.032	2.162 (1.095–6.542)	0.041
Traumatic intracranial hemorrhage				
No	1		1	
Yes	3.595 (1.329–9.247)	0.008	2.854 (1.241–10.372)	0.024
Previously diagnosed headache				
No	1		1	
Yes	1.921 (1.056–4.247)	0.046	1.677 (0.896–5.331)	0.097

CI confidence interval, *OR* odds ratio

Conclusions

The course of headache in patients with mild TBI continuously improved until 36-months follow-up. However, 13.1% of patients for whom post-traumatic seizure and traumatic intracranial hemorrhage might be risk factors still suffered from moderate-to-severe headache at 36-month follow-up.

Abbreviations

CI: Confidence interval; CT: Computed tomography; GCS: Glasgow Coma Scale; LOC: Loss of consciousness; MRI: Magnetic resonance image; mRS: Modified Rankin Scale; NRS: Numeric rating scale; TBI: Traumatic brain injury

Acknowledgements

None.

Funding

There is no financial support related to this study and we have no conflict of interest.

Authors' contributions

CKH conceived and designed the study, acquired, interpreted and analyzed data, drafted and revised the manuscript. JYJ, YSS and SYS acquired and interpreted data, revised the manuscript. MAK and YBK interpreted and analyzed data. JC conceived, designed and supervised the study, acquired and interpreted data, drafted and revised the manuscript. All authors read and approved the final manuscript.

Competing interests

The authors declare that they have no competing interests.

Author details

[1]Department of Neurosurgery, Gangnam Severance Hospital, Yonsei University College of Medicine, 211, Eonjuro, Gangnam-gu, Seoul 135-720, Republic of Korea. [2]Severance Institute for Vascular and Metabolic Research, Yonsei University, Seoul, Republic of Korea. [3]Department of Neurosurgery, Inha University School of Medicine and Hospital, Incheon, Republic of Korea. [4]Department of Neurosurgery, Inje University Seoul Paik Hospital, Seoul, Republic of Korea. [5]Department of Neurological Surgery, Rush University Medical Center, 1725 W. Harrison St., Professional Building Suite 855, Chicago, IL 60612, USA.

References

1. Lew HL, Lin PH, Fuh JL, Wang SJ, Clark DJ, Walker WC (2006) Characteristics and treatment of headache after traumatic brain injury: a focused review. Am J Phys Med Rehabil 85:619–627
2. Dikmen S, Machamer J, Fann JR, Temkin NR (2010) Rates of symptom reporting following traumatic brain injury. J Int Neuropsychol Soc 16:401–411
3. Nampiaparampil DM (2008) Prevalence of chronic pain after traumatic brain injury: a systematic review. JAMA 300:711–719
4. Headache Classification Subcommittee of the International Headache Society (2004) The international classification of headache disorders. Cephalalgia 24(Suppl 1):9–160
5. Headache Classification Committee of the International Headache Society (HIS) (2013) The international classification of headache disorders, 3rd edition (beta version). Cephalalgia 33:629–808
6. Saatman KE, Duhaime AC, Bullock R, Maas AI, Valadka A, Manley GT (2008) Classification of traumatic brain injury for targeted therapies. J Neurotrauma 25:719–738
7. Mild Traumatic Brain Injury Committee of the Head Injury Interdisciplinary Special Interest Group of the American Congress of Rehabilitation Medicine (1993) Definition of mild traumatic brain injury. J Head Trauma Rehabil 8:86–87
8. Iverson GL, Lange RT, Waljas M, Liimatainen S, Dastidar P, Hartikainen KM, Soimakallio S, Ohman J (2012) Outcome from complicated versus uncomplicated mild traumatic brain injury. Rehabil Res Pract 2012:415740
9. Gu DQ, Duan CZ, Li XF, He XY, Lai LF, Su SX (2013) Effect of endovascular treatment on headache in elderly patients with unruptured intracranial aneurysms. AJNR Am J Neuroradiol 34:1227–1231
10. Hong CK, Joo JY, Kim YB, Shim YS, Lim YC, Shin YS et al (2015) The course of headache in patients with moderate-to-severe headache due to aneurysmal subarachnoid hemorrhage: A retrospective cross-sectional study. Headache 55:992–999
11. Kwong WJ, Pathak DS (2007) Validation of the eleven-point pain scale in the measurement of migraine headache pain. Cephalalgia 27:336–342
12. Hoffman JM, Lucas S, Dikmen S, Braden CA, Brown AW, Brunner R et al (2011) Natural history of headache after traumatic brain injury. J Neurotrauma 28:1719–1725
13. Lucas S, Hoffman JM, Bell KR, Dikmen S (2014) A prospective study of prevalence and characterization of headache following mild traumatic brain injury. Cephalalgia 34:93–102
14. Stacey A, Lucas S, Dikmen S, Temkin N, Bell KR, Brown A et al (2017) Natural history of headache five years after traumatic brain injury. J Neurotrauma [Epub ahead of print]. doi:10.1089/neu.2016.4721
15. Smith-Seemiller L, Fow NR, Kant R, Franzen MD (2003) Presence of post-concussion syndrome symptoms in patients with chronic pain vs mild traumatic brain injury. Brain Inj 17:199–206
16. Uomoto JM, Esselman PC (1993) TBI and chronic pain: differential types and rates by head injury severity. Arch Phys Med Rehabil 74:61–64
17. Burch RC, Loder S, Loder E, Smitherman TA (2015) The prevalence and burden of migraine and severe headache in the United States: updated statistics from government health surveillance studies. Headache 55:21–34
18. Sakai F, Igarashi H (1997) Prevalence of migraine in Japan: a nationwide survey. Cephalalgia 17:15–22
19. Bekkelund SI, Salvesen R (2003) Prevalence of head trauma in patients with difficult headache: the North Norway Headache Study. Headache 43:59–62
20. Finkel AG, Yerry J, Scher A, Choi YS (2012) Headaches in soldiers with mild traumatic brain injury: findings and phenomenologic descriptions. Headache 52:957–965
21. Theeler BJ, Erickson JC (2012) Posttraumatic headache in military personnel and veterans of the Iraq and Afghanistan conflicts. Curr Treat Options Neurol 14:36–49
22. Walker WC, Seel RT, Curtiss G, Warden DL (2005) Headache after moderate to severe traumatic brain injury; a longitudinal analysis. Arch Phys Med Rehabil 86:1793–1800
23. Formisano R, Bivona U, Catani S, D'Ippolito M, Buzzi MG (2009) Post-traumatic headache: facts and doubts. J Headache Pain 10:145–152
24. Beetar JT, Guilmette TJ, Sparadeo FR (1996) Sleep and pain complaints in symptomatic TBI and neurologic populations. Arch Phys Med Rehabil 77:1298–1302
25. Finkel AG, Yerry JA, Klaric JS, Ivins BJ, Scher A, Choi YS (2016) Headache in military service members with a history of mild traumatic brain injury: a cohort study of diagnosis and classification. Cephalalgia. [Epub ahead of print].
26. Lucas S, Hoffman JM, Bell KR, Walker W, Dikmen S (2012) Characterization of headache after traumatic brain injury. Cephalalgia 32:600–606
27. Ponsford JL, Downing MG, Olver J, Ponsford M, Acher R, Carty M et al (2014) Longitudinal follow-up of patients with traumatic brain injury: outcome at two, five, and ten years post-injury. J Neurotrauma 31:64–77

16

Prevalence and burden of headache disorders in Lithuania and their public-health and policy implications: a population-based study within the Eurolight Project

Daiva Rastenytė[1], Dalia Mickevičienė[1], Lars Jacob Stovner[2,3], Hallie Thomas[2], Colette Andrée[4] and Timothy J Steiner[2,5*]

Abstract

Background: The Eurolight project assessed the impact of headache disorders in ten EU countries, using the same structured questionnaire but varying sampling methods. In Lithuania, sample selection employed methods in line with consensus recommendations for population-based burden-of-headache studies.

Methods: The survey was cross-sectional. We identified, from the Residents' Register Service, a sample of inhabitants of Kaunas city and surrounding Kaunas region reflecting age (in the range 18–65 years), gender and rural/urban distributions of Lithuania. Medical students called unannounced at their homes and conducted face-to-face interviews employing a structured questionnaire.

Results: Of 1137 people in the pre-identified sample, 573 (male 237 [41.4%], female 336 [58.6%]; mean age 40.9 ± 13.8 years) completed interviews (participation proportion: 50.4%). Gender-adjusted 1-year prevalences were: any headache 74.7%; migraine 18.8%; tension-type headache (TTH) 42.2%; all headache on ≥15 days/month 8.6%; probable medication-overuse headache (pMOH) 3.2%. Migraine (OR: 3.6) and pMOH (OR: 2.9) were associated with female gender. All headache types except TTH were associated with significantly diminished quality of life. Migraine caused a mean 4.5% loss in paid worktime per affected male and 3.5% per affected female. Lost per-person times due to TTH were much less, but to pMOH and other headache on ≥15 days/month much higher. Among the entire workforce, lost productivity to migraine was estimated at 0.7%, to TTH 0.3% and to pMOH or other headache on ≥15 days/month 0.5%. The total of 1.5% may translate directly into lost GDP. Alternative calculations based on headache yesterday (with little recall error) produced, for all headache, a corroborating 1.7%. Similar losses from household work would also drain the nation's economy. Our findings were comparable to those from earlier studies using similar methods in Russia and Georgia.

(Continued on next page)

* Correspondence: t.steiner@imperial.ac.uk
[2]Department of Neuromedicine and Movement Science, Faculty of Medicine and Health Sciences, NTNU Norwegian University of Science and Technology, Trondheim NO-7941, Norway
[5]Division of Brain Sciences, Imperial College London, London, UK
Full list of author information is available at the end of the article

(Continued from previous page)

Conclusions: The multiple burdens from headache in Lithuania indicate substantial ill-health and unmet need for health care. The heavy burdens on individuals are matched by heavy economic burden. Of particular concern is the high prevalence of headache on ≥15 days/month, seen also in Russia and Georgia. Health policy in Lithuania must heed WHO's advice that effective treatment of headache, clearly desirable for its health benefits, is also expected to be cost-saving.

Keywords: Migraine, Tension-type headache, Medication-overuse headache, Burden, Disability, Lost productivity, Population-based study, Public health, Health policy, Global campaign against headache, Lithuania

Background

The World Health Organization (WHO) recognised headache disorders as major contributors to public ill health, and therefore a public-health priority, in 2000 [1, 2]. Among these disorders, migraine and tension-type headache (TTH) are often lifelong illnesses which, as well as causing pain and disability, also diminish productivity, hinder family and social relationships and impoverish quality of life (QoL). Medication-overuse headache (MOH), usually a *sequela* of migraine or TTH caused by mistreatment of one or the other, occurs by definition on most days and is especially damaging to QoL.

Epidemiologically, many published studies demonstrate that headache disorders are ubiquitous and common [3]. Most of these studies, however, have focused on prevalence to the exclusion of burden. Consequently, they provide data of only limited value for purposes of health policy.

The Global Campaign against Headache was launched in 2004 [4]. Conducted by *Lifting The Burden* (LTB), a UK-registered non-governmental organisation in official relations with WHO [5], its first priority was to fill the major gaps in knowledge of the global burden of headache [6, 7]. For this purpose, LTB developed standardised methodology for population-based studies [8, 9], supported such studies in countries around the world [10], and contributed the data to various iterations of the Global Burden of Disease (GBD) study [11–13]. Migraine became recognized as the sixth highest cause of disability worldwide [12] (third in men and women aged under 50 years [14, 15]), MOH as 18th and headache disorders collectively as third [12, 14]. TTH, relatively non-disabling, is nonetheless now known to be the second most prevalent disorder in the world [12].

In Europe, meanwhile, despite many studies reporting migraine prevalence, there were still major knowledge gaps regarding TTH and MOH, and for all headache types there were few published data on headache-attributed burden [16, 17]. Furthermore, eastern Europe, and especially the countries of the former USSR, were very poorly represented among these [16, 17]. LTB addressed this with population-based studies in Georgia [18, 19] and Russia [20, 21], and Lithuania was included in the Eurolight Project [22].

Eurolight commenced in May 2007 as a partnership activity within the Global Campaign against Headache. Its purpose was to inform policy in the European Union (EU) by assessing the impact of headache. It looked at the EU as a whole, and applied modified cluster-sampling to it with samples drawn from 10 countries [22]. Multiple scientific and lay organisations collaborated with headache experts in these countries, and not all were able to draw population-based samples. In Lithuania alone, the survey was conducted in a sample drawn from public records to be representative of the national population, with each selected participant visited at home. These procedures came close to matching the recommended methodology for population-based burden-of-headache studies [8]. For this reason, we present the Lithuania findings as national estimates.

Methods

Study design

The detailed methods of the Eurolight Project have been published elsewhere [22]. We summarise them here. Eurolight was a cross-sectional survey of randomly-selected adults aged 18–65 years, using a structured questionnaire.

The survey in Lithuania was conducted from 1st December, 2009 to 31st March, 2010.

Sampling

In Lithuania, the survey was population-based, conducted among inhabitants of Kaunas city, the second largest city of Lithuania, and the surrounding areas of Kaunas region in the central part of the Republic. The population of Kaunas region exceeds 420,000 (about 14% of the national population), of whom >90% are ethnic Lithuanians; 80% live in the city and 20% in its surroundings. From the Residents' Register Service, at the time under the auspices of the Ministry of the Interior but now the Ministry of Justice [23], we identified a sample ($N = 1{,}137$) reflecting age (in the range 18–65 years) and gender distributions in Lithuania and the proportions living in rural (33%) or urban (67%) areas.

Seven trained medical students from the Lithuanian University of Health Sciences visited the home of each person in this sample, calling unannounced ("cold-calling"). At each house, only the person who had been pre-identified was eligible to participate. Interview was subject to that person's availability and willingness to participate; if the eligible person was not found during the first visit, at least one additional attempt was made to conduct the interview before that person was regarded as a non-participant.

Questionnaire

The development, content and validation of the Eurolight structured questionnaire, a close derivative of the HARDSHIP questionnaire [9], have been described previously [24]. The original English version was translated into Lithuanian following LTB's translation protocol for lay documents [25].

Demographic questions were followed by neutral screening questions for headache ("Have you ever had a headache?" and "Have you had a headache during the last year?") and, in those screening positively, by headache-diagnostic questions based on ICHD-II [26]. We also asked about headache on the preceding day ("headache yesterday" [HY]). Finally, there were several question sets addressing various components of burden, including symptom burden. As part of the enquiry into burden, we incorporated the HALT questionnaire [27] and WHOQoL-8 [28] as modules in our questionnaire. We applied WHOQoL-8 to all participants, whether reporting headache or not.

Burden enquiry focused primarily on the preceding 3 months (except WHOQoL-8, which addressed the preceding 4 weeks). Additionally, in order to obviate recall error [8, 9], we assessed burden on the preceding day: in respect of HY, we enquired into duration and intensity of the headache, and lost productivity as a consequence of it.

Diagnosis

Only one headache type was diagnosed in each participant (the most bothersome when more than one was identified).

According to the algorithm used to convert questionnaire responses to diagnoses [9], headache occurring on ≥15 days/month was first set aside from episodic headaches (frequency <15 days/month), and diagnosed according to reported acute medication consumption either as probable MOH (pMOH) or other headache on ≥15 days/month. To the episodic headaches, definite migraine criteria were first applied, then, in order, those of definite TTH, probable migraine and probable TTH [26]. For purposes of prevalence and burden estimations, definite and probable migraine were considered together as migraine, as were definite and probable TTH as TTH. A small minority of headaches remained unclassifiable.

When a participant reporting HY described one type of headache only, we assumed HY was of this type. Of those describing more than one type, we asked whether HY was of the same type as the most bothersome headache. Otherwise there was no diagnostic enquiry into HY, because this is problematic for a single episode.

Analysis and statistics

Analyses were performed using SPSS/PC version 20.0 software packages for statistical analysis (SPSS, INC, Chicago, IL) and Excel Professional Plus 2010 Version 14.0.7166.5000.

We described categorical variables in terms of frequency (n) and proportions (%), with 95% confidence intervals (CIs) where appropriate. We summarised continuous variables as means ± standard deviations (SDs), with medians and quartiles when distributions were highly skewed. We recorded gender, age, employment, marital status and incomes of participants, the last in Lithuanian litas (LTL) which we converted to United States dollars (USD) at the exchange rate of the time (USD 1.00 = LTL 2.22). We recorded headache frequency in days/month, duration in hours (for HY only, this was categorized as <1, 1–4, 5–12 and >12 h), and intensity in terms meaning "mild", "moderate" or "severe", which we converted to a numerical rating scale of 1–3 (0 being no pain) and treated as continuous data. We calculated headache-attributed disability at individual level as the product of time in ictal state (itself a product of frequency and duration) and the disability weight (DW) from GBD2013 [29] for the disorder in question. We measured lost productivity from HALT in whole days/3 months, equating, according to accepted methodology [9, 27], "less than half achieved" to "nothing achieved" and counterbalancing this by equating "more than half" to "everything". We calculated these losses as proportions of total productive time available. For HY, we reckoned productivity yesterday as either zero (less than half or nothing achieved) or 100% (more than half or everything achieved). We analysed WHOQoL-8 by summing the scores for the eight questions (each 1–5, higher scores indicating better QoL).

We calculated odds ratios (ORs) for gender- and age-related differences. We used chi-squared or Student's *t* test (one-sided) to assess significance of differences. We regarded $p < 0.05$ as significant.

Results

Of the 1137 pre-identified participants in the sample, all presumed to be eligible, 573 were available and willing and completed their interviews (participation proportion: 50.4%). There were more female participants (336 [58.6%]) than male (237 [41.4%]; chi-squared =

8.4448; $p = 0.0037$), necessitating gender-adjustments to observed prevalences. Mean age of participants was 40.9 ± 13.8 years; there was approximately even spread between 18 and 65, albeit with a non-significant preponderance (26.4%) among those aged 46–55 (OR: 1.3 [95% CI: 0.98–1.7]. Of those responding to the relevant questions, 62.8% were in paid employment or self-employment and 65.3% were married or living with a partner. The great majority (546 [95.3%]) were native Lithuanian speakers; only 27 (4.7%) were Russian-speaking, and only 12 of these (2.1%) were using Russian as their language at home.

Information on annual income was provided by 445 participants (77.7%). Of these, almost two thirds (292 [65.6%]) reported incomes below LTL 20,000 (USD 9000), including 170 (38.2%) below LTL 12,000 (USD 5400).

Headache prevalence

Of the 573 participants, 497 reported headache ever in their lives (lifetime prevalence: 86.7% [83.7–89.3%]). Headache in the preceding year was reported by 437 participants (76.3%), more commonly by females than males (OR: 2.7 [1.8–3.9]; $p < 0.0001$) (Table 1). The gender-adjusted 1-year prevalence of any headache was 74.7%.

Prevalence of any headache was highest (83.6%) in those aged 26–45 years (Table 1). In comparison with all other ages, prevalence fell significantly (to 62.1%) after 55 years (OR: 0.43 [0.27–0.69]; $p = 0.0014$).

HY was reported by 70 participants (12.2%) (Table 1). Females were twice as likely as males to report HY (OR: 2.4 [1.4–4.3]; $p = 0.0025$). The gender-adjusted 1-day prevalence of any headache was 11.5%. Probability of HY increased steadily with age after 35 years, doubling by 56–65 years from just over 9 to 17.9% (Table 1; OR: 2.2 [1.1–4.3], $p = 0.0307$).

Headache type

TTH (41.9%) was reported twice as commonly as migraine (20.4%); pMOH (3.5%) and other headache on ≥15 days/month (5.2%) were relatively uncommon (Table 1). There were 30 cases (5.2%) of unclassified headache among those characterised by headache on <15 days/month.

Table 1 also shows each headache type by gender and by age. Both migraine (OR: 3.6 [2.2–5.9]; $p < 0.0001$) and pMOH (OR: 2.9 [1.0–8.8]; $p = 0.0588$) were 3-fold more common among females than males, the latter not quite significantly. TTH (OR: 1.1 [0.8–1.6]) and other headache on ≥15 days/month (OR: 1.3 [0.6–2.6] were reported more commonly, but insignificantly so, by males. The gender-adjusted 1-year prevalences were 18.8% for migraine, 42.2% for TTH, 3.2% for pMOH and 5.4% for other headache on ≥15 days/month.

All headache types varied with age. Migraine increased in prevalence after age 25 years (OR: 2.9 [1.3–6.1]; $p = 0.0066$) and decreased again after 55 years (OR: 0.5 [0.3–1.0]; $p = 0.0521$). TTH declined with age from 35 years onwards, and was significantly less frequent after 55 years (OR: 0.4 [0.2–0.65]; $p = 0.0007$). pMOH showed a trend of increasing prevalence with age after 35 years (maximally among those aged 46–55 years: OR: 7.0 [0.9–55.8]; $p = 0.0677$). Numbers were too small to divide age groups by gender.

Burden attributable to headache

Symptom burden

The mean frequency of all headache was 5.0 (median 2.5) days/month), mean intensity (on the scale 1–3) was 1.7 (mild to moderate), and mean duration was 10.0 (median 2.0) hours.

Table 2 shows "usual" frequency, intensity and duration by headache type and, for migraine and TTH, by gender. Migraine was reportedly more frequent than TTH (4.4 *versus* 2.7 days/month), and also more intense (mean 2.1 [moderate pain] *versus* 1.4 [mild pain]) and longer lasting (13.0 *versus* 6.7 h, although with wide variation). The only significant gender difference was in migraine duration (males 4.5 h, females 12.6; Student's *t*-test, 2-sided: $p = 0.0003$).

Both pMOH and other headache on ≥15 days/month were, of course, far more frequent (Table 2). Intensity of pMOH was moderate to severe (mean 2.4) and of other headache on ≥15 days/month somewhat less (mean 1.8), but both types were moderate in most cases (median 2).

Disability

Mean duration of all headache was 10.0 h. Coupled with a mean frequency of 5.0 days/month, this meant that, on average, people affected by headache spent 6.9% of their total time ([5.0/30]*[10.0/24]*100) in the ictal state (*ie*, with headache).

For migraine, these values were (4.4/30)*(11.0/24)*100, equating to 6.7%. Applying the disability weight (DW) of 0.441 for migraine from GBD2013 [29], we can calculate a mean disability per person with migraine of 3.0% (that is, each person loses the equivalent of 3.0/100 healthy life years). For TTH, with a DW of 0.037 [29], we can similarly calculate a much lower mean disability per person with the disorder of 0.09% ([2.7/30]*[6.7/24]*100*0.037). For pMOH (DW 0.217 [29]), estimated disability (based on small numbers) is much higher at 6.7% ([18.5/30]*[12.1/24]*100*0.217).

Loss productive time

The HALT questionnaire captured headache-attributed lost time from paid and household work (calculated as whole days: see Methods), and missed social occasions,

Table 1 Observed and gender-adjusted prevalences (1-year) of headache types by gender and age, and of headache yesterday (1-day)

	All headache* ($n = 437$)	Migraine ($n = 117$)	Tension-type headache ($n = 240$)	Probable MOH ($n = 20$)	Other headache on ≥15 d/m ($n = 30$)	Any headache yesterday ($n = 70$)
Observed prevalences (% [95% CI])						
All ($N = 573$)	76.3 [72.6–79.6]	20.4 [17.3–23.9]	41.9 [37.9–46.0]	3.5 [2.3–5.3]	5.2 [3.7–7.4]	12 2 [9.8–15.2]
Gender						
Male ($n = 237$)	65.8 [59.6–71.6]	9.7 [5.9–13.4]	43.9 [37.6–50.2]	1.7 [0.1–3.4]	5.9 [2.9–8.9]	7.2 [3.9–10.4]
Female ($n = 336$)	83.6 [79.3–83.2]	28.0 [23.2–32.8]	40.5 [35.2–45.8]	4.8 [2.5–7.1]	4.8 [2.5–7.1]	15.8 [11.9–19.7]
Age (years)						
18–25 ($n = 108$)	75.9 [67.1–83.0]	10.2 [4.5–15.9]	50.9 [41.5–60.3]	0.9 [0–2.7]	6.5 [1.9–11.2]	9.3 [3.8–14.8]
26–35 ($n = 110$)	83.6 [75.6–89.3]	24.5 [16.5–32.5]	50.9 [41.6–60.2]	0.9 [0–2.7]	1.8 [0–4.2]	9.1 [3.7–14.5]
36–45 ($n = 108$)	82.4 [74.1–88.4]	22.2 [14.3–30.0]	49.1 [39.7–58.5]	4.6 [0.7–8.6]	3.7 [0.1–7.2]	10.2 [4.5–15.9]
46–55 ($n = 151$)	76.2 [68.8–82.3]	26.5 [19.5–33.5]	32.5 [25.0–40.1]	6.0 [2.2–9.8]	7.3 [3.2–11.5]	14.6 [9.0–20.2]
56–65 ($n = 95$)	61.1 [51.0–70.2]	15.8 [8.5–23.1]	27.4 [18.4–36.4]	4.2 [0.2–8.2]	6.3 [1.4–11.2]	17.9 [10.2–25.6]
Gender-adjusted prevalences (% [95% CI])						
All ($N = 573$)	74.7 [71.0–78.1]	18.8 [15.9–22.3]	42.2 [38.3–46.3]	3.2 [2.0–4.9]	5.4 [3.8–7.6]	11.5 [9.2–14.4]

*Including unclassified headache ($n = 30$); *MOH* medication-overuse headache, *d/m* days/month

Table 2 Symptom burden by headache type and, for migraine and tension-type headache, by gender

	All headache (*n* = 437)	Migraine (*n* = 117)			Tension-type headache (*n* = 240)			pMOH (*n* = 20)	Other headache on ≥15 d/m (*n* = 30)
		All	Male	Female	All	Male	Female		
Frequency (d/m)									
Mean ± SD	5.0 ± 6.5	4.4 ± 5.3	3.8 ± 2.8	4.6 ± 5.8	2.7 ± 3.7	2.7 ± 4.1	2.8 ± 3.4	18.5 ± 5.2	20.8 ± 6.0
Median	2.5	3.0	3.0	3.0	2.0	1.0	2.0	15.0	20.0
Quartiles 1, 3	1.0, 5.0	1.2, 5.3	2.0, 5.0	1.0, 5.6	0.8, 3.0	0.5, 3.0	1.0, 4.0	15.0, 20.0	15.0, 28.5
Intensity (scale 1–3)									
Mean ± SD	1.7 ± 0.7	2.1 ± 0.5	2.0 ± 0.4	2.1 ± 0.6	1.4 ± 0.5	1.4 ± 0.5	1.4 ± 0.5	2.4 ± 0.5	1.8 ± 0.5
Median	2	2	2	2	1	1	1	2	2
Quartiles 1, 3	1, 2	2, 2	2, 2	2, 2.5	1, 2	1, 2	1, 2	2, 3	1, 2
Duration (hr)									
Mean ± SD	10.0 ± 32.8	11.0 ± 16.3	4.5 ± 5.5	12.6 ± 17.7	6.7 ± 25.1	7.1 ± 34.4	6.5 ± 14.0	12.1 ± 9.8	9.1 ± 9.8
Median	2	4	2.75	5	2	2	2	11	3
Quartiles 1, 3	1, 6	2, 12	2, 3.75	2, 19.5	1, 3	1, 3	1, 4	3, 24	2, 24

pMOH probable medication-overuse headache; d/m: days/month

during the preceding 3 months [27]. Table 3 shows the findings from this enquiry by headache type and gender.

Here it should be noted that all but four of the 24 medians were 0, indicating on the one hand that most participants with headache lost no productive time and missed no social occasions and on the other that distributions among those who did were highly skewed, with especially badly-affected minorities. This said, mean total lost productive time from migraine was 7.3 days in males and 6.8 days in females; losses from TTH were much less (1.7 and 2.1 days respectively). Gender differences were generally small (numbers with pMOH and other headache on ≥15 days/month were too small to draw conclusions).

Assuming there were 65 (5*13) paid workdays in the preceding 3 months, the lost times from paid work attributable to migraine represented 4.5% (2.9/65) of all paid workdays in males and 3.5% (2.3/65) in females. Proportions lost from household work are less easily calculated: arguably there are 90 (3*30) potential days of household work in 3 months, but, if 65 of these are counted among paid workdays, it is also arguable that there are only 25. In the former case, losses were 4.7% (4.2/90) and 5.0% (4.5/90); in the latter 16.8% (4.2/25) and 18.0% (4.5/25). Lost times from paid work attributable to TTH were only 0.7% in both males and females. Much higher losses of 8–22 days were attributed to pMOH and other headache

Table 3 Lost productive time in whole days during the preceding 3 months, by headache type

	All headache (*n* = 437)		Migraine (*n* = 117)		Tension-type headache (*n* = 240)		Probable MOH (*n* = 20)		Other headache on ≥15 d/m (*n* = 30)	
	Male (*n* = 156)	Female (*n* = 281)	Male (*n* = 23)	Female (*n* = 94)	Male (*n* = 104)	Female (*n* = 136)	Male (*n* = 4)	Female (*n* = 16)	Male (*n* = 14)	Female (*n* = 16)
Lost paid workdays										
Mean ± SD	1.2 ± 4.5	1.5 ± 4.7	2.9 ± 7.9	2.3 ± 5.2	0.5 ± 2.9	0.5 ± 2.2	1.0 ± 2.0	6.1 ± 11.8	3.8 ± 6.6	2.2 ± 4.9
Median	0	0	0	0	0	0	0	0	0	0
Lost household workdays										
Mean ± SD	2.9 ± 8.8	3.7 ± 8.0	4.2 ± 7.6	4.5 ± 6.4	1.2 ± 3.0	1.6 ± 3.7	7.5 ± 15.0	15.6 ± 22.8	12.9 ± 23.2	7.4 ± 9.0
Median	0	0	0	2.3	0	0	0	6.0	6.0	5.0
Total mean lost workdays	4.1	5.2	7.1	6.8	1.7	2.1	8.5	21.7	16.7	9.6
Lost social occasions										
Mean ± SD	0.3 ± 1.7	0.4 ± 1.3	0.3 ± 0.8	0.7 ± 1.6	0.1 ± 0.3	0.1 ± 0.4	0	1.5 ± 2.8	1.9 ± 5.5	0.4 ± 1.0
Median	0	0	0	0	0	0	0	0	0	0

MOH medication-overuse headache; d/m: days/month

on ≥15 days/month. Lost times from paid work attributable to all headache were 1.8% (1.2/65) in males and 2.3% (1.5/65) in females.

Lost social occasions were few, although these numbers were dependent on social occasions being planned in the first place (data not collected).

Headache yesterday

Of the 70 reports of HY, one third were in participants with pMOH ($n = 10$) or other headache on ≥15 days/month ($n = 13$). We could identify headache type in 37 others (migraine $n = 19$, TTH $n = 18$), either because the participants had only one headache type or because HY was typical of their most bothersome (and therefore diagnosed) headache. These numbers were insufficient to support burden estimates from HY by headache type.

HY was mostly moderate (mean intensity 1.9 on the scale 1–3) and mostly of short duration (<4 h), although 11 participants reported >12 h. Nevertheless, HY was associated with substantial lost productivity: 30 (42.9%) of the participants with HY achieved less than half, or nothing, of whatever they had planned. Counting yesterday in such cases as a wholly lost day, these amounted to an overall lost productivity yesterday of 5.2% (30/573). Of the 33 participants with HY for whom yesterday had been a workday, 10 (30.3%) had achieved less than half or nothing of what they had expected (four taking sick leave for the whole day). These cases amounted to lost productivity from paid work yesterday of 1.7% (10/573).

Quality of life

Participants reporting no headache in the preceding year had a mean WHOQoL-8 summed score of 29.3 ± 5.8 (possible range 8–40). All headache types were associated with diminutions, which were significant for all but TTH. Participants with migraine scored 27.1 ± 6.0 (Student's t-test, 2-sided: $p = 0.0025$ *versus* no headache), those with TTH 28.4 ± 6.0 ($p = 0.126$), those with pMOH 25.8 ± 4.8 ($p = 0.0048$) and those with other headache on ≥15 days/month 24.9 ± 4.8 ($p < 0.0001$).

Discussion

As has been the case with all LTB studies, this population-based survey has revealed a lot of headache and much attributed burden. Almost three quarters (74.7%) of the Lithuanian population have a headache disorder of some type: migraine in 18.8% and TTH in 42.2%. These findings are considerably higher than global estimates of 14.7 and 20.8% from GBD studies [11–13], but within the ranges of studies using similar methodology [10] supported by LTB (15.6–25.6% for migraine, with China [9.3%] and Nepal [34.7%] outlying, and 20.6–44.6% for TTH, with China again outlying [10.8%]). We note that the GBD estimates are lowered by inclusion of studies using variable and sometimes questionable methods, and in some cases different diagnostic criteria [15]. In other words, these disorders are as common in Lithuania as everywhere else.

The relationships between headache and age are in line with expectations: both migraine and TTH are significantly less prevalent after 55 years. Migraine is strongly associated with female gender, again as expected. Migraine attacks reportedly lasted for much longer in females than in males (12.6 *versus* 4.5 h), a difference probably due largely to menstrually-related attacks. However, the medians were only 5 and 2.75 h respectively, and lower quartiles only 2 h in both genders, suggesting many attacks were truncated by treatment.

Notably, and of clear public-health concern, 3.2% of the population have pMOH. Although the prevalence of pMOH varies widely around the world, this is double the best global estimate of about 1.5% [30]; as will be seen, however, it is not an outlier. This disorder, too, is associated with female gender. More alarmingly, a total of 8.6% of the population have headache on ≥15 days/month – very high, but again not an outlier. These types of highly-frequent headache contribute substantially to the probability of HY and, in our sample, 11.5% reported HY. There was nothing special about "yesterday": it was the day before the interviewer happened to call, and might have been any day since the interviewers worked all days of the week; therefore, this finding implies that, on any day in Lithuania, a similar proportion, about one person in nine, have headache.

To add to their public-health significance, all headache types except TTH are associated with significantly diminished QoL. They are the cause of a range of other ill-health burdens. Although headache was moderate overall, mean duration was 10.0 h. People affected by headache spend 6.9% of all their time – more than one day in every 15 – in the ictal state (*ie*, with headache). For migraine it is a similar 6.7%, with an attendant disability equivalent to the loss of 3.0/100 healthy life years. Disability from TTH is much lower (0.09%), but from pMOH it is, as expected (although this estimate is based on small numbers), much higher (equivalent to the loss of 6.7/100 healthy life years).

For migraine and pMOH, these are very important penalties in lost years, incurred by those affected. Furthermore, disability translates into lost productivity. While most participants lost no productive time due to headache, and missed no social occasions, there were badly-affected minorities whose losses were substantial. As a result, mean per-person lost times from paid work attributable to migraine were 4.5% in males and 3.5% in females. These are somewhat higher than the 3.0% disability estimate, and considerable. Proportions of time lost from household work were even higher (4.7–16.8% and 5.0–18.0% respectively, depending on how these were calculated), probably reflecting the more optional nature of household work compared with paid work. The finding that lost productivity exceeds disability estimated from time spent with headache is usual, and suggests that the disabling effect of migraine in fact outlasts headache.

These individual losses allow estimates of the corresponding losses at population level. Males with migraine, losing on average 4.5% of their paid worktime, and being 9.7% of all males aged 18–65 years (effectively the working population), consequently account for 0.44% (4.5%*9.7%) lost productivity among the entire male workforce. Females with migraine, being 28.0% of all females of this age, likewise account for 1.0% (3.5%*28.0%) lost productivity among the entire female workforce. If the two genders are in equal numbers among the workforce, the losses overall are 0.7%, which may translate directly into lost gross domestic product (GDP).

The other (household) work losses to migraine are similar if based on a denominator of 90 days: 0.46 and 1.4% among all males and all females respectively. But if the denominator is 25 days, they are 1.6 and 5.0%. It is never clear what exactly people include in "household work", or how time engaged in it should be valued in comparison with paid worktime, but it certainly contributes to a nation's economy.

Lost times at individual level due to TTH were much less, but to pMOH and other headache on ≥15 days/month much greater. At population level, lost paid worktime for those with TTH can likewise be estimated at 0.3% (0.7*42.2%) overall, and those for pMOH or other headache on ≥15 days/month (very approximately from small numbers) at 0.5%. In total, from all headache types, lost productivity among the entire workforce was 1.2% (1.8%*65.8%) for males and 1.9% (2.3%*83.6%) for females. The average of 1.5% is the total potential loss to GDP from all headache.

HY offers an alternative and corroborating means of estimation. In the first place, its reported prevalence of 12.2% can be directly compared with the predicted 1-day prevalence of headache, which is the product of the observed 1-year prevalence (76.3%) and the mean probability of headache on any particular day among those with a headache disorder. The latter is calculated from the mean frequency: 5.0 days/month indicates a probability of 0.17 (5.0/30). The product of 12.7% is highly compatible with the reported prevalence of HY, suggesting very little recall error in the reporting of frequency over the last 3 months. In the second place, we calculated lost productivity from paid work yesterday of 1.7%. As noted above, there was nothing special about "yesterday", so this finding for HY seems likely to apply to every workday. This lost-productivity estimate is based on relatively small numbers, but its very close similarity to the 1.5% above generates confidence in the latter.

The limitations of this study are, to some extent, those of the Eurolight Project itself, which was "a very large and organizationally complex study, involving multiple collaborating partners (academic and lay) in ten countries [*making*] pragmatic methodological compromises in order to complete it" [31]. Eurolight also had considerable strengths: a questionnaire closely derived from the HARDSHIP questionnaire [9], and therefore validated in many different countries, cultures and translations; neutral screening questions expected to lead to better ascertainment than questions incorporating degrees of frequency or severity [8]; and diagnoses made according to a standard algorithm also widely used [9]. Nevertheless, Eurolight could not undertake further diagnostic validation in each of the translations it used, so diagnostic accuracy was not directly assessed. This was one limitation here, although we believe the instrument was reliable in view of its successful use elsewhere [9, 10], and cite, as evidence of this, the expected gender differential observed in migraine and pMOH but not TTH. The use of different sampling methods in Eurolight [22, 31] was not a limitation here, since sampling in Lithuania was population-based. While we sampled only from Kaunas region, Lithuania is a small and rather homogeneous country. More problematic was the rather small sample size of 1137, further diminished to 573 by participation of only 50.4%. Non-participants included those who had been selected but were not present on at least two visits to the household, and those declining to be interviewed (we did not seek reasons for refusal). The final value of N is above the 500 advised minimum for burden-of-headache studies [8], but the penalty is that estimates have relatively wide CIs. Additionally, although participation was much better in Lithuania than in Eurolight as a whole (27.5% on average, in those countries in which it was calculable [31]), there was still some probability of participation bias [8]. Nonetheless, the participating sample were representative for age, gender and rural/urban distribution of Lithuania's population.

With these limitations in mind, which may not be so important to health policy, it is worth comparing Lithuania with Russia. This nearby country differs ethnically from the very much smaller Lithuania, but LTB's nationwide population-based study in Russia used similar methodology and the HARDSHIP questionnaire [20, 21]. It was a larger study ($N = 2{,}725$), with a participating proportion of 74.3% ($n = 2{,}025$) [20]. The gender-adjusted 1-year prevalences were 20.8% for migraine (compared with 18.8% for Lithuania), 30.8% for TTH (42.2% for Lithuania) and 10.4% for all headache on ≥15 days/month (8.6% for Lithuania) [20]. Except for TTH, these differences are within the bounds of our uncertainty limits. The very high prevalence of headache on ≥15 days/month in Russia (10.4%) was largely behind the very high prevalence of HY (14.5%) [21]. A similar situation pertains in Lithuania: both these prevalences are only about 20% lower (8.6% and 12.2%). Where the countries differ is in pMOH: among the 10.4% in Russia with headache on ≥15 days/month, 68.1% were overusing acute medication [20], giving rise to an estimated prevalence of pMOH of 7.1% against Lithuania's 3.2%. Cost of headache to GDP in Russia was estimated at 1.75% [32], similar to (given the uncertainty limits), and supporting, the 1.5–1.7% suggested in Lithuania.

We can also compare with Georgia [18, 19], although the study here (the first supported by LTB) uniquely used a different questionnaire [33]. Like Lithuania, Georgia is a small European country, formerly part of the USSR, but it otherwise differs from Lithuania historically, ethnically and culturally. Furthermore, unlike Lithuania, which has developed rapidly since 2000 to high-income status, Georgia has remained in the lower-middle income category of countries [34]. Georgia had a larger participating sample of 1145, of whom 15.6% were diagnosed with migraine, 37.3% with TTH and 7.6% with any headache on ≥15 days/month (including, perhaps, 0.9% with pMOH) [18]. These numbers are all lower than those in Lithuania, but (except for pMOH, which may have been underestimated in Georgia [unpublished data]) only by small and non-significant margins, and these may be attributable to the different diagnostic instrument. All three countries (Lithuania, Russia and Georgia) are remarkable for the high prevalence of headache on ≥15 days/month, which calls for investigation.

Conclusions

Eurolight is not, generally, a source of reliable epidemiological data, and not designed to generate national estimates [31]. This population-based survey from Lithuania, however, was by far the most methodologically sound of the studies contributing to it. Despite the limitations mentioned, it does therefore provide a picture of headache in the country. As elsewhere, it is not a happy picture. The symptom, disability, lost-productivity and impaired-QoL burdens signal substantial ill-health, and therefore unmet need for health care [14]. This is a message that has been repeated to policy-makers in countries all over the world [34], but here, from this study, is empirical evidence to underpin it in Lithuania.

As in other countries, the high impact on individuals is matched by high economic burden; both are unmitigated by failures in health care. Health policy in Lithuania must take note of these findings, and of WHO's advice that effective treatment of headache is desirable not only for its health benefits but also because it is likely to be cost-saving [35]. There are recommendations, for Europe, on the organisation of headache services to meet need [36].

Acknowledgements
The Eurolight Project was funded by the European Agency for Health and Consumers (EAHC), Fonds National Luxembourg (FNR), with additional support from *Lifting The Burden*.
We are grateful to the medical students from the Lithuanian University of Health Sciences, Kaunas, who collected the data for this survey by visiting the households of participants.

Authors' contributions
D Rastenytė was principal investigator in Lithuania. She contributed to development of the specific methodology employed in Lithuania, to patient enrolment and data collection, and to manuscript preparation. D Mickevičienė contributed to patient enrolment and data collection. LJ Stovner was a member of the Eurolight Steering Committee and in part responsible for the design of the Eurolight Project. He contributed to development of the specific methodology employed in Lithuania, to data interpretation and to manuscript preparation. H Thomas performed the data analysis. C Andrée was instigator and project leader of the Eurolight Project. TJ Steiner was a member of the Eurolight Steering Committee, and in part responsible for the design of the Eurolight Project. He contributed to data analysis, was primarily responsible for data interpretation and drafted the manuscript. All authors reviewed and approved the final manuscript.

Competing interests
LJ Stovner and TJ Steiner are Directors and Trustees of *Lifting The Burden*. No other competing interests were declared.

Author details
[1]Lithuanian University of Health Sciences, Kaunas, Lithuania. [2]Department of Neuromedicine and Movement Science, Faculty of Medicine and Health Sciences, NTNU Norwegian University of Science and Technology, Trondheim NO-7941, Norway. [3]Norwegian Advisory Unit on Headache, St Olavs University Hospital, Trondheim, Norway. [4]Department of Pharmaceutical Sciences, University of Basel, Basel, Switzerland. [5]Division of Brain Sciences, Imperial College London, London, UK.

References

1. World Health Organization (2000) Headache disorders and public health. Education and management implications. WHO, Geneva
2. World Health Organization (2001) The World Health Report 2001. WHO, Geneva
3. Stovner L, Hagen K, Jensen R, Katsarava Z, Lipton R, Scher A, Steiner T, Zwart JA (2007) The Global burden of headache: a documentation of headache prevalence and disability worldwide. Cephalalgia 27:193–210
4. Steiner TJ (2004) Lifting the burden: the global campaign against headache. Lancet Neurol 3:204–205
5. Steiner TJ, Birbeck GL, Jensen R, Katsarava Z, Martelletti P, Stovner LJ (2011) The Global Campaign, World Health Organization and *Lifting The Burden*: collaboration in action. J Headache Pain 12:273–274
6. Steiner TJ (2005) *Lifting The Burden*: the global campaign to reduce the burden of headache worldwide. J Headache Pain 6:373–377
7. Steiner TJ, Birbeck GL, Jensen R, Katsarava Z, Martelletti P, Stovner LJ (2010) *Lifting The Burden*: the first 7 years. J Headache Pain 11:451–455
8. Stovner LJ Al Jumah M, Birbeck GL, Gururaj G, Jensen R, Katsarava Z, Queiroz LP, Scher AI, Tekle-Haimanot R, Wang SJ, Steiner TJ (2014) The methodology of population surveys of headache prevalence, burden and cost: principles and recommendations from the Global Campaign against Headache. J Headache Pain 15:5
9. Steiner TJ, Gururaj G, Andrée C, Katsarava Z, Ayzenberg I, Yu SY, Al Jumah M, Tekle-Haimanot R, Birbeck GL, Herekar A, Linde M, Mbewe E, Manandhar K, Risal A, Jensen R, Queiroz LP, Scher AI, Wang SJ, Stovner LJ (2014) Diagnosis, prevalence estimation and burden measurement in population surveys of headache: presenting the HARDSHIP questionnaire. J Headache Pain 15:3

10. *Lifting The Burden*. Current priority localities and countries. At: http://www.l-t-b.org/index.cfm/spKey/on_locality_national_fronts.current_priority_localities_countries.html. Accessed 5 Feb 2017.
11. Vos T, Flaxman AD, Naghavi M, Lozano R, Michaud C, Ezzati M, Shibuya K, Salomon JA, Abdalla S, Aboyans V, Abraham J, Ackerman I, Aggarwal R, Ahn SY, Ali MK, Alvarado M, Anderson HR, Anderson LM, Andrews KG, Atkinson C, Baddour LM, Bahalim AN, Barker-Collo S, Barrero LH, Bartels DH, Basáñez MG, Baxter A, Bell ML, Benjamin EJ, Bennett D et al (2012) Years lived with disability (YLDs) for 1160 sequelae of 289 diseases and injuries 1990–2010: a systematic analysis for the Global Burden of Disease Study 2010. Lancet 380:2163–2196
12. Vos T, Barber RM, Bell B, Bertozzi-Villa A, Biryukov S, Bolliger I, Charlson F, Davis A, Degenhardt L, Dicker D, Duan L, Erskine H, Feigin VL, Ferrari AJ, Fitzmaurice C, Fleming T, Graetz N, Guinovart C, Haagsma J, Hansen GM, Hanson SW, Heuton KR, Higashi H, Kassebaum N, Kyu H, Laurie E, Liang X, Lofgren K, Lozano R, MacIntyre MF et al (2015) Global, regional, and national incidence, prevalence, and years lived with disability for 301 acute and chronic diseases and injuries in 188 countries, 1990–2013: a systematic analysis for the Global Burden of Disease Study 2013. Lancet 386:743–800
13. Vos T, Allen C, Arora M, Barber RM, Bhutta ZA, Brown A, Carter A, Casey DC, Charlson FJ, Chen AZ, Coggeshall M, Cornaby L, Dandona L, Dicker DJ, Dilegge T, Erskine HE, Ferrari AJ, Fitzmaurice C, Fleming T, Forouzanfar MH, Fullman N, Gething PW, Goldberg EM, Graetz N, Haagsma JA, Hay SI, Johnson CO, Kassebaum NJ, Kawashima T, Kemmer L, Khalil IA, Kinfu Y, Kyu HH, Leung J, Liang X et al (2016) Global, regional, and national incidence, prevalence, and years lived with disability for 310 diseases and injuries, 1990–2015: a systematic analysis for the Global Burden of Disease Study 2015. Lancet 388:1545–1602
14. Steiner TJ, Birbeck GL, Jensen RH, Katsarava Z, Stovner LJ, Martelletti P (2015) Headache disorders are third cause of disability worldwide. J Headache Pain 16:544
15. Steiner TJ, Stovner LJ, Vos T (2016) GBD 2015: migraine is the third cause of disability in under 50s. J Headache Pain 17:104
16. Stovner L, Andrée C, on behalf of the Eurolight Steering Committee (2008) Impact of headache in Europe: a review for the Eurolight project. J Headache Pain 9:139–146
17. Stovner LJ, Andrée C (2010) Prevalence of headache in Europe: a review for the Eurolight project. J Headache Pain 11:289–299
18. Katsarava Z, Dzagnidze A, Kukava M, Mirvelashvili E, Djibuti M, Janelidze M, Jensen R, Stovner LJ, Steiner TJ (2009) Primary headache disorders in the Republic of Georgia: prevalence and risk factors. Neurology 73:1796–1803
19. Katsarava Z, Dzagnidze A, Kukava M, Mirvelashvili E, Djibuti M, Janelidze M, Jensen R, Stovner LJ, Steiner TJ (2009) Prevalence of cluster headache in the Republic of Georgia: results of a population-based study and methodological considerations. Cephalalgia 29:949–952
20. Ayzenberg I, Katsarava Z, Sborowski A, Chernysh M, Osipova V, Tabeeva G, Yakhno N, Steiner TJ (2012) The prevalence of primary headache disorders in Russia: a countrywide survey. Cephalalgia 32:373–381
21. Ayzenberg I, Katsarava Z, Sborowski A, Obermann M, Chernysh M, Osipova V, Tabeeva G, Steiner TJ (2015) Headache yesterday in Russia: its prevalence and impact, and their application in estimating the national burden attributable to headache disorders. J Headache Pain 16:7
22. Andrée C, Stovner LJ, Steiner TJ, Barré J, Katsarava Z, Lainez JM, Lanteri-Minet M, Mick G, Rastenyte D, Ruiz de la Torre E, Tassorelli C, Vriezen P, Lampl C (2011) The Eurolight project: the impact of primary headache disorders in Europe. Description of methods. J Headache Pain 12:541–549
23. Lithuanian Ministry of Justice. State Enterprise Centre of Registers. At: http://www.registrucentras.lt/gr/index_en.php. Accessed 5 Feb 2017.
24. Andrée C, Vaillant M, Barré J, Katsarava Z, Lainez JM, Lair ML, Lanteri-Minet M, Lampl C, Steiner TJ, Stovner LJ, Tassorelli C, Sándor PS (2010) Development and validation of the EUROLIGHT questionnaire to evaluate the burden of primary headache disorders in Europe. Cephalalgia 30:1082–1100
25. Peters M, Bertelote JM, Houchin C, Kandoura T, Steiner TJ (2007) Translation protocols. J Headache Pain 8:S40–S47
26. International Headache Society Classification Subcommittee (2004) The international classification of headache disorders, 2nd edn. Cephalalgia 24:1–160
27. Steiner TJ (2007) The HALT and HART indices. J Headache Pain 8:S22–S25
28. The WHO QoL Group (1998) Development of the World Health Organization WHO QoL_BREF quality of life assessment. Psychol Med 28:551–558
29. Salomon JA, Haagsma JA, Davis A, Maertens de Noordhout C, Polinder S, Havelaar AH, Cassini A, Devleesschauwer B, Kretzschmar M, Speybroeck N, Murray CJL, Vos T (2015) Disability weights for the Global Burden of Disease 2013 study. Lancet Global Health 3:e712–e723
30. Westergaard ML, Hansen EH, Glumer C, Olesen J, Jensen RH (2014) Definitions of medication-overuse headache in population-based studies and their implications on prevalence estimates: a systematic review. Cephalalgia 34:409–425
31. Steiner TJ, Stovner LJ, Zaza Katsarava Z, Lainez JM, Lampl C, Lantéri-Minet M, Rastenyte D, Ruiz de la Torre E, Tassorelli C, Barré J, Andrée C (2014) The impact of headache in Europe: principal results of the Eurolight project. J Headache Pain 14:31
32. Ayzenberg I, Katsarava Z, Sborowski A, Chernysh M, Osipova V, Tabeeva G, Steiner TJ (2014) Headache-attributed burden and its impact on productivity and quality of life in Russia: structured health care for headache is urgently needed. Eur J Neurol 21:758–765
33. Kukava M, Dzagnidze A, Janelidze M, Mirvelashvili E, Djibuti M, Fritsche G, Jensen R, Stovner LJ, Steiner TJ, Katsarava Z (2007) Validation of a Georgian language headache questionnaire in a population-based sample. J Headache Pain 8:321–324
34. World Bank. At: http://www.worldbank.org/en/results. Accessed 6 Feb 2017.
35. World Health Organization (2011) Atlas of headache disorders and resources in the world 2011. WHO, Geneva
36. Steiner TJ, Antonaci F, Jensen R, Lainez JMA, Lanteri-Minet M, Valade D (2011) Recommendations for headache service organisation and delivery in Europe. J Headache Pain 12:419–426

17

Post-traumatic headache in patients with minimal traumatic intracranial hemorrhage after traumatic brain injury

Chang-Ki Hong[1,2], Yu Shik Shim[3], Sook Young Sim[4], Jin-Yang Joo[1], Min A Kwon[1], Yong Bae Kim[1] and Joonho Chung[1,2,5*]

Abstract

Background: No evidence is available on the risks of neurologically asymptomatic minimal traumatic intracranial hemorrhage (mTIH) in patients with traumatic brain injury (TBI) for post-traumatic headache (PTH). The purpose of this study was to investigate whether mTIH in patients with TBI was associated with PTH and to evaluate its risk factors.

Methods: Between September 2009 and December 2014, 1484 patients with TBI were treated at our institution, 57 of whom had mTIH after TBI and were include in this study. We performed propensity score matching to establish a control group among the 823 patients with TBI treated during the same period. Patients with TBI rated their headaches prospectively using a numeric rating scale (NRS). We compared NRS scores between mTIH group ($n = 57$) and non-mTIH group ($n = 57$) and evaluated risk factors of moderate-to-severe PTH (NRS ≥ 4) at the 12-month follow-up.

Results: Moderate-to-severe PTH was reported by 21.9% of patients (29.8% in mTIH group and 14.0% in non-mTIH group B, $p = 0.012$) at the 12-month follow-up. The mean NRS was higher in mTIH group than in non-mTIH group throughout the follow-up period (95% confidence interval [CI], 0.11 to 1.14; $p < 0.05$, ANCOVA). Logistic regression analysis showed that post-traumatic seizure (odds ratio, 1.520; 95% CI, 1.128–6.785; $p = 0.047$) and mTIH (odds ratio, 2.194; 95% CI, 1.285–8.475; $p = 0.039$) were independently associated with moderate-to-severe PTH at the 12-month follow-up.

Conclusions: Moderate-to-severe PTH can be expected after TBI in patients with mTIH and post-traumatic seizure. PTH occurs more frequently in patients with mTIH than in those without mTIH.

Keywords: Head trauma, Post-traumatic headache, Traumatic brain injury, Traumatic intracranial hemorrhage

Background

Patients with traumatic brain injury (TBI) can have only a brief change in mental status, such as confusion, disorientation, loss of memory, or loss of consciousness (LOC) for less than 30 min, without serious permanent neurological deficits even if they have abnormal radiological findings. Previously, studies that addressed patients with neurologically asymptomatic minimal traumatic intracranial hemorrhage (mTIH) received little attention as the clinical course of most patients with mTIH is good, without morbidity or mortality. However, they frequently experience post-traumatic headache (PTH) that may affect the quality of life [1]. Little is known about PTH in patients with mTIH as, ultimately, achieving a good clinical outcome (to minimize morbidity and mortality) in patients with severe intracranial findings is of higher importance than PTH.

PTH refers to a headache that develops within 1 week after head trauma. During the first 3 months from onset, PTH is considered acute. Persistent PTH was described as headache of greater than 3 months' duration caused by traumatic injury to the head. The term persistent has

* Correspondence: ns.joonho.chung@gmail.com
[1]Department of Neurosurgery, Gangnam Severance Hospital, Yonsei University College of Medicine, 211, Eonjuro, Gangnam-gu, Seoul 06273, Republic of Korea
[2]Severance Institute for Vascular and Metabolic Research, Yonsei University, Seoul, Republic of Korea
Full list of author information is available at the end of the article

been adopted in place of chronic [2]. Although most PTHs resolve within 6 to 12 months after injury, approximately 18–33% of PTHs persist beyond 12 months [3]. PTH is known to be related to other problems, such as depression, cognitive dysfunction, or insomnia [4]. However, risk factors for development of PTH in patients with mTIH after TBI have not been determined. The incidence of PTH and its impact may be different in patients with mTIH than in those with without mTIH. Therefore, the purpose of this matched case-control study was therefore to investigate whether mTIH in patients with TBI was associated with PTH and to evaluate its risk factors.

Methods

This study, a retrospective case-control study from a prospectively collected database, was approved by our institutional review board, and informed consent was waived. Between September 2009 and December 2014, 1484 patients with TBI rated their headaches prospectively using a numeric rating scale (NRS). Among these patients, 57 (mTIH group) were included in the present study as they met the following criteria: (1) presence of headache due to head trauma; (2) presence of traumatic intracranial hemorrhage on radiographic images (computed tomography [CT] or magnetic resonance image [MRI]); (3) age ≥ 15 years; (4) initial Glasgow Coma Scale (GCS) ≥ 13; and (5) transient LOC ≤ 30 min. Of the 1427 remaining patients with TBI in the database, 604 were excluded for the following reasons: (1) initial GCS < 13 (n = 235); (2) initial or follow-up modified Rankin Scale (mRS) ≥ 3 (n = 45); (3) history of neurosurgery (craniotomy due to any cause) (n = 29); (4) TBI due to any cerebrovascular disease (n = 81); (5) history of previously diagnosed intracranial disease (n = 34); (5) post-traumatic amnesia >24 h (n = 22); (6) delayed hemorrhage (>24 h) (n = 22); (7) combined spinal cord injury (n = 74); (8) incomplete NRS score data (n = 14) and (9) loss to follow-up (n = 48). Among the remaining 823 patients, we performed propensity score matching to establish a proper control group (n = 57, non-mTIH group). All of them have experienced headache due to head trauma. Our inclusion/exclusion criteria have contained the definition of mild TBI since mild TBI, in general, is defined as TBI resulting in GCS ≥ 13, LOC ≤ 30 min, and post-traumatic amnesia ≤24 h [5, 6]. According to the GCS scoring system, moderate TBI is defined as a GCS of 9 to 12 and severe TBI is defined as a GCS of 3 to 8.p-h.

Three independent investigators blinded to the data retrospectively reviewed the clinical and radiographic data of the included patients using their medical records. Variables evaluated and compared between groups were age, gender, initial GCS score, cause of TBI, mechanism of TBI, type of mTIH, initial symptoms and signs (LOC, vomiting, tinnitus, visual symptoms, confusion, post-traumatic amnesia, and post-traumatic seizure), previously physician-diagnosed headache (treated by medications), and use of antiplatelet agent and/or anticoagulant. Anticonvulsant agents including topiramate or valproate have been given to all patients who experienced post-traumatic seizures.

Intensity of headache was assessed with the NRS, an 11-point numeric scale for rating pain intensity. The quantitative scale ranges from 0 to 10, with 0 meaning "no headache at all" and 10 meaning "the worst possible headache." This 11-point scale has been previously applied to headache assessment [7–9]. We defined NRS scores of 1 to 3, 4 to 6, and 7 to 10 as mild, moderate, and severe headache, respectively. Mild headache was described as nagging, annoying, or interfering little with active daily living. Moderate headache was described as interfering significantly with active daily living. Severe headache was described as disabling or interfering to the point that patients were unable to perform active daily activities. Thus, we defined an NRS score ≥ 4 as significant. All included patients visited the emergency department or the outpatient office within 48 h of onset. NRS score was determined every 8 h (three times per day) during a patient's hospitalization and twice during each outpatient visit. Analgesics were prescribed to patients with headache. Patient NRS scores were collected and averaged for the on initial visit and at 1-week, 1-month, 3-month, 6-month, and 12-month follow-ups. We compared the NRS and its changes between groups and evaluated risk factors of moderate-to-severe PTH (NRS ≥ 4) at the 12-month follow-up.

Propensity score matching was performed using multiple logistic regression to match patients who had mTIH with those that did not have mTIH with respect to age, gender, initial GCS score, and cause of TBI. After patient matching by estimated propensity scores via a conditional logistic regression method, multiple logistic regression analysis was performed. Using the logit estimated from the log odds of the propensity score of each patient, we matched the selected cases with controls who had the nearest estimated logit value by 1:1 matching. Balance between mTIH group and non-mTIH group for each variable was evaluated by propensity score distributions and absolute standardized differences (ASD) before and after matching were calculated (Fig. 1). An ASD < 0.10 implies good balance between the two groups. A complete set of baseline data is essential to develop a propensity model. Thus, we replaced missing data values with the mean for that variable instead of excluding patients with missing data.

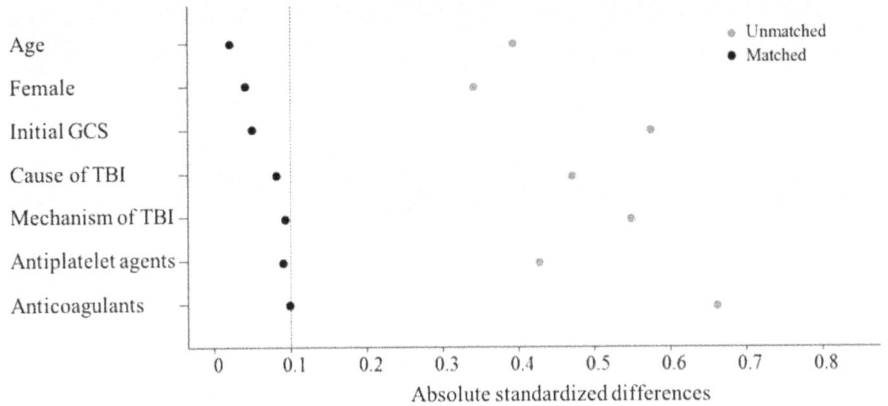

Fig. 1 Absolute standardized difference (ASD) before and after propensity score matching. ASD < 0.10 implies good balance between the two groups. GCS, Glasgow Coma Scale; TBI, traumatic brain injury

Statistical analysis

All statistical analyses were consulted with a biostatistician and were performed using R language ver. 3.01 (R Foundation for Statistical Computing, Vienna, Austria). Student's t tests were used for numeric variables. Chi-square tests were used for nominal variables. An ANCOVA with a general linear model, with group and follow-up time point as fixed factors, was used to compare the average NRS scores at each follow-up period between the two groups. Logistic regression analysis was performed to determine the independent risk factors of moderate-to-severe PTH at the 12-month follow-up. Multiple logistic regression analysis was performed on variables with an unadjusted effect and a *p*-value <0.10 on simple logistic regression analysis. Statistical significance was defined by a *p*-value <0.05 with a 95% confidence interval.

Results

The clinical characteristics of propensity score-matched subjects in both groups are presented in Table 1. Mean age was 34.7 ± 11.2 years in mTIH group and 34.4 ± 11.9 years in non-mTIH group (p = 0.916). There were 25 (43.9%) females in mTIH group and 26 (45.6%) in non-mTIH group (p = 0.864), while 43.9% of patients in mTIH group and 47.4% in non-mTIH group had an initial GCS score of 15 (p = 0.838). Motor vehicle accident (59.6% in mTIH group and 57.9% in non-mTIH group) was the most frequent cause of TBI (p = 0.782). Head striking an object (68.4% in mTIH group and 63.2% in non-mTIH group) was the most frequent mechanism of TBI, followed by head being struck (19.3% in mTIH group and 21.1% in non-mTIH group) and whiplash (12.3% in mTIH group and 15.8% in non-mTIH group) (p = 0.705). In mTIH group, subarachnoid hemorrhage was the most frequent mTIH (68.4%), followed by subdural hemorrhage (49.1%), epidural hemorrhage (29.8%), intraventricular hemorrhage (7.0%), and contusional hemorrhage (3.5%).

More patients experienced LOC after trauma in mTIH group (68.4%) than in non-mTIH group (42.6%, p = 0.046). Six (10.5%) of the 57 patients in mTIH group and one (1.8%) of the 57 patients in non-mTIH group experienced post-traumatic seizure, which was a significant difference (p = 0.005). Among the six patients with post-traumatic seizure in mTIH group, two patients had contusional hemorrhage and subarachnoid hemorrhage together in the frontal lobe, one had subdural hemorrhage and subarachnoid hemorrhage together in the fronto-temporal lobe, two had subdural hemorrhage in the fronto-parietal lobe, and one had epidural hemorrhage in the parietal lobe. An initial moderate-to-severe headache occurred in 71.1% of patients overall (75.4% in mTIH group and 66.7% in non-mTIH group, p = 0.079). At the 12-month follow-up, moderate-to-severe PTH occurred in 21.9% of all patients. Seventeen (29.8%) of the 57 patients in mTIH group had moderate-to-severe PTH, while eight (14.0%) of the 57 patients in non-mTIH group had moderate-to-severe PTH (p = 0.012). When the two groups were assessed throughout the 12-month follow-up period, the difference in NRS scores was statistically significant (95% confidence interval, 0.11 to 1.14; $p < 0.05$, ANCOVA), which was consistent over time (Fig. 2).

Multiple logistic regression analysis showed that post-traumatic seizure (odds ratio, 1.520; 95% CI, 1.128–6.785; p = 0.047) and mTIH (odds ratio, 2.194; 95% CI, 1.285–8.475; p = 0.039) were independently associated with moderate-to-severe PTH (NRS ≥ 4) at the 12-month follow-up (Table 2). Initial headache intensity had a *p*-value of 0.044 in simple logistic regression analysis, but was not statistically significant after adjustment (p = 0.094).

Table 1 Clinical characteristics of propensity score-matched subjects

	mTIH (*n* = 57)	non-mTIH (*n* = 57)	*p* value
Age (mean ± SD)	34.7 ± 11.2	34.4 ± 11.9	0.916
Female (n, %)	25 (43.9)	26 (45.6)	0.864
Initial GCS score (n, %)			0.838
15	25 (43.9)	27 (47.4)	
14	21 (36.8)	21 (36.8)	
13	11 (19.3)	9 (15.8)	
Cause of traumatic brain injury (n, %)			0.782
Motor vehicle accident	34 (59.6)	33 (57.9)	
Fall from height	12 (21.1)	12 (21.1)	
Direct hit on the head	11 (19.3)	12 (21.1)	
Mechanism of traumatic brain injury (n, %)			0.705
Whiplash	7 (12.3)	9 (15.8)	
Head being struck	11 (19.3)	12 (21.1)	
Head striking an object	39 (68.4)	36 (63.2)	
Type of traumatic intracranial hemorrhage (n, %)			-
Subarachnoid	39 (68.4)	-	
Contusional	2 (3.5)	-	
Epidural	17 (29.8)	-	
Subdural	28 (49.1)	-	
Intraventricular	4 (7.0)	-	
Loss of consciousness (n, %)	39 (68.4)	23 (42.6)	0.046
Vomiting (n, %)	19 (33.3)	13 (22.8)	0.194
Tinnitus (n, %)	4 (7.0)	7 (12.3)	0.341
Visual symptoms (n, %)	5 (8.8)	3 (5.3)	0.436
Confusion (n, %)	13 (22.8)	9 (15.8)	0.208
Post-traumatic amnesia (n, %)	15 (26.3)	10 (17.5)	0.145
Post-traumatic seizure (n, %)	6 (10.5)	1 (1.8)	0.005
Previously diagnosed headache (n, %)	9 (15.8)	14 (24.6)	0.172
Antiplatelet agent (n, %)	4 (7.0)	5 (8.8)	0.734
Anticoagulant (n, %)	1 (1.8)	0 (0)	0.681
Initial headache intensity (n, %)			0.079
Mild (NRS 0–3)	14 (24.6)	19 (33.3)	
Moderate-to-Severe (NRS 4–10)	43 (75.4)	38 (66.7)	
PTH at 12-month follow-up (n, %)			0.012
Mild (NRS 0–3)	40 (70.2)	49 (86.0)	
Moderate-to-Severe (NRS 4–10)	17 (29.8)	8 (14.0)	

Abbreviations: *GCS* Glasgow Coma Scale, *mTIH* minimal traumatic intracranial hemorrhage, *NRS* numeric rating scale, *PTH* post-traumatic headache, *SD* standard deviation

Discussion

Patients with mTIH after TBI were more likely to experience LOC and post-traumatic seizure than were patients without mTIH. Throughout the 12-month follow-up, NRS scores in patients with mTIH were significantly higher than in those without mTIH. The overall occurrence rate of moderate-to-severe PTH was 21.9% at the 12-month follow-up. Moderate-to-severe PTH might be expected in patients with post-traumatic seizure and mTIH after TBI.

The reported prevalence of PTH due to TBI ranges between 20 and 89% [2, 10–12]. Two recent studies examined the rate of headache longitudinally among a large cohort during the first year after TBI [13, 14]. The

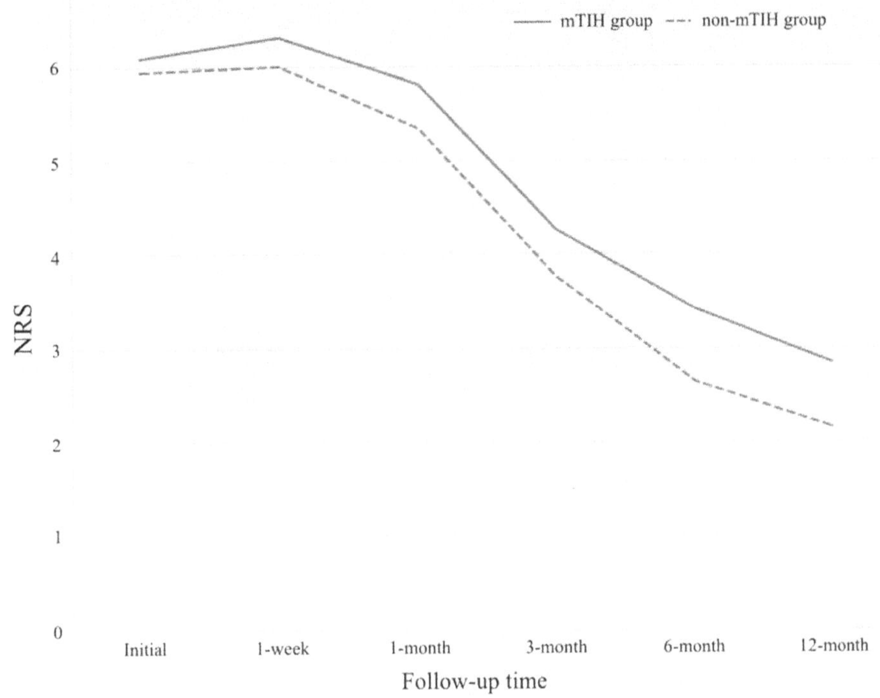

Fig. 2 Mean numeric rating scale (NRS) scores of both groups. The difference in NRS scores between mTIH groups and non-mTIH group was statistically significant (95% confidence interval, 0.11 to 1.14; $p < 0.05$, ANCOVA)

incidence at baseline was 44–54%, and the cumulative incidence of headache over 1 year was 71–91%. More than one-third of the subjects reported persistent headache throughout the follow-up period. In the present study, the prevalence of PTH (mild, moderate, and severe PTH) was 57.9% at the 12-month follow-up, which seemed to be higher than the previously reported prevalence. We focused on moderate-to-severe PTH, which might have more clinical relevance, because mild PTH (NRS 1 to 3) was described as interfering little with activities of daily living, while moderate-to-severe PTH (NRS 4 to 10) interfered with or prevented activities of daily living.

Pathophysiology and characteristics of PTH in patients with mTIH after TBI are not well understood. Consequently, the best treatment options for PTH remain unclear. Although PTH affects patient quality of life, patients with mTIH after TBI tends to be neglected in the real world because the clinical focus is to achieve a good outcome (to minimize morbidity and mortality) in patients with severe intracranial findings. However, we felt that it was worthwhile to study the incidence and risk factors of PTH in patients with mTIH after TBI. We identified two risk factors, mTIH and post-traumatic seizure, that were related to moderate-to-severe PTH at the 12-month follow-up in patients with mTIH after TBI. These data may allow providers to educate their patients about what they may expect with regards to PTH after mTIH.

Presence of mTIH after TBI suggests a greater impact force on the brain than absence of mTIH after TBI. This may explain why mTIH group had more patients who experienced LOC, post-traumatic seizure, and PTH than non-mTIH group in the present study. Post-traumatic seizure is more likely to occur in more severe injuries. Post-traumatic seizure that occurs immediately after TBI is thought to be a direct reaction to the injury. This happens because the force from the injury stimulates brain tissue that has a low threshold for seizures when stimulated [15, 16]. Early post-traumatic seizure can be caused by factors such as intracranial hemorrhage or cerebral contusion [15, 17]. Since we have not analyzed the relationship between post-traumatic seizure and types of mTIH, it was not clear if post-traumatic seizure was related to any type of mTIH in the present study. It is known that PTH after TBI can be caused by axonal shear, resulting in incomplete neuronal transmission, or by induction of trigeminal nociception, which subsequently results in cortical spreading depression [18]. The impact force of the trauma that produced the mTIH might provoke PTH by inducing incomplete neuronal transmission or cortical spreading depression. In the same context, 54.4% (62/114) of LOC (68.4% in mTIH group and 42.6% in non-mTIH group) in the present study, that seemed a bit high for patients with mild TBI, can be understood. The initial impact to the head could be more severe in patients of the present study than

Table 2 Risk factors for moderate-to-severe headache at the 12-month follow-up

	Simple logistic regression		Multiple logistic regression	
	OR (95% CI)	*p* value	OR (95% CI)	*p* value
Age in years				
<35	1			
≥35	1.407 (0.529–3.106)	0.748		
Gender				
Female	1			
Male	0.912 (0.478–2.106)	0.649		
Initial GCS				
15	1			
<15	1.794 (0.593–3.377)	0.573		
Cause of traumatic brain injury				
Motor vehicle accident	1			
Fall from height	2.975 (0.636–4.647)	0.443		
Direct hit on the head	0.846 (0.743–3.226)	0.384		
Mechanism of traumatic brain injury				
Whiplash	1			
Head being struck	1.839 (0.475–7.552)	0.751		
Head striking an object	2.883 (0.748–3.424)	0.395		
Loss of consciousness				
No	1		1	
Yes	2.174 (0.944–3.806)	0.078	2.311 (0.839–4.394)	0.162
Vomiting				
No	1			
Yes	2.082 (0.624–4.771)	0.736		
Tinnitus				
No	1			
Yes	0.859 (0.344–1.176)	0.611		
Visual symptoms				
No	1			
Yes	1.075 (0.525–3.239)	0.522		
Confusion				
No	1			
Yes	1.742 (0.438–2.262)	0.704		
Post-traumatic amnesia				
No	1			
Yes	2.242 (0.748–5.680)	0.663		
Post-traumatic seizure				
No	1		1	
Yes	1.779 (1.205–4.430)	0.035	1.520 (1.128–6.785)	0.047
Previously diagnosed headache				
No	1		1	
Yes	1.835 (0.806–4.704)	0.082	1.503 (0.724–5.960)	0.179

Table 2 Risk factors for moderate-to-severe headache at the 12-month follow-up *(Continued)*

Initial headache intensity				
Mild (NRS 0–3)	1		1	
Moderate-to-Severe (NRS 4–10)	2.927 (1.348–4.612)	0.044	2.154 (0.925–6.319)	0.094
mTIH				
No	1		1	
Yes	2.883 (1.038–6.124)	0.021	2.194 (1.285–8.475)	0.039

Abbreviations: *CI* confidence interval, *GCS* Glasgow Coma Scale, *mTIH* minimal traumatic intracranial hemorrhage, *NRS* numeric rating scale, *OR* odds ratio

those with mild TBI in general because a half of our patients had visible abnormalities on structural neuroimaging. Beetar et al. have previously reported that 62.9% (127/202) of their patients with mild TBI had LOC [19].

Based on our findings, brain CTs to detect mTIH in patients with TBI may be important because mTIH was associated with moderate-to-severe PTH throughout the 12-month follow-up period. There is significant disagreement about the indications for brain CT scan in such patients after TBI because of the cost, time, and probable complications of radiation [20]. Symptoms such as headache, vomiting, LOC, amnesia, post-traumatic seizure, skull fracture, contusion, raccoon sign, alcohol intoxication, coagulopathy, and age more than 60 years have been proposed as risk indicators of abnormalities in brain CT scans of patients with TBI; if any patient has these indicators following TBI, the patient should be considered to be at high-risk for abnormal CT findings [21]. However, no consensus has been achieved in the indications for brain CT scan. Nevertheless, headache by itself, as an initial symptom, can be used as a guide to predict the probability of an abnormal brain CT scan related to TBI [22, 23]. In our institution, we performed brain CT scans of as many patients with newly developed headache after head trauma as possible, but not in all patients. This is one of the limitations of our study and is described in detail below. We could not include some patients with mTIH because they did not have radiographic images. Patients with neurologically asymptomatic mTIH after TBI require close observation not only because of aggravation of hematoma and edema in the acute period, but because of PTH during the follow-up period. Risk factors of PTH should not be neglected, and appropriate medications should be prescribed for patients with mTIH who develop PTH after TBI.

There are several limitations to this study. First, this was a retrospective study with a small number of patients; therefore, there is potential for selection bias even though we performed propensity score matching. We did not have a database of patients who did not undergo CT scan after head injury. Because we required radiographic evidence of traumatic intracranial hemorrhage, we could not include those patients who did not have radiographic images. These patients may have had mTIH initially or PTH afterward, which could have altered our findings. Second, we also did not compare headache characteristics, such as type, onset, duration, or frequency, between groups. The most frequent types of PTH are migraine, tension-type headache, and cervicogenic headache [13]. Our results may have been different if we had evaluated PTH characteristics. However, our focus was headache intensity as assessed by a subjective score (NRS score), because we were interested in PTH in general and its potential effects on activities of daily living. In addition, we included patients who did not have neurological disability with GCS ≥ 13 because disability could affect PTH. We, also, excluded patients with spinal cord injury because some patients with TBI could have headaches secondary to spinal cord injury. Third, we did not obtain sufficient information about headache medications. Although medications may be an important factor affecting headache improvement, it was very difficult to analyze when or how medications were used, preventing such an analysis. However, we attempted to evaluate the correlation between previously physician-diagnosed headache treated by medication and moderate-to-severe PTH at the 12-month follow-up. Fourth, we could not have defined the type of post-traumatic seizures (generalized tonic-clonic, partial, or partial complex seizures) nor have had the results of electroencephalogram in all patients who experienced post-traumatic seizure since our database only has clinical signs of post-traumatic seizure. Finally, we did not evaluate symptoms related to cognitive, behavioral, or emotional dysfunction. We only evaluated and focused on a single physical symptom, PTH. Cognitive symptoms may result from dysfunctions of attention, concentration, memory, processing speed, judgment, and executive functioning. Behavioral or emotional symptoms may include depression, anxiety, agitation, irritability, and aggression. It is believed that those cognitive, behavioral, and emotional symptoms resulting from mTIH after TBI are inter-related; alleviation of one symptom often leads to improvement in others [24]. Consequently, aggressive treatment of any comorbid psychiatric illness may help to improve PTH, and vice versa. Thus, these symptoms may be risk factors of PTH after TBI and have important clinical implications. Future research is needed to evaluate the role of these kinds of symptoms in the development of PTH.

Conclusions

Moderate-to-severe PTH might occur after TBI in patients with mTIH and post-traumatic seizure. PTH appears to occur more frequently in patients with mTIH than in those without mTIH. In patients with mTIH, letting them be aware of what they can expect with regards to PTH after mTIH might be necessary.

Abbreviations

ASD: Absolute standardized differences; CI: Confidence interval; CT: Computed tomography; GCS: Glasgow Coma Scale; LOC: Loss of consciousness; MRI: Magnetic resonance image; mRS: Modified Rankin Scale; mTIH: Minimal traumatic intracranial hemorrhage; NRS: Numeric rating scale; PTH: Post-traumatic headache; TBI: Traumatic brain injury

Acknowledgements

None.

Funding

There is no financial support related to this study and we have no conflict of interest.

Authors' contributions

CKH conceived and designed the study, acquired, interpreted and analyzed data, drafted and revised the manuscript. YSS, SYS and JYJ acquired and interpreted data, revised the manuscript. MAK and YBK interpreted and analyzed data. JC conceived, designed and supervised the study, acquired and interpreted data, drafted and revised the manuscript. All authors read and approved the final manuscript.

Competing interests

All authors declare that they have no competing interests.

Author details

[1]Department of Neurosurgery, Gangnam Severance Hospital, Yonsei University College of Medicine, 211, Eonjuro, Gangnam-gu, Seoul 06273, Republic of Korea. [2]Severance Institute for Vascular and Metabolic Research, Yonsei University, Seoul, Republic of Korea. [3]Department of Neurosurgery, Inha University School of Medicine and Hospital, Incheon, Republic of Korea. [4]Department of Neurosurgery, Inje University Seoul Paik Hospital, Seoul, Republic of Korea. [5]Department of Neurological Surgery, Rush University Medical Center, 1725 W. Harrison St., Professional Building Suite 855, Chicago, IL 60612, USA.

References

1. Headache Classification Subcommittee of the International Headache Society (2004) The International classification of headache disorders. Cephalalgia 24(Suppl. 1):9–160
2. Headache Classification Committee of the International Headache Society (HIS) (2013) The International classification of headache disorders, 3rd edition (beta version). Cephalalgia 33:629–808
3. Lew HL, Lin PH, Fuh JL, Wang SJ, Clark DJ, Walker WC (2006) Characteristics and treatment of headache after traumatic brain injury: a focused review. Am J Phys Med Rehabil 85:619–627
4. Minen MT, Boubour A, Walia H, Barr W (2016) Post-concussive syndrome: a focus on post-traumatic headache and related cognitive, phychiatric, and sleep issues. Curr Neurol Neurosci Rep 16:100
5. Saatman KE, Duhaime AC, Bullock R, Maas AI, Valadka A, Manley GT (2008) Classification of traumatic brain injury for targeted therapies. J Neurotrauma 25:719–738
6. Mild Traumatic Brain Injury Committee of the Head Injury Interdisciplinary Special Interest Group of the American Congress of Rehabilitation Medicine (1993) Definition of mild traumatic brain injury. J Head Trauma Rehabil 8:86–87
7. Hong CK, Joo JY, Kim YB, Shim YS, Lim YC, Shin YS et al (2015) The course of headache in patients with moderate-to-severe headache due to aneurysmal subarachnoid hemorrhage: a retrospective cross-sectional study. Headache 55:992–999
8. Gu DQ, Duan CZ, Li XF, He XY, Lai LF, Su SX (2013) Effect of endovascular treatment on headache in elderly patients with unruptured intracranial aneurysms. AJNR Am J Neuroradiol 34:1227–1231
9. Kwong WJ, Pathak DS (2007) Validation of the eleven-point pain scale in the measurement of migraine headache pain. Cephalalgia 27:336–342
10. Nampiaparampil DM (2008) Prevalence of chronic pain after traumatic brain injury: a systematic review. JAMA 300:711–719
11. Smith-Seemiller L, Fow NR, Kant R, Franzen MD (2003) Presence of post-concussion syndrome symptoms in patients with chronic pain vs mild traumatic brain injury. Brain Inj 17:199–206
12. Uomoto JM, Esselman PC (1993) TBI and chronic pain: differential types and rates by head injury severity. Arch Phys Med Rehabil 74:61–64
13. Lucas S, Hoffman JM, Bell KR, Dikmen S (2014) A prospective study of prevalence and characterization of headache following mild traumatic brain injury. Cephalalgia 34:93–102
14. Hoffman JM, Lucas S, Dikmen S, Braden CA, Brown AW, Brunner R et al (2011) Natural history of headache after traumatic brain injury. J Neurotrauma 28:1719–1725
15. Annegers JF, Hauser WA, Coan SP, Rocca WA (1998) A population-based study of seizures after traumatic brain injuries. N Engl J Med 338:20–24
16. Chiaretti A, De Benedictis R, Polidori G, Piastra M, Iannelli A, Di Rocco C (2000) Early post-traumatic seizures in children with head injury. Childs Nerv Syst 16:862–866
17. Temkin NR (2009) Preventing and treating posttraumatic seizures: the human experience. Epilepsia 50(Suppl.2):10–13
18. Piovesan EJ, Kowacs PA, Oshinsky ML (2003) Convergence of cervical and trigeminal sensory afferents. Curr Pain Headache Rep 7:377–383
19. Beetar JT, Guilmette TJ, Sparadeo FR (1996) Sleep and pain complaints in symptomatic TBI and neurologic populations. Arch Phys Med Rehabil 77:1298–1302
20. Stein SC, Burnett MG, Glick HA (2006) Indication for CT scanning in mild traumatic brain injury: a cost-effectiveness study. J Trauma 61:558–566
21. Sharif-Alhoseini M, Khodadadi H, Chardoli M, Rahimi-Movaghar V (2011) Indications for brain computed tomography scan after minor head injury. J Emerg Trauma Shock 4:472–476
22. Miller EC, Holmes JF, Derlet RW (1997) Utilizing clinical factors to reduce head CT scan ordering for minor head trauma patients. J Emerg Med 15:453–457
23. Haydel MJ, Preston CA, Mills TJ, Luber S, Blaudeau E, DeBlieux PM (2000) Indications for computed tomography in patients with minor head injury. N Engl J Med 343:100–105
24. Blyth BJ, Bazarian JJ (2010) Traumatic alterations in consciousness: traumatic brain injury. Emerg Med Clin North Am 23:571–594

18

Insomnia in tension-type headache

Jiyoung Kim[1], Soo-Jin Cho[2], Won-Joo Kim[3], Kwang Ik Yang[4], Chang-Ho Yun[5] and Min Kyung Chu[6*]

Abstract

Background: Tension-type headache (TTH) represents the most common type of headache among the general population. Although such headaches are usually mild in severity, some individuals with TTH experience severe symptoms and psychiatric comorbidities. Such patients may also experience sleep disturbances, which have been associated with headache exacerbation. Nevertheless, information regarding the prevalence and impact of insomnia among individuals with TTH in a population-based setting is limited. Therefore, the aim of the present study was to evaluate the prevalence and impact of insomnia among individuals with TTH using data from the Korean Headache-Sleep Study (KHSS).

Methods: We analysed data from the KHSS—a nation-wide, cross-sectional, population-based survey on headache and sleep involving Korean adults aged 19 to 69 years. Insomnia was defined as an Insomnia Severity Index score ≥ 10.

Results: Among 2695 participants, 570 (21.2%) and 290 (10.8%) were classified as having TTH and insomnia, respectively. Among individuals with TTH, 113 (19.8%) met the criteria for probable migraine (PM). The prevalence of insomnia among individuals with TTH was significantly higher than that among individuals without headache (13.2% vs. 5.8%, $p < 0.001$). However, among the TTH group, the prevalence of insomnia did not significantly differ between participants fulfilling PM criteria and those not fulfilling PM criteria (14.2% vs. 12.9%, $p = 0.725$). Among individuals with TTH, headache frequency [median and interquartile range (IQR): 1.0 (0.3–3.0) vs. 0.4 (0.2–1.0), $p = 0.002$], visual analogue scale scores for headache intensity [median and IQR: 5.0 (4.0–7.0) vs. 4.0 (3.0–6.0), $p < 0.001$], Headache Impact Test-6 scores [median and IQR: 46.0 (40.0–52.0) vs. 42.0 (38.0–46.0), $p < 0.001$], anxiety prevalence (28.0% vs. 6.7%, $p < 0.001$), and depression prevalence (21.3% vs. 1.6%, $p < 0.001$) were significantly higher in those with insomnia than in those without insomnia.

Conclusions: Our findings indicate that insomnia is prevalent among individuals with TTH. Moreover, insomnia was associated with exacerbation of headache symptoms and psychiatric comorbidities. Therefore, identification of insomnia among individuals with TTH is required to improve the management of headache symptoms in such patients.

Keywords: Anxiety, Depression, Headache, Insomnia, Tension-type headache

Background

Tension-type headache (TTH) is the most common form of primary headache among the general population, with a lifetime prevalence ranging from 20 to 87% [1]. TTH is usually associated with mild symptoms, and has been regarded as relatively non-severe since the condition is not life-threatening. However, some individuals with TTH experience frequent and severe headaches, which can decrease the ability to function at work, school, or home. Due to its high prevalence, the Global Campaign against Headache—a collaborative effort among the World Health Organization and three non-governmental organisations—has reported that the rate of disability due to TTH is greater than that due to migraine [1]. Therefore, the identification of factors associated with TTH represents an important public health issue.

Individuals who experience frequent headaches, including those with TTH, often report experiencing insomnia as well. Research has demonstrated that both lack of sleep and excessive sleep can trigger TTH [2, 3],

* Correspondence: chumk@hallym.ac.kr
[6]Department of Neurology, Kangnam Sacred Heart Hospital, Hallym University College of Medicine, 1 Singil-ro, Yeongdeungpo-gu, Seoul 07441, Korea
Full list of author information is available at the end of the article

and that sleep disturbances are associated with an increased risk of chronic tension-type headache (CTTH) among individuals with frequent episodic tension-type headaches (ETTH) [4].

Insomnia is a relatively common condition, affecting 10–30% of the general population [5]. Individuals with insomnia tend to exhibit limited functional capacity and decreased quality of life due to a variety of symptoms, including headaches [6, 7]. Cross-sectional studies have revealed that individuals with headaches exhibit increased odds ratios (ORs) for insomnia relative to those for individuals without headache [8, 9]. Additional research has indicated that the prevalence of insomnia is higher in patients with TTH than in individuals without headache [10]. Longitudinal studies have demonstrated that patients with migraine (OR =1.7) and non-migraineous headache (OR =1.4) are at increased risk for insomnia at the 11-year follow-up. Furthermore, individuals with insomnia exhibited an increased risk for TTH (relative risk [RR] = 1.4) and migraine (RR =1.4) at the 11-year follow-up [11, 12]. Several clinical studies have demonstrated an association between insomnia and exacerbation of TTH symptoms [13, 14]. Nevertheless, information regarding the impact of insomnia on the clinical presentation of TTH in a population-based setting is limited. We hypothesised that, among individuals with TTH, those with insomnia experience more severe symptoms than those without insomnia. Therefore, the objectives of the present study were as follows: 1) to evaluate the prevalence of insomnia and TTH in a general population-based sample, 2) to assess clinical characteristics and comorbidities of TTH according to the presence of insomnia, and 3) to investigate the association between TTH and insomnia including covariates such as sociodemographic factors, sleep time, sleep quality, and psychiatric comorbidities.

Methods

Survey

The present study utilised data from the Korean Headache-Sleep Study (KHSS), the design and methods of which have been described in detail in a previous report [15]. Briefly, a two-stage clustered random-sampling method was adopted for all Korean territories except Jeju-do, proportional to population distribution. The survey was performed via door-to-door visits and face-to-face interviews. The questionnaire utilised during these interviews exhibited sensitivity and specificity values of 86.2 and 75.5% for TTH diagnosis, respectively [16]. All interviewers were non-medical employees of Gallup Korea. The study protocol was approved by the Institutional Review Board and Ethics Committee of Hallym University Sacred Heart Hospital (Approval No. 2011-I077). Informed consent was obtained from each participant prior to each interview.

Assessment of TTH

Diagnoses of TTH were based on criteria B to D for infrequent TTH (code 2.1) as listed in the third edition of the International Classification of Headache Disorders, beta version (ICHD-3 beta) (B: attack duration ranging from 30 min to 7 days; C: any two of four typical headache characteristics [i.e., bilateral location, non-pulsating quality, mild-to-moderate pain intensity, and no aggravation with movement]; D: attacks associated with both of the following: no nausea or vomiting and no more than either photophobia or phonophobia). Participants fulfilling all criteria were classified as having TTH. In accordance with ICHD-3 beta criteria, participants meeting criteria for both TTH and probable migraine (PM) were considered to have TTH.

Assessment of insomnia

The self-reported Insomnia Severity Index (ISI) was used to evaluate the presence and severity of insomnia [17]. Participants with ISI scores of 10 or more were classified as having insomnia [18].

Assessment of sleep time and sleep quality

Data regarding typical sleep times on workdays and free days during the previous month were collected and analysed. Average sleep time was defined as follows: [(workday sleep time × 5) + (free-day sleep time × 2)] / 7. Short sleep time was defined as an average sleep time ≤ 6 h per day. The Pittsburgh Sleep Quality Index (PSQI) was used to evaluate the quality of sleep in the present study. The PSQI is a self-administered questionnaire composed of 19 questions designed to assess seven components of perceived sleep status, including subjective sleep quality, sleep latency, sleep duration, habitual sleep insufficiency, sleep disturbance, use of sleep medications, and daytime dysfunction. Poor sleep quality was defined as a global PSQI score of 6 or more [19].

Assessment of anxiety and depression

The Goldberg Anxiety Scale (GAS) was used to assess the prevalence of anxiety among participants. The GAS comprises four screening items and five supplementary items [20]. Participants who responded positively to two or more screening items and five or more total items were considered to have anxiety. The present study utilised the Korean version of the GAS, which has a sensitivity of 82.0% and a specificity of 94.4% for the diagnosis of anxiety [21]. The Korean version of the Patient Health Questionnaire-9 (PHQ-9), which has a sensitivity of 81.1% and specificity of 89.9% for the diagnosis of depression, was used to screen for depression in the present study [22, 23]. PHQ-9 scores of 10 or more were considered indicative of depression.

Data analyses

The Kolmogorov–Smirnov test was used to evaluate the normality of the distribution. After confirming the normality of the distribution, Student's t-tests and Chi-square tests were utilised to compare prevalence rates where appropriate. If the normality of the distribution was not confirmed, Mann-Whitney *U* tests were used to compare data between two groups. All statistical analyses were performed using Statistical Package for Social Sciences version 22.0 (SPSS 22.0; IBM, Armonk, NY, USA). The significance level was set at $p < 0.05$ for all analyses.

Univariable and multivariable analyses were performed to determine factors contributing to insomnia among individuals with TTH. Among individuals with TTH, factors exhibiting significant differences between those with insomnia and those without insomnia were considered for univariable analyses. For multivariable analyses, three models were developed to examine the association between insomnia and TTH. Model 1—which included sociodemographic variables (age, sex, size of residential area, and educational level), anxiety, and depression—was used to investigate the association between insomnia and psychiatric conditions. Model 2—which included sociodemographic variables, short sleep time, and poor sleep quality as covariates—was used to investigate the association between insomnia and sleep-related parameters. Finally, Model 3—which included sociodemographic variables, anxiety, depression, short sleep time, and poor sleep quality as covariates—was used to investigate the association among insomnia, psychiatric conditions, and sleep-related parameters. Missing data occurred only with regard to educational level. All reported results are based on available data. Imputation techniques were not used to minimise non-response effects [24].

Results

Survey

Among 7430 individuals contacted by our interviewer, a total of 3114 provided consent for the survey, including the 2695 individuals who had completed the survey (cooperation rate: 36.2%, Fig. 1). No significant differences in the distributions of age, sex, size of residential area, or level of education were observed between the study population and the general population in Korea (Table 1).

Prevalence of TTH, non-headache controls, and insomnia

Among the 2695 participants, 570 (21.2%) experienced TTH during the previous year, while 1422 (52.8%) did not. Among individuals with TTH, 113 (19.8%) also met the criteria for PM. The prevalence of TTH was not significantly affected by age, sex, or educational level. However, the prevalence of TTH was higher in rural areas than in large or small-to-medium cities (Table 1). A total of 290 (10.8%) participants were classified as having insomnia. Insomnia was more prevalent among women than men, and among those with lower levels of education (middle school or less) than those with higher levels of education. The prevalence of insomnia tended to increase with increasing age (Table 1). Sociodemographic characteristics of individuals with TTH and those without headache are summarised in Additional file 1: Table S1.

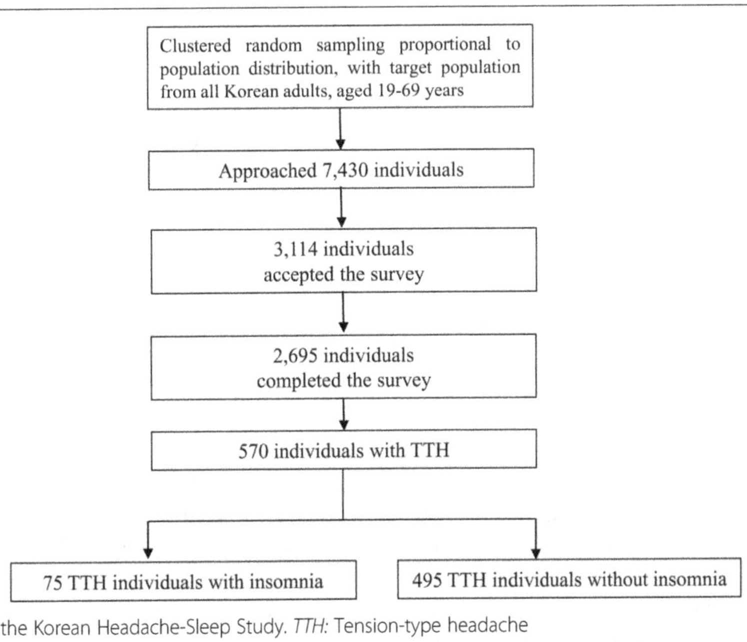

Fig. 1 Patient flow chart in the Korean Headache-Sleep Study. *TTH:* Tension-type headache

Table 1 Sociodemographic characteristics of survey participants and total Korean population and cases identified as having TTH or insomnia

	Survey participants N (%)	Total population N (%)	P	Tension-type headache N, % (95% CI)	P	Insomnia N, % (95% CI)	P
Sex							
Men	1345 (49.3)	17,584,365 (50.6)	0.854[a]	268, 19.9 (17.8–22.0)	0.120[b]	117, 8.7 (7.2–1.2)	0.001[c]
Women	1350 (50.7)	17,198,350 (49.4)		302, 22.3 (20.1–24.6)		173, 12.4 (11.0–14.6)	
Age							
19–29	542 (20.5)	7,717,947 (22.2)	0.917[a]	119, 22.0 (18.5–25.5)	0.971[b]	59, 10.9 (8.3–13.5)	0.427[c]
30–39	604 (21.9)	8,349,487 (24.0)		127, 21.0(17.8–24.3)		53, 8.8 (6.5–11.0)	
40–49	611 (23.1)	8,613,110 (24.8)		131, 21.4 (18.2–24.7)		66, 10.8 (8.3–13.3)	
50–59	529 (18.9)	6,167,505 (17.7)		107, 20.2 (16.8–23.7)		63, 11.9 (9.1–14.7)	
60–69	409 (15.6)	3,934,666 (11.3)		86, 21.0 (17.1–25.0)		49, 12.0 (8.8–15.1)	
Size of residential area							
Large city	1248 (46.3)	16,776,771 (48.2)	0.921[a]	251, 20.1 (17.9–22.4)	0.004[b]	136, 10.9 (9.2–12.6)	0.943[c]
Medium-to-small city	1186 (44.0)	15,164,345 (43.6)		243, 20.5 (18.2–22.8)		125, 10.5 (8.8–12.2)	
Rural area	261 (9.7)	2,841,599 (8.2)		76, 29.1 (23.6–34.7)		29, 11.1 (7.3–14.9)	
Education level							
Middle school or less	393 (14.9)	6,608,716 (19.0)	0.752[a]	96, 24.5 (20.1–28.7)	0.327[b]	62, 15.8 (12.1–19.4)	0.006[c]
High school	1208 (44.5)	15,234,829 (43.8)		247, 20.5 (18.2–22.7)		116, 9.6 (7.9–11.3)	
College or more	1068 (39.6)	12,939,170 (37.2)		223, 20.9 (18.4–23.3)		109, 10.2 (8.4–12.0)	
Not responded	26 (1.0)			4, 15.4 (0.5–30.2)		3, 11.5 (0.0–24.7)	
Total	2695 (100.0)	34,782,715 (100.0)		570, 21.2 (19.6–22.7)		290, 10.8 (9.6–11.9)	

N number, *CI* confidence interval, *TTH* tension-type headache
[a]Comparison of sex, age group, size of residential area, and educational level distributions between the sample in the present study and the total population of Korea
[b]Comparison of sex, age group, size of residential area, and educational level distributions among survey participants
[c]Comparison of sex, age group, size of residential area, and educational level distributions among survey participants

Prevalence of anxiety, depression, short sleep time and poor sleep quality

A total of 268 (9.9%) participants exhibited symptoms of anxiety, while 116 (4.3%) exhibited symptoms of depression. The prevalence of anxiety (9.5% vs. 5.3%, $p = 0.001$) and depression (4.2% vs. 1.8%, $p = 0.001$) was significantly higher among individuals with TTH than among individuals without headache. A total of 469 (17.4%) participants reported an average sleep duration ≤6 h, and were thus classified as having short sleep time. Poor sleep quality was noted in 715 (26.5%) participants.

Prevalence of insomnia among individuals with TTH

Among the 570 participants with TTH, 75 (13.2%) were classified as having insomnia. The prevalence of insomnia among participants with TTH was significantly higher than that among participants without headache (13.2% vs. 5.8%, $p < 0.001$).

Previous studies have demonstrated a significant association between insomnia and migraine [12, 25]. Therefore, migrainous features may affect the prevalence of insomnia. We assessed the prevalence of insomnia among participants with TTH according to fulfillment of PM criteria. Among participants with TTH, the prevalence of insomnia did not significantly differ between those fulfilling PM criteria and those not fulfilling PM criteria (14.2% vs. 12.9%, $p = 0.725$). The prevalence of insomnia was significantly higher among participants with TTH not fulfilling PM criteria than among individuals without headache (12.9% vs. 5.8%, $p < 0.001$) (Fig. 2). We then analysed the prevalence of insomnia according to headache frequency. The prevalence of insomnia was significantly higher among participants with 1–10 TTH attacks per month than among those with < 1 TTH attack per month (17.1% vs. 10.4%, $p = 0.022$). However, the prevalence of insomnia did not significantly differ between participants with > 10 TTH attacks per month and those with < 1 TTH attack per month (14.3% vs. 10.4%, $p = 0.575$).

Demographic characteristics and clinical presentation of TTH according to the presence of insomnia

Among individuals with TTH, those with insomnia exhibited significantly higher headache frequency per month, visual analogue scale (VAS) scores for headache intensity, and Headache Impact Test-6 scores than those

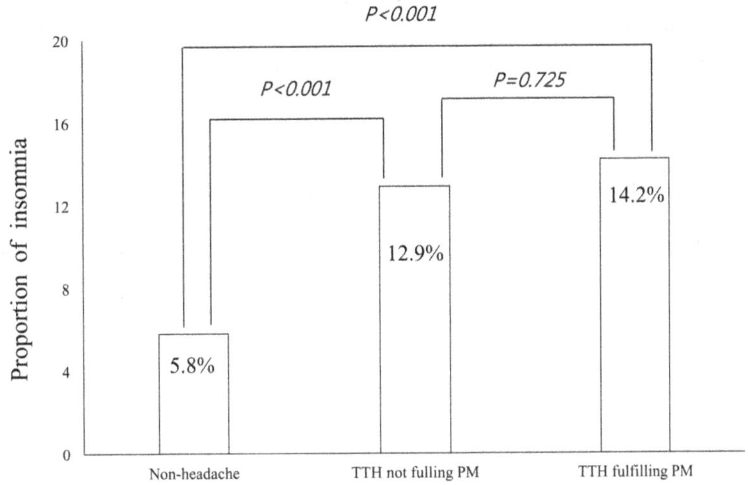

Fig. 2 Prevalence of insomnia among individuals without headache, those with TTH fulfilling PM criteria, and those with TTH not fulfilling PM criteria. *PM,* probable igraine; *TTH,* tension-type headache

without insomnia. Anxiety and depression were more prevalent among individuals with TTH and insomnia than among those without insomnia (Table 2).

Univariable and multivariable analyses for factors contributing to insomnia among individuals with TTH

Univariable analyses revealed that anxiety [OR = 5.4, 95% Confidence interval (CI): 2.9–10.0], depression (OR = 16.5, 95% CI: 6.8–40.2), short sleep time (OR = 3.1, 95% CI: 1.9–5.3), and poor sleep quality (OR = 12.8, 95% CI: 7.1–23.0) were associated with an increased risk of insomnia among individuals with TTH. Multivariate analyses including sociodemographic variables, anxiety and depression (Model 1) indicated that patients with anxiety (OR = 3.9, 95% CI: 2.0–8.0) and depression (OR = 14.8, 95% CI: 5.5–39.7) exhibited increased ORs for insomnia. In Model 2 (including sociodemographic variables, short sleep time, and poor sleep quality), poor sleep quality (OR = 13.4, 95% CI: 7.1–25.3) was significantly associated with insomnia status. In Model 3 (including sociodemographic variables, anxiety, depression, short sleep time, and poor sleep quality), anxiety

Table 2 Demographics and clinical presentation of individuals with TTH according to the presence of insomnia

	TTH with insomnia, *N* = 75	TTH without insomnia, *N* = 495	*P*
Demographics			
Age, Mean ± SD (years)	44.5 ± 13.7	42.5 ± 13.7	0.236
Women, N (%)	43 (57.3)	259 (52.3)	0.418
Headache characteristics			
Bilateral pain, N (%)	45 (60.0)	329 (66.5)	0.272
Non-pulsating quality, N (%)	29 (38.7)	198 (40.0)	0.824
Mild-to-moderate severity, N (%)	73 (97.3)	490 (99.0)	0.225
Non-aggravation by movement, N(%)	58 (77.3)	393 (79.4)	0.682
Associated symptoms			
Photophobia, N (%)	6 (8.0)	40 (8.1)	0.981
Phonophobia, N (%)	31 (41.3)	150 (30.3)	0.056
Headache frequency, Median (IQR)	1.0 (0.3–3.0)	0.4 (0.2–1.0)	0.002[a]
VAS score, Median (IQR)	5.0 (4.0–7.0)	4.0 (3.0–6.0)	< 0.001[a]
HIT-6 score, Median (IQR)	46.0 (40.0–52.0)	42.0 (38.0–46.0)	< 0.001[a]
Anxiety, N (%)	21 (28.0)	33 (6.7)	< 0.001
Depression, N (%)	16 (21.3)	8 (1.6)	< 0.001

N number, *SD* standard deviation, *IQR* interquartile range
[a]Mann-Whitney U test

(OR = 3.0, 95% CI: 1.4–6.7), depression (OR = 5.8, 95% CI: 2.0–16.3), and poor sleep quality (OR = 9.9, 95% CI: 5.1–19.2) were significantly associated with insomnia status (Table 3).

Discussion

The main findings of the present study were as follows: 1) The prevalence of insomnia was significantly higher among individuals with TTH than among individuals without headache; 2) headache frequency, headache intensity, and impact of headache on functioning were significantly greater among participants with TTH and insomnia than among those without insomnia; and 3) anxiety, depression, and poor sleep quality were significant risk factors for insomnia among participants with TTH.

Previous studies have demonstrated a significant association between insomnia and TTH. For example, a community-based study in Hong Kong revealed that individuals with TTH exhibit increased ORs for insomnia relative to those for individuals without headache (OR = 2.2) [26]. A population-based study conducted in Norway further reported that the prevalence of insomnia is 1.8 times higher in individuals with TTH than in those without headache [10]. The findings of the present study are in agreement with the results of these previous studies, as our analyses indicated that the prevalence of insomnia was approximately two times higher among individuals with TTH than among those without headache. Therefore, our findings support the association between TTH and insomnia, and the similarity between our data and values reported in previous studies suggests that the methods of the present study were appropriate for evaluating this association.

One possible explanation for the observed association between insomnia and TTH involves the shared comorbidities of anxiety and depression. Indeed, anxiety and depression are common among patients with insomnia, and previous studies have indicated that both anxiety and depression are closely associated with the clinical presentation of insomnia [27]. Furthermore, insomnia symptoms tend to worsen as the severity of anxiety and/or depression [28]. Anxiety and depression are common among patients with headache [29, 30]. Although the prevalence of anxiety and depression among patients with TTH is lower

Table 3 Univariable and multivariable logistic regression analyses for contributing factors of insomnia among individuals with tension-type headache (*N* = 570)

	Univariable analysis OR, 95% CI, *P-value*	Multivariable analysis Model 1	Multivariable analysis Model 2	Multivariable analysis Model 3
Sex				
	1.2 (0.8–2.0), *p = 0418*	1.2 (0.7–2.0), *p = 0.609*	1.3 (0.8–2.4), *p = 0.305*	1.2 (0.7–2.2), *p = 0.528*
Age				
20s	Reference			
30s	0.8 (0.3–1.8), *p = 0.556*	0.7 (0.2–1.6), *p = 0.360*	0.6 (0.2–1.5), *p = 0.256*	0.5 (0.2–1.4), *p = 0.220*
40s	1.1 (0.5–2.4), *p = 0.772*	1.1 (0.5–2.5), *p = 0.833*	1.1 (0.5–2.6), *p = 0.836*	1.1 (0.4–2.6), *p = 0.910*
50s	1.6 (0.8–3.4), *p = 0.206*	1.7 (0.7–4.2), *p = 0.246*	0.8 (0.3–2.1), *p = 0.704*	1.0 (0.4–2.8), *p = 0.931*
60s	1.3 (0.6–3.0), *p = 0.485*	1.2 (0.4–3.5), *p = 0.689*	0.9 (0.3–2.6), *p = 0.789*	0.9 (0.3–3.0), *p = 0.928*
Size of residential area				
Large city	Reference			
Medium-to-small city	1.2(0.7–2.0), *p = 0.508*	1.2 (0.7–2.1), *p = 0.566*	1.4(0.8–2.4), *p = 0.295*	1.3(0.7–2.4), *p = 0.395*
Rural area	0.5(0.2–1.2), *p = 0.125*	0.5 (0.2–1.5), *p = 0.244*	0.5(0.2–1.6), *p = 0.268*	0.6(0.2–1.8), *P = 0.340*
Education level				
Middle school or less	Reference			
High school	0.9(0.5–1.7), *p = 0.732*	0.9(0.4–2.0), *p = 0.716*	0.6(0.2–1.5), *p = 0.260*	0.6(0.2–1.4), *p = 0.215*
College or more	0.7(0.3–1.3), *p = 0.226*	0.8(0.3–2.1), *p = 0.622*	0.5(0.2–1.4), *p = 0.190*	0.5(0.2–1.6), *p = 0.250*
Not responded	1.8(0.2–18.5), *p = 0.621*	2.1(0.2–22.2), *p = 0.543*	1.9(0.1–28.8), *p = 0.626*	2.3(0.2–32.9), *p = 0.539*
Anxiety	5.4 (2.9–10.0), *p < 0.001*	3.9(2.0–8.0), *p < 0.001*		3.0 (1.4–6.7), *p = 0.006*
Depression	16.5 (6.8–40.2), *p < 0.001*	14.8(5.5–39.7), *p < 0.001*		5.8 (2.0–16.3), *p = 0.001*
Short sleep time	3.1 (1.9–5.3), *p < 0.001*		1.2(0.7–2.3), *p = 0.538*	1.2 (0.6–2.4), *p = 0.570*
Poor sleep quality	12.8 (7.1–23.0), *p < 0.001*		13.4(7.1–25.3), *p < 0.001*	9.9 (5.1–19.2), *p < 0.001*

Model 1 included sociodemographic variables (sex, age, size of residential area, level of education), anxiety, and depression
Model 2 included sociodemographic variables, short sleep time (≤6 h), and poor sleep quality (PSQI ≥ 6)
Model 3 included sociodemographic variables, anxiety, depression, short sleep time, and poor sleep quality

than among patients with migraine, a significant proportion of individuals with TTH experience anxiety and depression [31]. In the present study, anxiety and depression were identified as significant risk factors for insomnia among individuals with TTH, even after adjusting for potential covariates. Alternatively, insomnia may trigger TTH [32]. Taken together, these findings indicate that the prevalence of TTH may be higher among individuals with insomnia than among those without insomnia. However, previous studies have reported that sleep deprivation and interruption of slow wave sleep can reduce pain threshold and cause hyperalgesia [33, 34]. Thus, insomnia may induce frequent headaches (including TTH) by decreasing the pain threshold.

Previous studies regarding the association between insomnia and TTH have not examined the impact of insomnia on the clinical presentation of TTH. In the present study, we observed that, among individuals with TTH, those with insomnia exhibited a higher frequency of headache and increased impact of headache on daily function than those without insomnia. In accordance with our findings, previous studies have indicated that individuals with a high frequency of TTH may experience increased disability, decreased quality of life, and a higher rate of comorbidities than those with low frequency of TTH [13]. Therefore, proper identification and management of insomnia may reduce the impact of headache among individuals with TTH. While pharmacological treatments for insomnia have demonstrated efficacy in randomised controlled trials, research has indicated that non-pharmacological alternatives such as cognitive behavioral therapy (CBT) are also effective [35].

In the present study, anxiety and depression were more common among individuals with TTH and insomnia than among those with TTH only (Table 2). Multivariable regression analyses revealed that anxiety and depression were significant contributing factors for insomnia among individuals with TTH (Table 3). Anxiety and depression often co-occur and have been closely associated with insomnia in previous studies [28, 36, 37]. Therefore, anxiety and depression may underlie the association between insomnia and TTH. However, further studies are required in order to clarify the associations among anxiety, depression, insomnia, and TTH.

Although there was no significant difference in the prevalence of insomnia between individuals with TTH fulfilling PM criteria and those not fulfilling PM criteria, the prevalence of insomnia among those fulfilling PM criteria was numerically higher than that among those not fulfilling PM criteria (Fig. 2). Considering that the prevalence of insomnia among individuals with migraine is much higher than that among those with TTH, our findings indicate that migrainous features may be substrates for the development of insomnia among individuals with TTH [9, 10, 25]. Further studies involving larger sample sizes are required to more fully elucidate the association between migrainous features and insomnia among individuals with TTH.

The present study possesses some limitations of note. First, polysomnography (PSG) was not performed to evaluate for sleep disorders such as sleep-disordered breathing. Some patients with sleep-disordered breathing present with symptoms of chronic insomnia [38]. Second, our study did not investigate the rate of chronic pain disorders such as fibromyalgia among participants. Since chronic pain disorders are also associated with psychiatric comorbidities, future studies should investigate the association between chronic pain disorders and anxiety/depression in patients with headaches. Third, we did not evaluate the use of antidepressants, hypnotics, anxiolytics, or preventive medications for TTH, and were thus unable to examine the effects of such agents on TTH and insomnia. Fourth, although our study utilised a large sample size, the statistical power for executing some subgroup analyses was limited. That is, the lack of significant findings in certain subgroup analyses may have been due to the limited sample size.

Despite these limitations, our study possesses several strengths. First, the distributions of sex, age, size of residential area, and level of education for the study population reflected those observed in the general population, indicating that our findings may be applicable to the general population. Second, the characteristics of headache and psychiatric comorbidities were compared according to the presence of insomnia in patients with TTH. Third, we examined the association among TTH, insomnia, and closely related psychiatric comorbidities (i.e., anxiety and depression).

Conclusion

Our findings indicate that insomnia is more prevalent among individuals with TTH than among those without headache. Moreover, among individuals with TTH, those with insomnia experienced more frequent headaches, increased rates of psychiatric comorbities, and more severe disability due to headache. Our findings suggest that insomnia represents an important comorbidity among individuals with TTH. Therefore, proper identification and management of insomnia may reduce the impact of headache among individuals with TTH.

Abbreviations

CBT: Cognitive behavioral therapy; CI: Confidence interval; CM: Chronic migraine; CTTH: Chronic tension-type headache; ETTH: Episodic tension-type headache; GAS: Goldberg Anxiety Scale; ICHD: International Classification of

Headache Disorders; KHSS: Korean Headache-Sleep Study; OR: Odds ratio; PHQ-9: Patient Health Questionnaire-9; PM: Probable migraine; PSG: Polysomnography; PSQI: Pittsburgh Sleep Quality Index score; RR: Relative risk; TTH: Tension-type headache; VAS: Visual analogue scale

Acknowledgements
The authors would like to thank Gallup Korea for providing technical support for the Korean Headache-Sleep Study.

Funding
This Study was Supported by a 2011-Grant from Korean Academy of Medical Sciences.

Authors' contributions
JYK conceptualized and designed the study, analyzed data, and wrote the manuscript. SJC, WJK, KIY, and CHY conceptualized and collected data. MKC conceptualized and designed the study, collected data, analyzed data, and wrote the manuscript. All authors read and approved the final manuscript.

Competing interests
The authors declare that they have no competing interests.

Author details
[1]Department of Neurology, Bio Medical Research Institute, Pusan National University Hospital, Pusan National University School of Medicine, Busan, Korea. [2]Department of Neurology, Dongtan Sacred Heart Hospital, Hallym University College of Medicine, Hwaseong, Korea. [3]Department of Neurology, Gangnam Severance Hospital, Yonsei University, College of Medicine, Seoul, Korea. [4]Department of Neurology, Soonchunhyang University College of Medicine, Cheonan Hospital, Cheonan, Korea. [5]Department of Neurology, Bundang Clinical Neuroscience Institute, Seoul National University Bundang Hospital, Seongnam, Korea. [6]Department of Neurology, Kangnam Sacred Heart Hospital, Hallym University College of Medicine, 1 Singil-ro, Yeongdeungpo-gu, Seoul 07441, Korea.

References

1. Stovner L, Hagen K, Jensen R, Katsarava Z, Lipton R, Scher A, Steiner T, Zwart JA (2007) The global burden of headache: a documentation of headache prevalence and disability worldwide. Cephalalgia 27(3):193–210
2. Spierings EL, Ranke AH, Honkoop PC (2001) Precipitating and aggravating factors of migraine versus tension-type headache. Headache 41(6):554–558
3. Rains JC, Davis RE, Smitherman TA (2015) Tension-type headache and sleep. Curr Neurol Neurosci Rep 15(2):520
4. Lyngberg AC, Rasmussen BK, Jorgensen T, Jensen R (2005) Prognosis of migraine and tension-type headache: a population-based follow-up study. Neurology 65(4):580–585
5. Morin CM, LeBlanc M, Daley M, Gregoire JP, Merette C (2006) Epidemiology of insomnia: prevalence, self-help treatments, consultations, and determinants of help-seeking behaviors. Sleep Med 7(2):123–130
6. Daley M, Morin CM, LeBlanc M, Gregoire JP, Savard J, Baillargeon L (2009) Insomnia and its relationship to health-care utilization, work absenteeism, productivity and accidents. Sleep Med 10(4):427–438
7. Bolge SC, Doan JF, Kannan H, Baran RW (2009) Association of insomnia with quality of life, work productivity, and activity impairment. Qual Life Res 18(4):415–422
8. Kim K, Uchiyama M, Liu X, Shibui K, Ohida T, Ogihara R, Okawa M (2001) Somatic and psychological complaints and their correlates with insomnia in the Japanese general population. Psychosom Med 63(3):441–446
9. Sutton DA, Moldofsky H, Badley EM (2001) Insomnia and health problems in Canadians. Sleep 24(6):665–670
10. Odegard SS, Engstrom M, Sand T, Stovner LJ, Zwart JA, Hagen K (2010) Associations between sleep disturbance and primary headaches: the third Nord-Trondelag health study. J Headache Pain 11(3):197–206
11. Odegard SS, Sand T, Engstrom M, Zwart JA, Hagen K (2013) The impact of headache and chronic musculoskeletal complaints on the risk of insomnia: longitudinal data from the Nord-Trondelag health study. J Headache Pain 14:24
12. Odegard SS, Sand T, Engstrom M, Stovner LJ, Zwart JA, Hagen K (2011) The long-term effect of insomnia on primary headaches: a prospective population-based cohort study (HUNT-2 and HUNT-3). Headache 51(4):570–580
13. Ong JC, Stepanski EJ, Gramling SE (2009) Pain coping strategies for tension-type headache: possible implications for insomnia? J Clin Sleep Med 5(1): 52–56
14. Sancisi E, Cevoli S, Vignatelli L, Nicodemo M, Pierangeli G, Zanigni S, Grimaldi D, Cortelli P, Montagna P (2010) Increased prevalence of sleep disorders in chronic headache: a case-control study. Headache 50(9):1464–1472
15. Cho SJ, Chung YK, Kim JM, Chu MK (2015) Migraine and restless legs syndrome are associated in adults under age fifty but not in adults over fifty: a population-based study. J Headache Pain 16:554
16. Kim B-K, Chu MK, Lee TG, Kim J-M, Chung C-S, Lee K-S (2012) Prevalence and impact of migraine and tension-type headache in Korea. J Clin Neurol 8(3):204–211
17. Bastien CH, Vallieres A, Morin CM (2001) Validation of the insomnia severity index as an outcome measure for insomnia research. Sleep Med 2(4):297–307
18. Morin CM, Belleville G, Belanger L, Ivers H (2011) The insomnia severity index: psychometric indicators to detect insomnia cases and evaluate treatment response. Sleep 34(5):601–608
19. Buysse DJ, Reynolds CF 3rd, Monk TH, Berman SR, Kupfer DJ (1989) The Pittsburgh sleep quality index: a new instrument for psychiatric practice and research. Psychiatry Res 28(2):193–213
20. Goldberg D, Bridges K, Duncan-Jones P, Grayson D (1988) Detecting anxiety and depression in general medical settings. BMJ 297(6653):897–899
21. Lim JY, Lee SH, Cha YS, Park HS, Sunwoo S (2001) Reliability and validity of anxiety screening scale. J Korean Acad Fam Med 22(8):1224–1232
22. Pignone MP, Gaynes BN, Rushton JL, Burchell CM, Orleans CT, Mulrow CD, Lohr KN (2002) Screening for depression in adults: a summary of the evidence for the U.S. Preventive Services Task Force. Ann Intern Med 136(10):765–776
23. Choi HS, Choi JH, Park KH, Joo KJ, Ga H, Ko HJ, Kim SR (2007) Standardization of the Korean version of patient health questionnaire-9 as a screening instrument for major depressive disorder. J Korean Acad Fam Med 28(2):114–119
24. Little RJ, Rubin DB (2014) Statistical analysis with missing data. New York: John Wiley & Sons
25. Lateef T, Swanson S, Cui L, Nelson K, Nakamura E, Merikangas K (2011) Headaches and sleep problems among adults in the United States: findings from the National Comorbidity Survey-Replication study. Cephalalgia 31(6):648–653
26. Yeung WF, Chung KF, Wong CY (2010) Relationship between insomnia and headache in community-based middle-aged Hong Kong Chinese women. J Headache Pain 11(3):187–195
27. Jansson-Frojmark M, Lindblom K (2008) A bidirectional relationship between anxiety and depression, and insomnia? A prospective study in the general population. J Psychosom Res 64(4):443–449
28. Johnson EO, Roth T, Breslau N (2006) The association of insomnia with anxiety disorders and depression: exploration of the direction of risk. J Psychiatr Res 40(8):700–708
29. Serafini G, Pompili M, Innamorati M, Gentile G, Borro M, Lamis DA, Lala N, Negro A, Simmaco M, Girardi P, Martelletti P (2012) Gene variants with suicidal risk in a sample of subjects with chronic migraine and affective temperamental dysregulation. Eur Rev Med Pharmacol Sci 16(10):1389–1398
30. Houle TT, Butschek RA, Turner DP, Smitherman TA, Rains JC, Penzien DB (2012) Stress and sleep duration predict headache severity in chronic headache sufferers. Pain 153(12):2432–2440
31. Song TJ, Cho SJ, Kim WJ, Yang KI, Yun CH, Chu MK (2016) Anxiety and depression in tension-type headache: a population-based study. PLoS One 11(10):e0165316
32. Wang J, Huang Q, Li N, Tan G, Chen L, Zhou J (2013) Triggers of migraine and tension-type headache in China: a clinic-based survey. Eur J Neurol 20(4):689–696
33. Onen SH, Alloui A, Gross A, Eschallier A, Dubray C (2001) The effects of total sleep deprivation, selective sleep interruption and sleep recovery on pain tolerance thresholds in healthy subjects. J Sleep Res 10(1):35–42

34. Lentz MJ, Landis CA, Rothermel J, Shaver JL (1999) Effects of selective slow wave sleep disruption on musculoskeletal pain and fatigue in middle aged women. J Rheumatol 26(7):1586–1592
35. Geiger-Brown JM, Rogers VE, Liu W, Ludeman EM, Downton KD, Diaz-Abad M (2015) Cognitive behavioral therapy in persons with comorbid insomnia: a meta-analysis. Sleep Med Rev 23:54–67
36. Ohayon MM, Roth T (2003) Place of chronic insomnia in the course of depressive and anxiety disorders. J Psychiatr Res 37(1):9–15
37. Oh K, Cho SJ, Chung YK, Kim JM, Chu MK (2016) Erratum to: combination of anxiety and depression is associated with an increased headache frequency in migraineurs: a population-based study. BMC Neurol 16:51
38. American Academy of Sleep Medicine (2014) International classification of sleep Sisorders—third edition (ICSD-3). American Academy of Sleep Medicine Resource Library Avialble via DIALOG. http://www.aasmnet.org/library/default.aspx. Accessed 20 Aug 2017.

19

Sphenopalatine ganglion stimulation for cluster headache, results from a large, open-label European registry

Mads Barloese[1,2*], Anja Petersen[2], Philipp Stude[3], Tim Jürgens[4], Rigmor Højland Jensen[2] and Arne May[5]

Abstract

Background: Cluster headache (CH) is a disabling primary headache disorder characterized by severe periorbital pain. A subset of patients does not respond to established pharmacological therapy. This study examines outcomes of a cohort of mainly chronic CH patients treated with sphenopalatine ganglion (SPG) stimulation.

Methods: Patients were followed in an open-label prospective study for 12 months. Ninety-seven CH patients (88 chronic, 9 episodic) underwent trans-oral insertion of a microstimulator targeting the SPG. Patients recorded stimulation effect prospectively for individual attacks. Frequency, use of preventive and acute medications, headache impact (HIT-6) and quality of life measures (SF-36v2) were monitored at clinic visits. Per protocol, frequency responders experienced ≥ 50% reduction in attack frequency and acute responders treated ≥ 50% of attacks. HIT-6 responders experienced an improvement ≥ 2.3 units and SF-36 responders ≥ 4 units vs. baseline.

Results: Eighty-five patients (78 chronic, 7 episodic) remained implanted and were evaluated for effectiveness at 12 months. In total, 68% of all patients were responders, 55% of chronic patients were frequency responders and 32% of all patients were acute responders. 67% of patients using acute treatments were able to reduce the use of these by 52% and 74% of chronic patients were able to stop, reduce or remain off all preventive medications. 59% of all patients were HIT-6 responders, 67% were SF-36 responders.

Conclusions: This open-label registry corroborates that SPG stimulation is an effective therapy for CH patients providing therapeutic benefits and improvements in use of medication as well as headache impact and quality of life.

Keywords: Cluster headache, Sphenopalatine ganglion, Neurostimulation, Neuromodulation, Long term effectiveness

Background

Cluster headache (CH) is a primary headache manifesting as unilateral attacks of severe pain with increased cranial parasympathetic outflow lasting 15–180 min [1]. Attacks may occur up to eight times per day and it has been described as one of the most painful sensations humans can experience. CH exists as episodic CH (eCH), where attacks occur in clusters lasting weeks-months separated by attack-free intervals > 1 month, and chronic CH (cCH) with no periods of remission lasting > 1 month for > 1 year. Around 85% of patients suffer from the episodic form but CH is by no means a static condition and patients may transition between the two forms. There are no known differences in pathophysiology and in both eCH and cCH impairment is high with reduced quality of life [2] and high direct and indirect costs [3].

Traditional treatment can be divided into acute and preventive strategies. Acute therapies consist of oxygen

* Correspondence: mads.christian.johannes.barloese@regionh.dk

The data in this manuscript has previously been presented in abstract form at EHMTIC, Glasgow, 15–18 September, 2016 and will be presented in abstract form at INS, Edinburgh, May 27 – June 1, 2017.

[1]Department of Clinical Physiology, Nuclear Medicine and PET, Rigshospitalet-Glostrup, Nordre Ringvej 57, 2600 Glostrup, Denmark
[2]Danish Headache Centre, Department of Neurology, Rigshospitalet-Glostrup, Nordre Ringvej 57, 2600 Glostrup, Denmark
Full list of author information is available at the end of the article

and injectable or nasal triptans taken as early as possible during the individual attacks. Preventive therapies are taken daily during the cluster period, or in cCH continuously, and consist of verapamil or lithium [4]. With up to eight attacks/day use of acute medications may exceed recommendations, and often doses of preventive medications higher than recommended are necessary, increasing the risk of side-effects [5]. To complicate management further, around 1% of patients are medically refractory [6]. Invasive neurostimulation, including deep brain and occipital nerve stimulation, is usually reserved for these patients. Consequently, the literature consists of reports of relatively small populations [7].

It is desirable to develop targeted treatments with no systemic side effects and no safety issues with repeated use. Sphenopalatine ganglion (SPG) stimulation using an implantable microstimulater (Pulsante™) has been evaluated in a randomized, controlled trial where 68% were therapeutic responders [8]. These results were subsequently confirmed in a 24-month follow-up study [9, 10].

The aim of this study is to evaluate the effectiveness of SPG stimulation through 12 months in an open label setting, in a large population including cCH and a limited number of eCH patients. As opposed to the previously mentioned forms of neurostimulation, ONS and DBS, SPG stimulation elicits both an acute and preventive effect which this study was specifically designed to capture.

Methods

The Pathway R-1 registry study is a post-market registry of the Pulsante™ SPG Microstimulator System (Autonomic Technologies, Inc., Redwood City, California, USA) to confirm safety and long-term effectiveness of SPG stimulation in a large population, where patients underwent trans-oral insertion of this SPG microstimulator [11, 12].

Patient selection

Selection criteria for this registry were patients who met CH criteria per CE -labeling for the Pulsante Microstimulation System. Patients should have cluster headaches for a minimum of 16 weeks (investigator opinion) and the ability to provide written informed consent. Exclusion criteria included changes in preventive medication in the month prior to enrollment and patients who have bony facial deformities, inappropriate surgical anatomy or have had facial surgery that would prevent the proper placement of the Pulsante Microstimulator. Given that previous studies established a good safety profile it was not a requirement that patients were medically refractory per established criteria [6], however, most had tried several or all pharmaceutical options and were considered difficult to treat with a high headache burden.

SPG microstimulator system

The SPG Microstimulator System is designed to fit in the facial anatomy with an integrated lead placed proximate to the SPG. The microstimulator communicates with a handheld remote control by radio-waves, is inductively powered and contains no battery. Using the remote control, patients apply on-demand SPG stimulation to treat individual cluster attacks and were advised to treat these for at least 15 min as soon as they were felt. Patients were also permitted to use SPG stimulation prophylactically without any sense of an impending or ongoing attack.

Data collection

Response to SPG stimulation during each treated attack was collected prospectively in an electronic headache diary incorporated into the remote control. Pain scores were reported using the Categorical Pain Scale (CPS; 0 = none, 1 = mild, 2 = moderate, 3 = severe, 4 = very severe). Headache pain was reported just prior to stimulation use and headache pain and acute medication were reported immediately following stimulation.

Average attack frequency, laterality and acute and preventive medication use were collected retrospectively at each clinic visit, with patients asked to recall their attack frequency and acute medication usage over the prior 4 week period. Headache Impact Test (HIT-6) and Short Form Health Survey (SF-36v2) questionnaires were completed at baseline and quarterly during the first year. Following microstimulator insertion, a patient experience questionnaire was completed quarterly. Adverse events were collected throughout the study.

Outcomes and analyses

Per protocol analyses included percent change in attack frequency, percent of attacks achieving effective therapy, the number of patients achieving acute and/or frequency effect, changes in acute and preventive medication, characterization of HIT-6 headache disability and SF-36v2 quality of life and patient evaluation of therapy using the patient experience questionnaire. Due to the different nature of eCH and cCH additional frequency analyses were performed separately for chronic and episodic patients. Surgical outcomes, including insertion of the microstimulator within the pterygopalatine fossa, explants and lead revision rates were collected.

Change in the frequency of attacks was analyzed as the change in attack frequency from baseline (4 weeks prior to enrollment) to the 12 month visit (4 weeks prior to the 12 month visit) where Frequency Responders experienced at least a 50% reduction.

Analysis of the acute response included all attacks where SPG stimulation was applied and for which the patient entered diary responses through the 12 month study visit. An Acute Responder is a patient able to achieve effective therapy in at least 50% of attacks.

Acute effective therapy was defined in the protocol as pain relief (decrease in categorical pain scale (CPS) from 2 (moderate) or higher to 1 (mild) or 0 (none)) without the use of acute medications or pain freedom (decrease in CPS from 1 (mild) or higher to 0 (none)) without the use of acute medications as evaluated immediately following the cessation of SPG stimulation.

Furthermore, therapeutic responders were defined as patients who were either acute responders, frequency responders, or both. An additional post hoc analysis was performed to evaluate therapeutic response at the 75% and 30% levels.

Change in acute medication use compared to baseline was calculated for all acute medication uses (average number of uses per week), as well as separately for triptans and oxygen. Preventive medication changes were characterized to identify patients who stopped, decreased dose, remained off, or added/increased doses of preventive medications.

Headache impact improvements were considered clinically meaningful when scores improved by at least 2.3 units relative to baseline [13]. Quality of life improvements were considered clinically meaningful if either the physical (PCS) or mental component score (MCS) improved by at least 4 units relative to baseline [14]. Responses to a patient experience questionnaire were characterized. In 8 patients, who missed their 12 month study visit, any missing data for frequency, medication, or questionnaire data were imputed from the preceding 9 month study visit. HIT-6 data was incomplete in 5 patients and 6 patients had incomplete SF-36v2 data. These were omitted from the respective analyses. With regards to study visits and duration, 28 days were considered a month. Some patients completed their 3, 6 or 12 month visit earlier or later than scheduled (see results) based on the protocol defined visit schedule and visit windows.

Statistics

For all quantitative comparisons against baseline (frequency, acute medication, headache disability, quality of life) a paired t-test was used to account for changes over time with $p < 0.05$ regarded as statistically significant. Results for stimulation usage for acute cluster headache pain, were analyzed using a generalized estimating equation with least squares means. Changes in use of medication were calculated as absolute changes using Wilcoxon signed ranks.

Results

Patient disposition, clinical characteristics, and surgical outcomes

Ninety-seven CH patients (88 chronic, 9 episodic) were enrolled at 12 centers (Germany: 10, Denmark: 1, Austria: 1) and underwent microstimulator insertion from September 2012 through March 2015 (Fig. 1, Table 1). None of these patients were included in previous studies of SPG stimulation. Four patients were not able to be implanted during the initial attempt, however two of the four underwent an additional insertion attempt and a microstimulator was successfully placed within the pterygopalatine fossa. Twelve patients did not complete the study through to the 12 month visit (Fig. 1). Two of these have some efficacy data available indicating non-response to therapy. The remaining 85 patients (78 chronic, 7 episodic) continued through the study to 12 months and are included in the present 12 month evaluation of effectiveness (average time from microstimulator insertion to 12 month study visit: 368 ± 42 days (range 245–475)). Of the 85 patients included in the final analysis at 12 months, 8 underwent lead repositioning prior to the 12 month time point. Seven of these were repositioned on the same day as the original surgery as post-op CT showed misplacement. The eighth patient was explanted 3 months after the original surgery and re-implanted 9 months later as lead placement was deemed to be suboptimal. Three patients (1 episodic, 2 chronic) had a frequency of 0 attacks/week at baseline. These patients were still implanted as they were very well characterized clinically, had CH for many years and logistics did not allow postponement.

Attack frequency, chronic patients

Fifty-five per-cent (43/78) of the cCH patients were frequency responders, defined as experiencing at least a 50% reduction in attack frequency. For these, frequency was significantly reduced at 12 months compared to baseline (Table 2).

In the 78 chronic patients evaluated, 23 (29%) reported no attacks at the 12 month visit. For these cCH patients experiencing no attacks, the preventive effect manifested 150 ± 102 (range 8–390) days after microstimulator insertion. In all chronic patients, the average frequency at 3 months, 6 months, 9 months and 12 months was 14.9 ± 17.6, 14.9 ± 18.9, 14.2 ± 17.4 and 14.9 ± 18.1, respectively. At the 12 M visit 9 cCH patients experienced an increase in frequency of $\geq 50\%$.

Transitional therapies (oral steroids and greater occipital nerve (GON) blocks) were permitted at any time. Three of the 48 frequency responders (6%) received transitional therapies between microstimulator insertion and the 12 month visit. One patient received oral steroids at the 12 month visit, another had a GON block at 7 months post baseline, and a third a GON block 1½ months after microstimulator insertion. Of the frequency non-responders, six (16%) received GON blocks (0–6 months before 12 month visit), and two received oral steroids (6 and 9 months before 12 month visit).

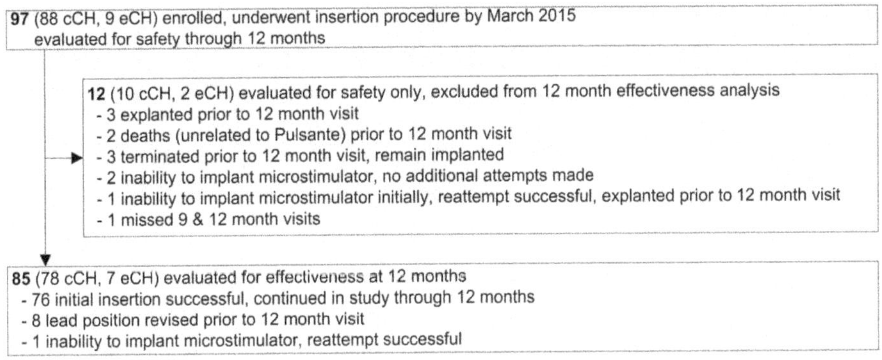

Fig. 1 Patient disposition for the Pathway R-1 study 12 month interim analysis

Acute effectiveness, episodic and chronic patients

Among all 85 patients, 13,600 attacks were treated with acute SPG stimulation (average 160 ± 245, median 82, range 0–1424 attacks per patient). Per protocol, 39% (5304/13600) of these attacks were effectively treated with SPG stimulation, with 26% (3534/13600) achieving pain freedom (Additional file 1: Figure S1). 32% (27/85) of patients were acute responders achieving effective therapy in at least 50% of their attacks. These acute responders were able to effectively treat 86% (4157/4811) of their attacks, with 57% (2750/4811) achieving pain freedom. Average SPG stimulation application for acute pain was 16.9 ± 12.1 min (0.02–127.3 min). Stimulation duration was not statistically different between attacks achieving effective therapy and those not (18.9 ± 15.7 and 15.7 ± 8.8 min, respectively, $p = 0.5024$).

Table 1 Baseline characteristics for the 97 patients included in the safety analysis. Data are presented as mean ± SD (range). In case of missing data, the number of evaluated patients is given in parentheses

Baseline characteristics ($n = 97$ evaluated for safety)	
Age	46.6 ± 11.7 (22–75)
Gender	71 Male/26 Female
Cluster headache subtype	88 Chronic/9 Episodic
Laterality of headache	56 Left/41 Right
Cluster headache duration (years)	13.4 ± 9.0 (1–44) ($n = 95$)
Cluster attack frequency (per week)	25.6 ± 20.9 (0–96) ($n = 95$)
HIT-6 score at baseline	64.4 ± 6.4 (41–78) ($n = 92$)
Preventive medications at baseline	28% (27/97) used no preventive medications 72% (70/97) used preventive medications Of these: 48% (47/97) used verapamil as monotherapy or part of polytherapy, 24% (23/97) used other medications[a]

HIT-6 Headache Impact Test
[a]Topiramate, valproic acid, gabapentin, lithium carbonate, melatonin, methysergide, ergotamine and indomethacin

Therapeutic endpoints, chronic patients

As described above, patients using SPG stimulation experience both acute and frequency effects, and therapeutic response was therefore defined as experiencing either acute and/or frequency response. In the chronic patients, 65% (51/78) were considered responders per protocol (achieving effective therapy in at least 50% of attacks or experiencing a 50% reduction in attack frequency or both). Seventeen patients (20%) experienced both an acute and frequency response per the protocol. Nearly half of the chronic patients (47% (37/78)) experienced a very strong ≥ 75% response to SPG stimulation. 74% (58/78) of patients experienced at least a 30% therapeutic response.

Acute and preventive medication use

Ninety-seven percent (82/85) of patients used acute treatments (triptans and/or oxygen) at baseline. All acute treatments were reduced by 52% from 22.0 ± 21.3 to 10.6 ± 17.6 uses/week ($p < 0.0001$, $n = 82$), triptan usage was reduced by 57% from 11.3 ± 13.3 to 5.0 ± 9.9 uses/week ($p < 0.0001$, n = 82), and oxygen usage was reduced by 54% from 9.8 ± 15.4 to 4.5 ± 11.3 uses/week ($p = 0.0024$, $n = 84$) (Fig. 2). Among those using acute medications at baseline, 67% (52/78) reduced all acute treatments, 87% (59/68) reduced triptan use, and 79% (34/43) reduced oxygen use by ≥50% compared to baseline.

At 12 months, for chronic patients only, improvements in preventive medication use were noted in 74% (58/78) with 18 stopping all, 19 stopping some and/or decreasing the dose of others, 20 remaining off all, and 1 experiencing a clinical improvement (per clinical judgment) in preventive medication use at 12 months versus baseline.

Episodic cluster headache patient outcomes

Seven patients with eCH were followed through the study and per protocol, two were acute responders. This study is not ideally suited to evaluate the frequency response in eCH patients, however, per protocol, 5 of

Table 2 Change in attack frequency (mean ± SD (range)) between baseline and 12 months post-microstimulator insertion

Analysis	All patients		Chronic patients only		Episodic patients only	
	Baseline frequency (attacks/week)	12 month frequency (attacks/week)	Baseline frequency (attacks/week)	12 month frequency (attacks/week)	Baseline frequency (attacks/week)	12 month frequency (attacks/week)
All patients	25.2 ± 20.3 (0–96)	14.4 ± 17.9 (0–70)	24.3 ± 18.2 (0–84)	14.9 ± 18.1 (0–70)	34.3 ± 37.7 (7–96)	9.1 ± 13.6 (0–30)
	$p < 0.0001$, $n = 85$		$p < 0.0001$, $n = 78$		$p = 0.1094$, $n = 7$	
Frequency responders	26.7 ± 22.4 (3–96)	3.3 ± 6.3 (0–28)	24.7 ± 19.1 (3–84)	2.9 ± 5.4 (0–25)	30.0 ± 37.8 (7–96)	10.0 ± 14.8 (0–30)
	$p < 0.0001$, $n = 48$		$p < 0.0001$, $n = 43$		$p = 0.0625$, $n = 5$	

these were frequency responders. These eCH patients also saw improvements in quality of life and headache impairment similar to chronic patients: HIT-6 baseline: 64.5 ± 6.7, 12 months: 54.6 ± 13.2, SF-36v2 PCS baseline: 39.7 ± 7.9, 12 months: 44.9 ± 12.9 and SF-36v2 MCS baseline: 29.7 ± 8.4, 12 months: 40.4 ± 13.2.

Headache disability, quality of life, and patient surveys

Fifty-nine percent (47/80) of all the patients that completed HIT-6 at baseline, and 74% (39/53) of therapeutic responders were HIT-6 responders, experiencing a reduction in headache disability of at least 2.3 points. 67% (53/79) of all the patients that completed the SF-36, and 73% (38/52) of therapeutic responders, were SF-36v2 responders, experiencing an improvement in PCS, MCS, or both in the SF-36v2 survey. In addition, HIT-6, SF-36v2 PCS, and SF-36v2 MCS scores were significantly improved at 12 months compared to baseline (Table 3).

Seventy percent (56/80) of all patients who completed the questionnaire and 86% (48/56) of therapeutic responders rated the Pulsante™ system as good or very good. 81% considered the sensation of stimulation tolerable, 83% found the inserted device comfortable or did not feel it, 81% found surgery effects tolerable, 86% would recommend the therapy to someone else, 80% would make the same decision again, and 76% found SPG stimulation useful for treating their attacks.

Safety

The occurrence of side-effects in this population was similar to previously published data [12] on this issue, which typically included sensory disturbances, post-operative pain and swelling (Additional file 2: Table S1). Briefly, 73% of patients experienced such postoperative sequelae and these were generally considered mild to moderate and resolved within 2–3 months (average: 68 days for resolved

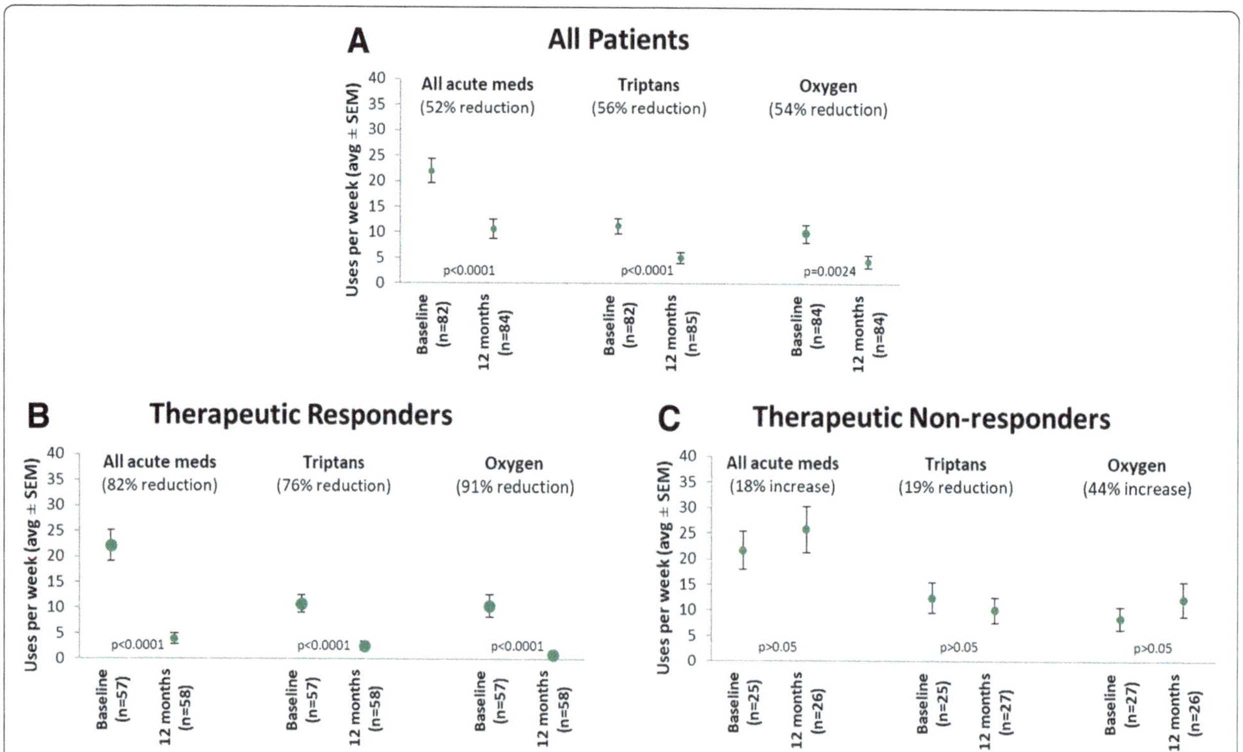

Fig. 2 Acute medications at 12 months as compared to baseline for (**a**) all patients, (**b**) therapeutic responders and (**c**) therapeutic non-responders

Table 3 Changes in headache disability (HIT-6) and quality of life (SF-36v2 physical component score (PCS) and mental component score (MCS)) from baseline to 12 months post-microstimulator insertion are provided (mean ± SD (range))

Analysis	HIT-6 headache disability		SF-36v2 quality of life – PCS		SF-36v2 quality of life – MCS	
	Baseline	12 months	Baseline	12 months	Baseline	12 months
All patients	64.3 ± 6.6 (41–78)	56.0 ± 11.1 (36–76)	40.4 ± 7.4 (23.9–57.6)	43.5 ± 10.1 (21.7–63.3)	32.2 ± 13.7 (6.0–59.7)	39.2 ± 15.0 (6.1–65.1)
	$p < 0.0001$, $n = 80$		$p = 0.0062$, $n = 79$		$p = 0.0003$, $n = 79$	
Therapeutic responders only	64.7 ± 6.9 (41–78)	53.2 ± 11.1 (36–74)	39.9 ± 7.7 (23.9–57.6)	45.2 ± 10.4 (22.3–63.3)	32.2 ± 12.6 (14.4–57.7)	40.8 ± 14.8 (6.1–65.1)
	$p < 0.0001$, $n = 53$		$p = 0.0001$, $n = 52$		$p = 0.0005$, $n = 52$	

Differences were statistically significant for all patients, as well as for therapeutic responders

events). There were no cases of device/lead migration after correct placement. There were no cases of lead fracture. Eight patients underwent lead revision after initial insertion due to suboptimal electrode placement.

Discussion

In this prospective study of 85 eCH and cCH patients treated with an implantable neurostimulator, we have demonstrated the effectiveness of SPG stimulation for attack frequency reductions and acute pain relief. At 12 months 55% of chronic patients were frequency responders and 32% of all patients were acute responders. At the per protocol defined level of ≥50%, 68% of all patients were therapeutic responders to SPG stimulation. 67% (52/78) of patients were able to reduce the use of acute medications by at least 50% and clinical improvements in the use of preventive medications were observed in 74% of patients. These clinical improvements were reflected in improved headache disability in 59% of all patients and 74% of responders.

Compared to deep brain stimulation and occipital nerve stimulation, SPG stimulation elicits both acute and preventive responses as supported by the reduction of both acute and preventive treatments in this population. Other studies in chronic headache have employed a responder level of 30% [15, 16]. If such a responder level were applied to this population, 76% of patients would be considered responders. However, some problems remain. For example, how the preventive response should be interpreted, given the possibility of spontaneous fluctuations [17]. The response to SPG stimulation appears stable over time as demonstrated in a previous 24 month study [9]. However, the difficulty in interpreting this response is underlined by results in the cCH group where the majority experienced reductions in frequency but a small subset *did* see an increase in the number of attacks compared to baseline. Further, in episodic CH, the frequency response cannot be solely attributed to treatment as the bout may be ending of its own accord. Longer baseline prospective attack diaries may be helpful in this regard, but given the dreadfulness of the disease, are impracticable and indeed unethical as it could delay effective treatment.

Overall, the data presented here is very similar to previously published results of SPG stimulation [8–10] with one exception: The proportion of acute uses of the stimulator achieving effective therapy was lower than previously reported (39% vs. 65%). This difference may be attributed to acute non-responders choosing the SPG stimulator over other acute treatments, despite it not being effective in them. This hypothesis may be supported by the fact that in the acute responders, the number of acute uses achieving effective therapy was similar in this study to that previously reported (86% vs. 78%, respectively). SPG stimulation is uniquely useful to CH patients as it is not associated with the daily limit in the number of uses as triptans which is especially important to patients with more than 2 daily attacks. Nor does it have the impracticality and stigmatization of oxygen, especially in the context of maintaining a professional life. Given that the use of acute medication is significantly reduced using SPG stimulation, this method also has an economical advantage [18].

As stated, SPG stimulation provides acute relief in some, a preventive effect in others, or both. This makes characterizing the efficacy challenging as reflected in previous studies [8, 9] where the preventive effect was unanticipated. However, this registry study was specifically designed to capture both signals. In the highly dynamic field of neurostimulation no official guidelines exist and there are only very few long-term neuromodulation studies of relatively small populations of CH patients. It should be noted that for want of a specific CH tool for measuring headache impact, the HIT-6, validated for migraine, was used. Although interventions with steroids were allowed per protocol, we believe these to have played a minor part in the overall results as only 3 of the 48 frequency responders were treated in this manner. A recall bias cannot be excluded, as the attack frequency was self-reported retrospectively at each study visit. Also, while a frequency effect is apparent, the effect of preventive simulation, i.e. stimulating without pain, is still unknown. At current, no positive or negative predictors for efficacy of SPG stimulation have been identified therefore patients with no immediate acute effect should keep stimulating as a preventive effect may manifest at a later point. An obvious possibility may be an influence of highly variant facial anatomy; however, other mechanisms should not be excluded. Additionally, stimulation duration and timing may play a role and future studies should investigate this and possible predictive factors.

Conclusion

In conclusion, SPG stimulation is an effective treatment for CH patients reducing their need for medications and improving quality of life and reducing headache impairment.

Abbreviations

cCH: Chronic cluster headache; CH: Cluster headache; CPS: Categorical pain scale; eCH: Episodic cluster headache; GON: Greater occipital nerve; HIT-6: Headache Impact Test; MCS: Mental component score; PCS: Physical component score; SF-36v2: Short Form Health Survey; SPG: Sphenopalatine ganglion stimulation

Acknowledgements

The authors would like to acknowledge all sub-investigators and site coordinators, and our surgical colleagues for their contributions to the Pathway R-1 study. The authors would also like to thank Anthony Caparso (former employee of ATI) and Dr. Amy Goodman (former employee of ATI) for their valuable contributions towards analyzing the data and writing the manuscript. The authors acknowledge the contributions of Tami Crabtree, PhD, (a consultant for ATI) for her assistance with the statistical analysis.

Funding

The study was funded by Autonomic Technologies, Inc., Redwood City, California.

Disclosures

MB, TPJ, and RJ are or have been (AM) consultants for ATI and have been paid for their services. All investigators but TPJ and AM have received per patient honoraria for the Pathway CH-1 trial. AP received a congress grant from ATI.

Authors' contributions

MB has concepted the study along with the coauthors, collected and analyzed the dataset, and drafted the manuscript. AP has collected the patients and the data from The Danish Headache Center and critically contributed to the manuscript. PS has collected the patients and the data from his center and critically contributed to the manuscript. TJ has co-concepted the study, collected and analyzed the dataset, and critically contributed to the manuscript. RHJ has contributed to the datacollection, co-concepted the study and contributed critically to the manuscript. AM has also co-concepted the study and contributed critically to the data analysis and the manuscript. All authors have read and approved the final manuscript.

Competing interests

The authors declare that they have no competing interests.

Author details

[1]Department of Clinical Physiology, Nuclear Medicine and PET, Rigshospitalet-Glostrup, Nordre Ringvej 57, 2600 Glostrup, Denmark. [2]Danish Headache Centre, Department of Neurology, Rigshospitalet-Glostrup, Nordre Ringvej 57, 2600 Glostrup, Denmark. [3]Schmerztherapie, Geriatrie und Palliativmedizin, Bochum, Kurt-Schumacher-Platz, 11-12 44787 Bochum, Germany. [4]Department of Neurology, University Medical Center Rostock, Gehlsherimer Str. 20, 18147 Rostock, Germany. [5]Department of Systems Neuroscience, Universitäts-Klinikum Hamburg-Eppendorf, Martinistraße 52, 20246 Hamburg, Germany.

References

1. Headache Classification Committee of the International Headache Society (IHS) (2013) The international classification of headache disorders, 3rd edition (beta version). Cephalalgia 33:629–808. https://doi.org/10.1177/0333102413485658
2. Jensen RM, Lyngberg A, Jensen RH (2007) Burden of cluster headache. Cephalalgia 27:535–541. https://doi.org/10.1111/j.1468-2982.2007.01330.x
3. Gaul C, Finken J, Biermann J, Mostardt S, Diener H-C, Müller O et al (2011) Treatment costs and indirect costs of cluster headache: a health economics analysis. Cephalalgia 31:1664–1672. https://doi.org/10.1177/0333102411425866
4. Matharu MS, Goadsby PJ (2008) Trigeminal autonomic Cephalalgias: diagnosis and management. In: Silberstein SD, Lipton R, Dodick D (eds) Wolff's headache other head pain, 8th edn. Oxford University Press, New York
5. Lanteri-Minet M, Silhol F, Piano V, Donnet A (2011) Cardiac safety in cluster headache patients using the very high dose of verapamil (≥720 mg/day). J Headache Pain 12:173–176. https://doi.org/10.1007/s10194-010-0289-x
6. Mitsikostas DD, Edvinsson L, Jensen RH, Katsarava Z, Lampl C, Negro A et al (2014) Refractory chronic cluster headache: a consensus statement on clinical definition from the European headache federation. J Headache Pain 15:79. https://doi.org/10.1186/1129-2377-15-79
7. Pedersen JL, Barloese M, Jensen RH (2013) Neurostimulation in cluster headache: a review of current progress. Cephalalgia 33:1179–1193. https://doi.org/10.1177/0333102413489040
8. Schoenen J, Jensen RH, Lantéri-Minet M, Láinez MJ, Gaul C, Goodman AM et al (2013) Stimulation of the sphenopalatine ganglion (SPG) for cluster headache treatment. Pathway CH-1: a randomized, sham-controlled study. Cephalalgia 33:816–830. https://doi.org/10.1177/0333102412473667
9. Jürgens TP, Barloese M, May A, Láinez JM, Schoenen J, Gaul C et al (2017) Long-term effectiveness of sphenopalatine ganglion stimulation for cluster headache. Cephalalgia 37:423–434. https://doi.org/10.1177/0333102416649092
10. Barloese MCJ, Jürgens TP, May A, Lainez JM, Schoenen J, Gaul C et al (2016) Cluster headache attack remission with sphenopalatine ganglion stimulation: experiences in chronic cluster headache patients through 24 months. J Headache Pain 17:67. https://doi.org/10.1186/s10194-016-0658-1
11. Jürgens TP, Schoenen J, Rostgaard J, Hillerup S, Láinez MJ, Assaf AT et al (2014) Stimulation of the sphenopalatine ganglion in intractable cluster headache: expert consensus on patient selection and standards of care. Cephalalgia 34:1100–1110. https://doi.org/10.1177/0333102414530524
12. Assaf AT, Hillerup S, Rostgaard J, Puche M, Blessmann M, Kohlmeier C et al (2016) Technical and surgical aspects of the sphenopalatine ganglion (SPG) microstimulator insertion procedure. Int J Oral Maxillofac Surg 45:245–254. https://doi.org/10.1016/j.ijom.2015.09.023
13. Smelt AFH, Assendelft WJJ, Terwee CB, Ferrari MD, Blom JW (2014) What is a clinically relevant change on the HIT-6 questionnaire? An estimation in a primary-care population of migraine patients. Cephalalgia 34:29–36. https://doi.org/10.1177/0333102413497599
14. Hays RD, Morales LS (2001) The RAND-36 measure of health-related quality of life. Ann Med 33:350–357
15. Silberstein S, Tfelt-Hansen P, Dodick DW, Limmroth V, Lipton RB, Pascual J et al (2008) Guidelines for controlled trials of prophylactic treatment of chronic migraine in adults. Cephalalgia 28:484–495. https://doi.org/10.1111/j.1468-2982.2008.01555.x
16. Dworkin RH, Turk DC, McDermott MP, Peirce-Sandner S, Burke LB, Cowan P et al (2009) Interpreting the clinical importance of group differences in chronic pain clinical trials: IMMPACT recommendations. Pain 146:238–244. https://doi.org/10.1016/j.pain.2009.08.019

20

The burden of headache is associated to pain interference, depression and headache duration in chronic tension type headache

Stella Fuensalida-Novo[1], Maria Palacios-Ceña[1,2], Juan J. Fernández-Muñoz[3], Matteo Castaldo[2,4,5], Kelun Wang[2], Antonella Catena[5], Lars Arendt-Nielsen[2] and César Fernández-de-las-Peñas[1,2*]

Abstract

Background: To investigate variables associated at one year (longitudinal design) with the physical or emotional component of burden in chronic tension type headache (CTTH).

Methods: One hundred and thirty ($n = 130$) individuals with CTTH participated in this longitudinal study. Clinical features were collected with a 4-weeks headache diary at baseline and 1-year follow-up. The burden of headache was assessed at baseline and one -year follow-up with the Headache Disability Inventory (HDI), physical (HDI-P) or emotional (HDI-E) component. Sleep quality (Pittsburgh Sleep Quality Index), anxiety and depression (Hospital Anxiety and Depression Scale-HADS), and quality of life (SF-36) were also assessed at baseline. Hierarchical regression analyses were conducted to determine the associations between the baseline variables and the headache burden at 1-year. Simple mediation models were also applied to determine the potential mediation effect of any intermediary variable.

Results: Regression analyses revealed that baseline pain interference and depression explained 32% of the variance in the emotional burden of headache, whereas baseline emotional burden of the headache, pain interference, and headache duration explained 51% of the variance in the physical burden of headache ($P < .01$) at 1-year. The mediation models observed that the effect of baseline pain interference on emotional burden of headache at 1-year was mediated through baseline depression, whereas the effect of baseline pain interference on the physical burden of headache at 1-year was mediated through baseline emotional burden of headache (both $P < .05$).

Conclusions: The current study found a longitudinal interaction between pain interference and depression with the burden of headache in individuals with CTTH.

Keywords: Tension type headache, Burden, Depression, Emotional, Pain

Background

Tension type headache is a common headache disorder showing a global prevalence of 42% in the general population [1] and an important socio-economic impact [2]. In the last Global Burden of Disease Study, headache was found to be the 3rd most prevalent pain condition in terms of global prevalence, the 6th in terms of global incidence and 28th in terms of years of life lived with disability [3]. The Eurolight project found that the burden of migraine and TTH in Europe is substantial, mostly related to lost days from work, lost days with household activity, lost family, social or leisure activities [4]. The general costs of headache, most related to migraine and TTH, in Europe in 2010 were €13.8 billion [5]. The Eurolight project estimated that indirect costs accounted for 92% of the financial burden of TTH [6]. In fact, recent data derived from the Eurolight project have confirmed that the burden of TTH is also substantial in middle-income

* Correspondence: cesarfdlp@yahoo.es
[1]Department Physical Therapy, Occupational Therapy, Rehabilitation, and Physical Medicine, Facultad de Ciencias de la Salud, University Rey Juan Carlos, Avenida de Atenas s/n, 28922 Alcorcón, Madrid, Spain
[2]Center for Sensory-Motor Interaction (SMI), Department of Health Science and Technology, Faculty of Medicine, Aalborg University, Aalborg, Denmark
Full list of author information is available at the end of the article

European countries such as Lithuania [7]. Similarly, headache burden is also similar in low-income countries, e.g., Ethiopia [8]. Therefore a better understanding of those potential variables associated with the burden of headache can assist clinicians in understanding which factors may play an important role in the management of TTH.

The concept of burden can be defined from different viewpoints. The Eurolight project focused, but not limited, the definition of burden in relation to work productivity [4, 6], although this project clearly shows that headache has negative impact on different aspects of life including education, career and earnings, family, or social life. Therefore, the term burden includes several components (physical or emotional) of an individual. Lampl et al. defined the term burden as "any loss of health or well-being attributable to a headache disorder" [9]. This definition of burden will be used in the current study.

It seems clear that headache can have physical and emotional repercussions on the life of the individual. Therefore, emotional factors may be crucial for the burden and perception of the disease. There is evidence suggesting that subjects with TTH exhibit co-morbid anxiety, depression [10], or sleep disturbances [11]. Some studies have previously investigated the association between depression and the burden of headache, but most of them included patients with migraine, but not TTH [12, 13]. Zebenholzer et al. observed that coexistence of depression and anxiety had a significant impact on the burden in patients with TTH and migraine [14]. It would be conceivable that different variables can interact at different levels to headache-associated burden. No study has previously investigated variables associated with the burden of headache in patients with TTH in a longitudinal design. Therefore, the purpose of the current study was to investigate potential variables associated at one year (longitudinal design) with the physical or emotional component of burden in a cohort of patients with chronic tension type headache (CTTH).

Methods

Study design

The current analysis is included as part of a multicenter international headache study. Some patients from the current study were also included in a previous part of the study which data have been already previously published [15]. This study presents new data by including new patients, different outcomes, different statistical analysis, and a different design since we had used a longitudinal desing, instead just only a cross-sectional design.

Participants

Patients with a diagnosis of TTH were recruited from three different university-based hospitals (Hospital Universitario Fundación Alcorcón-Spain, Aalborg University Hospital-Denmark, University Hospitals Parma Medical Center-Italy) from September 2014 to June 2016. Diagnosis was conducted according to the criteria of the International Classification of Headache Disorders, third edition (ICHD3 beta, 2013) down to third-digit level (codes 2.2, 2.3) by a neurologist expert in headaches [16]. They were excluded if presented: 1, epidosic headaches; 2, other primary or secondary headaches; 3, medication overuse headache as defined by the ICHD-III; 4, history of neck or head trauma; 5, any systemic degenerative disease; 6, diagnosis of fibromyalgia syndrome; 7, have received anesthetic blocks or botulinum toxin the previous 6 months; 8, have received physical treatment in the neck or head the previous 6 months; or, 8, pregnancy.

All participants read and signed a consent form prior to their participation. The local Ethics Committee approved the study (URJC 23/2014, HUFA 14/104, Aalborg N20140063, CESU 5/2015).

Headache diary

A headache diary for 4 weeks was used to substantiate the diagnosis and to record the headache clinical features [17]. This diary was recorded at baseline and at one-year follow-up. On the diary, patients registered the frequency of headaches (days per week), the headache intensity on an 11points numerical pain rate scale [18] (NPRS; 0: no pain, 10: the maximum pain), and the duration of each headache attack (hours per day).

Burden of headache

The Headache Disability Inventory (HDI) was used to assess the burden of headache. This questionnaire uses 25 items that inquire about the perceived impact of headache on emotional functioning and daily life activities [19]. Possible answers for each item include YES (4 points), SOMETIMES (2 points) and NO (0 points). Thirteen items assess the emotional burden (HDI-E, maximum score: 52) whereas the remaining 12 items assess the physical burden (HDI-P, maximum score: 48). A greater score suggests a greater burden of headache for each subscale. The HDI has exhibited good stability at short and long-term in patients with headache [20]. The HDI was assessed at baseline and at 1-year follow-up. The main outcome of this study was the burden of headache (HDI) at one-year follow-up.

Anxiety and depressive symptoms

The Hospital Anxiety and Depression Scale (HADS) is a 14-items self-report screening scale indicating the presence of anxiety and depressive symptom [21]. It consists of 7 items for evaluating anxiety (HADS-A) and 7 for depression (HADS-D). Each item scores on a Likert scale (0–3) giving a maximum score of 21 points for each subscale [22]. The HADS has shown good validity and internal consistency for being used in subjects with headache [23]. Anxiety and depressive symptoms were assessed at baseline.

Sleep quality

The Pittsburgh Sleep Quality Index (PSQI) as used to assess sleep quality [24]. This questionnaire assesses the quality of sleep over the previous month by including 19 self-rated questions and 5 questions answered by bedmates or roommates. Items use varying response categories recording usual bed time, usual wake time, number of actual hours slept, and number of minutes to fall asleep. All questions are answered on a Likert-type scale (0–3). The total score ranges from 0 to 21 where higher score indicates worse sleep quality. This questionnaire has good internal consistency and test-retest reliability [25, 26]. Sleep quality was assessed at baseline.

Health-related quality of life

Quality of life was assessed with the Medical Outcomes Study Short Form 36 (SF-36) questionnaire [27]. This questionnaire includes the following 8 domains: physical functioning, physical role, bodily pain (pain interference), general health, vitality, social function, role-emotional, and mental health. Total score range from 0 (the lowest quality of life) to 100 (the highest quality of life) [28]. Health-related quality of life was assessed at baseline.

Statistical analysis

Means and confidence intervals were calculated to describe the outcomes. The Kolmogorov-Smirnov test revealed that all data had a normal distribution ($P > .05$). To determine the relationship between the dependent measure (the emotional or physical burden of headache at one-year follow-up) and the independent outcomes (headache intensity, headache duration, headache frequency, sleep quality, HADS-D, HADS-A, physical functioning, physical role, pain interference, general health, vitality, social function, role-emotional, mental health at baseline), several Pearson product-moment correlation coefficients were first assessed. This correlational statistical analysis was used to check for multicollinearity and shared variance between the outcomes.

First, two regression models were used to assess the independent variables that contributed significantly to the variance in the emotional (HDI-E) and physical (HDI-P) burden of headache, separately. To examine the proportions of explained variance of the burden of headache, a hierarchical regression analysis was conducted. Changes in R^2 were reported after each step of the regression model to determine the association of the additional variables. Last, variables that significantly contributed to the score on the emotional or physical burden of headache were selected for inclusion into parsimonious final regression model. The significance criterion of the critical F value for entry into the regression equation was set at $P < .05$.

After the stepwise regression analyses, simple mediation models were applied to determine the potential mediation effect of depression (HADS-D) or emotional burden of headache (HDI-E) in the correlation between pain interference (bodily pain) and the emotional (HDI-E) or physical (HDI-P) burden of headache at 12 months, respectively. According to Baron and Kelly [29] in order to check a mediation hypothesis, previously it is necessary to develop several simple regression models between all variables included at the model for checking the following steps: 1, pain interference (bodily pain) as the predictable variable has a significant correlation with the emotional burden of headache (HDI-E) at one-year follow-up; 2, the predictive variable is related significantly with depression (HADS-D); 3, checking the mediated variable, in the first case, depression (HADS-D), is related with the criteria variable (the emotional burden of headache at 1-year) when the effect from the predictable variable is constant; and, 4, showing as the direct effect from pain interference (bodily pain) is significantly lower than when the mediated variable is included at the model (indirect effect) [30].

Results

Clinical data of the sample

A total of 200 individuals with headache were screened for possible eligibility criteria. Finally, 172 patients with CTTH (120 women, 50 men, mean age: 48 ± 15 years) satisfied all eligibility criteria, agreed to participate and signed the informed consent at baseline. Twenty-eight were excluded for the following reasons: co-morbid migraine ($n = 17$), episodic tension type headache ($n = 5$) previous whiplash ($n = 3$), fibromyalgia ($n = 2$) and medication overuse headache (n = 1). One hundred and thirty ($n = 130$, 76%, 95 women, 35 men, mean age: 47 ± 20 years) were also assessed at one-year follow-up and therefore included in the main analysis.

Correlation analysis

Pearson's correlation coefficients and the descriptive analysis between outcome variables are summarized in Table 1. Significant positive correlations were observed between the emotional burden of headache (HDI-E) at one-year and headache frequency ($r = .281$; $P = .015$), sleep quality ($r = .326$; $P = .004$), and depression ($r = .408$; $P < .001$) at baseline: the higher the frequency of the headaches, the worse the sleep quality, or the higher the depressive symptoms at baseline, the higher the emotional burden of the headache one year after. Significant negative correlations between the emotional burden of headache (HDI-E) at 1-year and pain interference ($r = -.508$;

Table 1 Pearson-Product Moment Correlation Matrix for Functional and Psychological Variables at Baseline Statistically Associated with the Physical or Emotional Burden of Headache at One Year

	Mean	95% CI	1	2	3	4	5	6	7	8	9
1. HDI-E at 12 months (0–52)	16.1	13.1–19.1									
2. HDI-P at 12 months (0–48)	20.5	17.7–23.3	.783**								
3. Headache Intensity (0–10)	5.7	5.4–6.0	n.s	228*							
4. Headache Duration (hours/day)	7.7	6.9–8.5	n.s	.376**	.335**						
5. Headache Frequency (days/month)	19.1	17.3–20.9	.281*	.306**	.247*	.245*					
6. Pittsburg Questionnaire (0 21)	8.8	7.9–9.7	.326**	.291*	.284**	n.s	.193*				
7. HADS-D (0–21)	9.5	8.6–10.4	.408**	.330**	.199*	n.s	.209*	.451**			
8. Bodily Pain (SF-36, 0–100)	47.3	42.3–52.3	−.508**	−.556**	−.190**	n.s	−.222**	−.362**	−.447**		
9. Vitality (SF-36, 0–100)	46.3	41.6–51.0	−.374**	−.453**	n.s	n.s	n.s	−.418**	−.615**	.608**	
10. Mental Health (SF-36, 0–100)	51.1	46.4–55.8	−.343**	−.254*	−.206*	n.s	n.s	−.386**	−.730**	.447**	.647**

95% CI 95% confidence interval, *HDI* Headache Disability Inventory (*E* Emotional, *P* Physical), *HADS* Hospital Anxiety and Depression Scale (*D* Depression)
*$P < 0.05$; **$P < 0.01$

$P < .001$), vitality ($r = -.374$; $P = .001$) or mental health ($r = -.343$; $P = .002$) at baseline were also found: the lower the vitality, pain interference or mental health score, i.e., the lower vitality, the higher experience of pain or the worse mental health, at baseline, the higher the emotional burden of the headache one year after.

Significant positive correlations were observed between the physical burden of headache (HDI-P) at 1-year and headache intensity ($r = .228$; $P = .045$), frequency ($r = .306$; $P = .008$) and duration ($r = .376$; $P = .009$), sleep quality ($r = .291$; $P = .01$), and depression ($r = .330$; $P = .004$) at baseline: the higher the headache frequency, the higher the intensity of headache, the longer the headache duration, the worse the sleep quality, or the higher the depressive symptoms at baseline, the higher the physical burden of the headache one year after. Finally, significant negative correlations between the physical burden of the headache (HDI-P) at one-year and pain interference ($r = -.556$; $P < .001$), vitality ($r = -.453$; P < .001) or mental health ($r = -.254$; $P = .03$) at baseline were also observed: the lower the vitality, the pain interference or mental health score, i.e., the lower vitality, the higher experience of pain or the worse mental health at baseline, the higher the physical burden of the headache one year after.

Regression analyses

Table 2 summarizes the hierarchical regression analysis conducted for the emotional burden of headache (HDI-E) at one-year. In this analysis, baseline pain interference (bodily pain) approximately contributed 27.2% ($P < .001$), whereas baseline depression (HADS-D) contributed an additional 5% (P < .001) to the variance of emotional burden of headache (HDI-E) at one-year follow-up. When combined, both variables explained 32.2% of the variance in the emotional burden of headache (r^2 adjusted: 0.322, F = 11.33, $P < .01$).

The hierarchical regression analysis conducted for the physical burden of headache (HDI-P) at one-year is summarized in Table 3. In this analysis, baseline emotional burden of headache (HDI-E) contributed 46% ($P < .001$), pain interference (bodily pain) an additional 6% ($P < .01$) and baseline headache duration an additional 3% ($P < .001$) of the variance of physical burden of headache (HDI-P) at one-year. When combined, all variables explained 51.1% of the variance in the physical burden of headache (r^2 adjusted: 0.511, F = 27.77, $P < .01$).

Mediation effects

Figure 1 summarizes the standardized effect of the first simple mediation model. First, the total effect from pain interference (bodily pain) on depression (HADS-D) was statistically significant (B = −0.18, $P < .001$). Second, the total direct effect from pain interference (bodily pain) on emotional burden of headache (HDI-E) at one-year was significant (B = −0.27, P < .001). Third, the total direct effect from depression (HADS-D) to the emotional burden of headache (HDI-E) at one-year was significant (B = 0.78, $P < .001$). Finally, the total indirect effect of pain interference on the emotional burden of headache

Table 2 Summary of Stepwise Regression Analyses to Determine Baseline Predictors of the Emotional Burden of Headache at One Year ($r^2 = 32.2\%$)

Independent Variable	*B*	SE B	β	t	F	P
Step 1						
Bodily Pain	−.272	.052	−.532	−5.246	27.51	<0.001
Step 2						
Bodily Pain	−.222	.057	−.433	−3.925	11.33	<0.01
HADS-D	.689	.342	.222	2.014		

$R^2 = .272$ for step 1; $R^2 = .322$ for step 2
HADS Hospital Anxiety and Depression Scale (*D* Depression)

Table 3 Summary of Stepwise Regression Analyses to Determine Baseline Predictors of the Physical Burden of Headache at One Year ($r^2 = 55.1\%$)

Independent Variable	*B*	SE B	Β	t	F	P
Step 1						
HDI-E	.598	.077	.678	7.721	59.61	<0.001
Step 2						
HDI-E	.453	.088	.514	5.143	37.54	<0.01
Bodily Pain	−.144	.048	−.297	−2.790		
Step 3						
HDI-E	.423	.087	.480	4.852	27.77	<0.01
Bodily Pain	−.148	.047	−.305	−3.124		
Headache Duration	.513	.243	.174	2.113		

$R^2 = .460$ for step 1 $R^2 = .521$ for step 2; $R^2 = .551$ for step 3
HDI Headache Disability Inventory (*E* Emotional)

(HDI-E) at one-year mediated through baseline depression (HADS-D) was also significant ($B = -0.07$, $P = .04$). To consider statistically significant the partial effect of mediation at this first model, Zobel test was significant ($z = -2.52$, $P = .01$) with a confidence level not including the value 0 (LLCI: -0.1546, ULCI: -0.0236).

The standardized effect of the second simple mediation model is shown in Fig. 2. First, the total effect from pain interference (bodily pain) on the emotional burden of headache (HDI-E) was statistically significant ($B = -0.28$, $P < .001$). Second, the total direct effect from pain interference (bodily pain) on the physical burden of headache (HDI-P) at one-year was also statistically significant ($B = -0.19$, $P = .04$). Third, the total direct effect from the baseline emotional burden of headache (HDI-E) on the physical burden of headache (HDI-P) at one-year was significant ($B = 0.47$, $P < .001$). Finally, the total indirect effect from pain interference (bodily pain) on the physical burden of headache at one-year mediated through the baseline emotional burden of headache (HDI-E) was also significant ($B = -0.13$, $P = .04$). Again, to consider the partial effect of mediation statistically significant at the second model, the Zobel test revealed that the model was significant ($z = -3.74$, $P = .002$) with a confidence level not including the value 0 (LLCI: -0.2200; ULCI: -0.0734).

Discussion

This is the first longitudinal study investigating the variables associated with the burden of headache in individuals with CTTH. We observed that the emotional burden of headache was associated to baseline pain interference and depression whereas the physical burden of headache was associated to baseline emotional aspects of the burden, pain interference, and headache duration. Baseline depression and the emotional burden mediated the effects of pain interference with the emotional or physical burden at one-year follow-up, respectively.

The findings from this study show two important aspects. First, pain interference was longitudinally associated with both emotional and physical components of burden; and second, a relevant role of emotional aspects in patients with CTTH since depression and emotional component of burden indirectly mediated the effect of pain inference on the headache burden. Our results support an important association of pain interference with burden, which would agree with the conception that pain is a dimension associated to burden perception. In fact, the duration of the headache attack was also independently associated to the physical component of burden; supporting that not only the presence of pain, but also its duration, is relevant for burden perception. This may be related to the fact that pain interference refers to limitations on daily life activities due to the presence of pain and headache duration is related to the time with pain; therefore, this outcome reveals two different spheres of the pain spectrum.

We also found that the effects of pain interference on the emotional burden were mediated by depression,

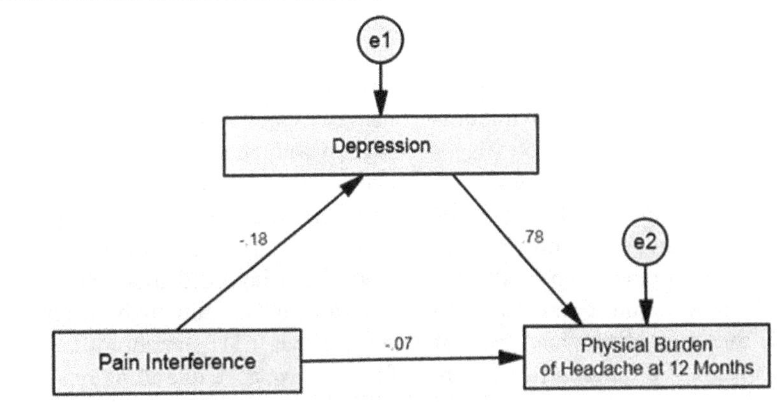

Fig. 1 Mediation Analysis of Pain Interference on Physical Burden of Headache at one-year through Depression

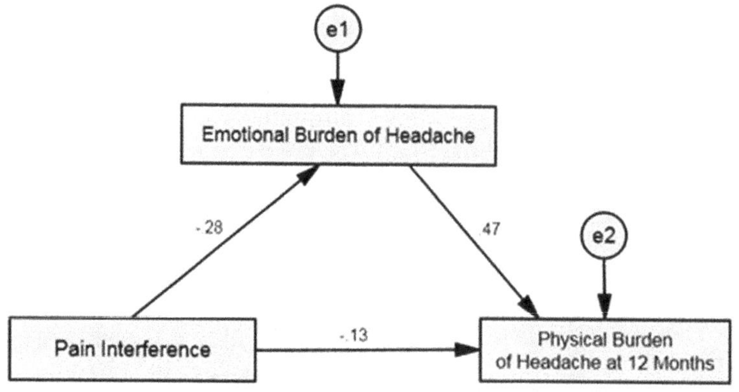

Fig. 2 Mediation Analysis of Pain Interference on Physical Burden of Headache at one-year through Emotional Burden of Headache

suggesting a relevant role of depression in patients with CTTH. It has been previously observed that depression has a marked impact on the burden in patients with chronic headaches since it increases the risk of feeling less understood by the family and friends as well as an increased risk of avoiding to tell other people about the headache [14]. In fact, it has been previously suggested that depression contributes to chronic pain via supra-spinal mechanisms and emotional modulation of pain [31]. Our results support this mechanism since depression mediated the effect of pain interference on the emotional burden of headache.

Similarly, the effect of pain interference on the physical burden was mediated by emotional aspects of burden, supporting a relevant role of emotional factors. It seems that emotional (stressful) factors are common precipitating factors of headache episodes in patients with TTH [32] since they may trigger hyperalgesic responses within the central nervous system [33]. Therefore, it is possible that emotional (stressful) factors can trigger more headache attacks inducing an increasing in the frequency of headaches, which would lead to worse pain interference and, therefore, higher self-perceived burden. In fact, the presence of mood disorders is more associated to the frequency of headaches rather than to headache diagnosis [34].

Uncertainty over biological mechanisms withstanding in these interactions, our results have clinical implications. Since emotional stress is the most common trigger for pain in subjects with TTH, proper management of emotional factors may be relevant for avoiding chronification and an increase of burden perception. In fact, emotional stress and depression represent two modifiable risk factors implicated in the progression from episodic to chronic headaches [35]; therefore, their management could also lead to better control of the headache burden. Our study found that depression and emotional aspects of burden were mediating factors in the association between pain interference and the burden of headache. Therefore, proper copying strategies for management of potential stressful emotional events and a reduction of depressive symptoms may be those factors associated with a reduction of the headache burden. Current findings would suggest that management of patients with CTTH should include therapeutic interventions targeted to decrease the emotional burden of headache (copying strategies or cognitive behavioral techniques) and to decrease depressive symptoms (i.e., psychological approaches) with the aim to decrease the burden of headache.

Although strengths of the current study include a large sample size, the inclusion of patients accordingly to the most updated diagnostic criteria, the use of diagnostic diaries and a longitudinal design, some limitations should be also recognized. First, we included patients with CTTH from a tertiary headache center; therefore, they may be not representative of the general population. Second, the impact of medication intake was not considered in the mediation models. Third, it should be noted that the HADS is a screening rather than diagnostic instrument for depressive symptoms with a tendency to underestimate its prevalence [36]. In fact, we noted that depression levels observed in our sample of CTTH patients were low; therefore, it is possible that the mediating effect between pain interference and the emotional burden of headache may be different in individuals experiencing higher levels of depression. Finally, we assessed the emotional or physical component of burden with the HDI. Previous studies assessing the burden of headache had used the HALT index which considers the days lost completely or partially because of headache in the preceding months and covers professional work, household activities or chores, and family, social or leisure activities. Although current and previous data [3] suggest that TTH should not be considered as a minimal form of headache due to its repercussions, current results should be considered in this context of headache burden, but not in the economic factor of headache.

Conclusions

The current study found that pain interference and depression were longitudinally associated to the emotional burden of headache whereas the emotional headache burden, pain interference, and headache duration were longitudinally associated to the physical burden of headache in individuals with CTTH. Baseline depression and the emotional burden mediated the effects of pain interference with the emotional or physical burden at one-year follow-up, respectively. This study suggests that emotional factors play a relevant role in the association between pain interference and burden in patients with CTTH.

Abbreviations

CTTH: Chronic tension type headache; HADS: Hospital Anxiety and Depression Scale; HDI: Headache Disability Inventory; ICHD3: International Classification of Headache Disorders, third edition; NPRS: Numerical Pain Rate Scale; PSQI: Pittsburgh Sleep Quality Index; SF-36: Health-related quality of life questionnaire; TTH: Tension type headache

Acknowledgements

Not applicable

Author' contributions

All authors contributed to the study concept and design. JJFM and CFdlP did the main statistical analysis and interpretation of data. SFN, MPC and CFdlP contributed to draft the report. LAN obtained funding. LAN, KW, MC, AC provided administrative, technical, and material support. LAN and CFdlP supervised the study. All authors revised the text for intellectual content and have read and approved the final version of the manuscript.

Funding

No funds were received for this study.

Disclosures

Financial disclosure statements have been obtained, and no conflicts of interest have been reported by the authors or by any individuals in control of the content of this article.

Competing interests

The authors declare that they have no competing interests.

Author details

[1]Department Physical Therapy, Occupational Therapy, Rehabilitation, and Physical Medicine, Facultad de Ciencias de la Salud, University Rey Juan Carlos, Avenida de Atenas s/n, 28922 Alcorcón, Madrid, Spain. [2]Center for Sensory-Motor Interaction (SMI), Department of Health Science and Technology, Faculty of Medicine, Aalborg University, Aalborg, Denmark. [3]Department of Psychology, Universidad Rey Juan Carlos, Alcorcón, Spain. [4]Master in Sport Physiotherapy, University of Siena, Siena, Italy. [5]Poliambulatorio Fisiocenter, Collecchio, (Parma), Italy.

References

1. Ferrante T, Manzoni GC, Russo M, Camarda C, Taga A, Veronesi L et al (2013) Prevalence of tension-type headache in adult general population: the PACE study and review of the literature. Neurol Sci 34:S137–S138
2. Dowson A (2015) The burden of headache: global and regional prevalence of headache and its impact. Int J Clin Pract Suppl 182:3–7
3. GBD 2016 Disease and Injury Incidence and Prevalence Collaborators (2017) Global, regional, and national incidence, prevalence, and years lived with disability for 328 diseases and injuries for 195 countries, 1990-2016: a systematic analysis for the global burden of disease study 2016. Lancet 390:1211–1259
4. Steiner TJ, Stovner LJ, Katsarava Z, Lainez JM, Lampl C, Lantéri-Minet M, Rastenyte D, Ruiz de la Torre E, Tassorelli C, Barré J, Andrée C (2014) The impact of headache in Europe: principal results of the Eurolight project. J Headache Pain 15:31
5. Raggi A, Leonardi M (2015) Burden and cost of neurological diseases: a European north-south comparison. Acta Neurol Scand 132:16–22
6. Linde M, Gustavsson A, Stovner LJ et al (2012) The cost of headache disorders in Europe: the Eurolight project. Eur J Neurol 19:703–711
7. Rastenytė D, Mickevičienė D, Stovner LJ, Thomas H, Andrée C, Steiner TJ (2017) Prevalence and burden of headache disorders in Lithuania and their public-health and policy implications: a population-based study within the Eurolight project. J Headache Pain 18:53
8. Zebenigus M, Tekle-Haimanot R, Worku DK, Thomas H, Steiner TJ (2017) The burden of headache disorders in Ethiopia: national estimates from a population-based door-to-door survey. J Headache Pain 18:58
9. Lampl C, Thomas H, Stovner LJ, Tassorelli C, Katsarava Z, Laínez JM, Lantéri-Minet M, Rastenyte D, Ruiz de la Torre E, Andrée C, Steiner TJ (2016) Interictal burden attributable to episodic headache: findings from the Eurolight project. J Headache Pain 17:9
10. Lampl C, Thomas H, Tassorelli C, Katsarava Z, Laínez JM, Lantéri-Minet M, Rastenyte D, Ruiz de la Torre E, Stovner LJ, Andrée C, Steiner TJ (2016) Headache, depression and anxiety: associations in the Eurolight project. J Headache Pain 17:59
11. Uhlig BL, Engstrøm M, Ødegård SS, Hagen KK, Sand T (2014) Headache and insomnia in population-based epidemiological studies. Cephalalgia 34:745–751
12. Rao AS, Scher AI, Vieira RV, Merikangas KR, Metti AL, Peterlin BL (2015) The impact of post-traumatic stress disorder on the burden of migraine: results from the national comorbidity survey-replication. Headache 55:1323–1341
13. Oh K, Cho SJ, Kim J, Chu MK (2014) Combination of anxiety and depression is associated with an increased headache frequency in migraineurs: a population-based study. BMC Neurol 14:238
14. Zebenholzer K, Lechner A, Broessner G, Lampl C, Luthringshausen G, Wuschitz A, Obmann SM, Berek K, Wöber C (2016) Impact of depression and anxiety on burden and management of episodic and chronic headaches - a cross-sectional multicentre study in eight Austrian headache centres. J Headache Pain 17:15
15. Palacios-Ceña M, Fernández-Muñoz JJ, Castaldo M, Wang K, Guerrero-Peral Á, Arendt-Nielsen L, Fernández-de-las-Peñas C (2017) The association of headache frequency with pain interference and the burden of disease is mediated by depression and sleep quality, but not anxiety, in chronic tension type headache. J Headache Pain 18:19
16. ICHD-III (2013) International classification of headache disorder: headache classification Subcommittee of the International Headache Society, 3nd edition. Cephalalgia 33:629–808
17. Jensen R, Tassorelli C, Rossi P, Allena M, Osipova V, Steiner T, Sandrini G, Olesen J, Nappi G, Basic Diagnostic Headache Diary Study Group (2011) A basic diagnostic headache headache diary (BDHD) is well accepted and useful in the diagnosis of headache. A multicentre European and Latin American study. Cephalalgia 31:1549–1560
18. Jensen MP, Turner JA, Romano JM, Fisher L (1999) Comparative reliability and validity of chronic pain intensity measures. Pain 83:157–162
19. Jacobson GP, Ramadan NM, Norris L, Newman CW (1994) The Henry ford hospital headache disability inventory. Neurology 44:837–842
20. Jacobson GP, Ramadan NM, Norris L, Newman CW (1995) Headache disability inventory (HDI): short-term test-retest reliability and spouse perceptions. Headache 35:534–539
21. Zigmond AS, Snaith RP (1983) The hospital anxiety and depression scale. Acta Psychiatr Scand 67:361–370

22. Herrmann-Lingen C, Buss U, Snaith R (2011) Hospital Anxiety and Depression Scale – Deutsche Version (HADS-D) Verlag Hans Huber, Bern
23. Juang KD, Wang SJ, Lin CH, Fuh JL (1999) Use of the hospital anxiety and depression scale as a screening tool for patients with headache. Zhonghua Yi Xue Za Zhi (Taipei) 62:749–755
24. Cole JC, Dubois D, Kosinski M (2007) Use of patient-reported sleep measures in clinical trials of pain treatment: a literature review and synthesis of current sleep measures and a conceptual model of sleep disturbance in pain. Clin Ther 29:2580–2588
25. Buysse DJ, Reynolds CF, Monk TH, Berman SR, Kupfer DJ (1989) The Pittsburgh sleep quality index: a new instrument for psychiatric practice and research. Psychiatry Res 28:193–213
26. Carpenter JS, Andrykowski M (1998) Psychometric evaluation of the Pittsburgh sleep quality index. J Psychosom Res 45:5–13
27. Ware JE, Sherbourne CD (1992) The MOS 36-item short-form health survey (SF-36). I. Conceptual framework and item selection. Med Care 30:473–483
28. McHorney CA, Ware JE, Raczek AE (1993) The MOS 36-item short-form health survey (SF-36): II. Psychometric and clinical tests of validity in measuring physical and mental health constructs. Med Care 31:247–263
29. Baron RM, Kenny DA (1986) The moderator-mediator variable distinction in social psychological research: conceptual, strategic and statistical considerations. J Personality Social Psychol 51:1173–1182
30. Hayes AF (2013) Introduction to mediation, moderation and conditional process analysis. A regression based approach. The Guilford Press, Nueva York
31. Terry EL, DelVentura JL, Bartley EJ, Vincent AL, Rhudy JL (2013) Emotional modulation of pain and spinal nociception in persons with major depressive disorder (MDD). Pain 154:2759–2768
32. Wang J, Huang Q, Li N, Tan G, Chen L, Zhou J (2013) Triggers of migraine and tension-type headache in China: a clinic-based survey. Eur J Neurol 20:689–696
33. Cathcart S, Petkov J, Winefield AH, Lushington K, Rolan P (2010) Central mechanisms of stress-induced headache. Cephalalgia 30:285–295
34. Zwart JA, Dyb G, Hagen K et al (2003) Depression and anxiety disorders associated with headache frequency: the Nord-Trøndelag health study. Eur J Neurol 10:147–152
35. Rains JC (2008) Chronic headache and potentially modifiable risk factors: screening and behavioral management of sleep disorders. Headache 48:32–39
36. Steel Z, Marnane C, Iranpour C, Chey T, Jackson JW, Patel V, Silove D (2014) The global prevalence of common mental disorders: a systematic review and meta-analysis 1980-2013. Int J Epidemiol 43:476–493

21

Headache following head injury: a population-based longitudinal cohort study (HUNT)

Lena Hoem Nordhaug[1*], Knut Hagen[1,3], Anne Vik[1,2], Lars Jacob Stovner[1,3], Turid Follestad[4], Torunn Pedersen[5], Gøril Bruvik Gravdahl[3] and Mattias Linde[1,3]

Abstract

Background: Headache is the most frequent symptom following head injury, but long-term follow-up of headache after head injury entails methodological challenges. In a population-based cohort study, we explored whether subjects hospitalized due to a head injury more often developed a new headache or experienced exacerbation of previously reported headache compared to the surrounding population.

Methods: This population-based historical cohort study included headache data from two large epidemiological surveys performed with an 11-year interval. This was linked with data from hospital records on exposure to head injury occurring between the health surveys. Participants in the surveys who had not been hospitalized because of a head injury comprised the control group. The head injuries were classified according to the Head Injury Severity Scale (HISS). Multinomial logistic regression was performed to investigate the association between head injury and new headache or exacerbation of pre-existing headache in a population with known pre-injury headache status, controlling for potential confounders.

Results: The exposed group consisted of 294 individuals and the control group of 25,662 individuals. In multivariate analyses, adjusting for age, sex, anxiety, depression, education level, smoking and alcohol use, mild head injury increased the risk of new onset headache suffering (OR 1.74, 95% CI 1.05–2.87), stable headache suffering (OR 1.70, 95% CI 1.15–2.50) and exacerbation of previously reported headache (OR 1.93, 95% CI 1.24–3.02). The reference category was participants without headache in both surveys.

Conclusion: Individuals hospitalized due to a head injury were more likely to have new onset and worsening of pre-existing headache and persistent headache, compared to the surrounding general population. The results support the entity of the ICHD-3 beta diagnosis "persistent headache attributed to traumatic injury to the head".

Keywords: Headache attributed to head injury, Head injury, Traumatic brain injury, Secondary headache disorders, Post-traumatic headache, Population-based

Background

Headache often has a major impact on the lives of the individuals affected, and constitutes a large social and economic burden for the global society [1–3].

Likewise, head injury is an important global health issue and a major cause of morbidity [4, 5]. Headache is the most frequent symptom following head injury, and it is manifested both as new onset and worsening of pre-existing headache [6–9]. The international classification of headache disorders (third edition, ICHD-3 beta) defines headache attributed to head injury (HAIH) as a headache with no defining clinical characteristics that starts within seven days of injury [10]. Persistent HAIH is of greater than 3 months' duration [10]. Long-term follow-up of headache after head injury entails methodological challenges. To investigate a causal relationship between head injury and subsequent headache, a control group for

* Correspondence: lena.h.nordhaug@ntnu.no
[1]Department of Neuromedicine and Movement Science (INB), Faculty of Medicine and Health Sciences, Norwegian University of Science and Technology, Postbox 8905, 7491 Trondheim, Norway
Full list of author information is available at the end of the article

comparison is vital, preferably through a population-based design. There are, to our knowledge, only two other population-based, controlled studies on this subject and their findings are inconsistent [11, 12]. Moreover, both studies have methodological limitations [11, 12]. Headache prevalence and severity have been reported to be greater in those with mild head injury compared to those with more severe head injury [13, 14]. This inverse dose-response relationship is paradoxical and needs further investigation.

In a previous population-based historical cohort study, which was based on the third wave of the Nord-Trøndelag Health Study (HUNT), we evaluated the relationship between previous head injury and headache phenotype [15]. The primary aim of the current study was to analyze headache data for those who participated in both the second and third waves of the HUNT Study, evaluating the impact on new onset headache or exacerbation of headache due to head injuries in a population with known pre-injury headache status, taking into account the head injury severity.

Methods

Study design

This historical cohort study included data on headache from the second and third HUNT surveys, two large epidemiological surveys performed with an 11-year interval. Headache data was linked with data from hospital records on exposure to head injury occuring between the surveys. The exposed group consisted of study participants hospitalized due to a head injury, the remaining participants were used as controls.

The HUNT-surveys

The HUNT Study is a longitudinal cohort study in which all inhabitants ≥20 years of age in Nord-Trøndelag were invited to participate. Participants were examined three times. The two last surveys, HUNT2 (1995–1997) and HUNT3 (2006–2008) covered a large number of health-related items. Details of these comprehensive surveys, including non-respondents, are described elsewhere [16, 17].

Headache categories

Both HUNT2 and HUNT3 questionnaires included the screening question "Have you suffered from headache during the last 12 months?" The answers to the screening questions were used to categorize the responders into four mutually exclusive groups with regard to headache suffering at the two time points: Stable non-sufferers (headache-free in both studies), past sufferer (headache in HUNT2 but not in HUNT3), stable headache sufferer (headache in both studies) and new sufferer (headache in HUNT3, but not in HUNT2).

Participants answering "yes" to the headache screening question also reported their headache frequency. This enabled categorization of the responders with headache suffering in both surveys into three mutually exclusive groups: less frequent headache (in HUNT3 compared to HUNT2), stable headache frequency (same headache frequency in HUNT3 as in HUNT2), more frequent headache (in HUNT3 compared to HUNT2). Alternatives available for the headache frequency question were < 7, 7–14 and > 14 days/month.

To examine exacerbation or improvement in headache status between HUNT2 and HUNT3 we merged the frequency variable with the screening question so that each participant could be categorized in one of the following four groups: no headache suffering, headache suffering < 7 days/month, headache suffering 7–14 days/month, headache suffering > 14 days/month. Exacerbation of headache was defined as new onset of headache or increased frequency of previously reported headache. Improvement was defined as absence of or decrease in frequency of previously reported headache. Stable headache frequency was defined as headache suffering in both surveys with the same headache frequency in both.

Pre-existing headache was classified into two mutually exclusive groups: Migraine and non-migrainous headache. The approach used in determining headache subtype is described and validated elsewhere [18].

The validities of the headache questionnaires in HUNT2 and HUNT3 have been reported previously [18, 19]. For any headache suffering in HUNT2, the sensitivity was 85% and specificity 83% (kappa 0.57, 95% CI 0.41–0.73). For any headache suffering in HUNT3, the sensitivity was 88% and specificity 86% (kappa 0.70, 95% CI 0.61–0.79). A personal interview by a neurologist was used as gold standard.

Head injury data collection

All participants who had answered the headache screening question in HUNT3 and who had also been hospitalized in the region due to a head injury during the period 1988–2008 were identified in 2012 by a computer-based search. Details on how this was performed have been reported previously [15].

Information regarding the head injuries was collected from medical records. If the same individual had more than one head injury within the period, up to three of the most recent head injuries were recorded. The head injuries were classified according to the Head Injury Severity Scale (HISS) [20].

Only participants who answered the headache screening question in both HUNT2 and HUNT3 were of interest for analyses. Participants with head injuries between participation in HUNT2 and HUNT3 were included in the exposed group. Participants with head injuries before HUNT2 were excluded.

Other measurements

The HUNT2 and HUNT3 surveys included many health-related items, and in the present study we used the following information about the participants in addition to headache status: age, sex, duration of education, smoking habits, total Hospital Anxiety and Depression Scale (HADS) score, self-reported health, BMI and CAGE score. The HADS is a fourteen item scale used to determine levels of anxiety and depression. The CAGE questionnaire is a widely used screening instrument for potential alcohol problems [21].

Statistical analysis

Demographic data for individuals with and without head injury are presented as means with standard deviations (continuous variables) and percentages (categorical data). In multivariate analyses, using multinomial logistic regression, we first examined the association between head injury and relative headache status in HUNT3 versus HUNT2 with regard only to suffering from headache and then the association between head injury and relative headache status in HUNT3 versus HUNT2 with regard both to suffering from headache and change in headache frequency. The results are presented as odds ratios (OR) with 95% confidence intervals (CI). OR's for which the 95% CI did not include 1 were considered statistically significant. Stable non-sufferers were used as reference category. The associations were investigated both with head injury as a binary variable (yes/no) and with head injury in four categories according to head injury severity (no head injury/minimal/mild/moderate head injury).

In the multivariate analyses we initially adjusted for age and sex. Subsequently, we also added the following potential confounding factors retrieved from the HUNT2 dataset: duration of education (≤ 9, 10–12 and ≥13 years) as proxy for socioeconomic status, daily smoking (yes/no), total HADS score (categorized from a continuous variable into three categories with score ≤ 16, 17–21 and ≥22) and CAGE score (0 or ≥1). In the logistic regression analyses missing data were handled by listwise deletion. Linearity of the continuous variables with respect to the logit of the dependent variable was assessed via the Box-Tidwell procedure [22]. The continuous variable age was found to fail the assumption of linearity and was split into categories with 10 year intervals. We investigated potential interactions between all covariates and head injury by including the product of the two variables into the multinomial logistic regression analyses. The interaction coefficients were tested using Wald statistics, with p-values less than 0.05 considered statistically significant. Because headache disorders in general are highly dependent on sex [17], separate analyses after stratifying for sex are common in research concerning headache. Consequently we chose to also do separate analyses after stratifying for sex. No formal adjustment for multiple testing was made.

The study was approved by the Regional Committee for Medical and Health Research Ethics and by the HUNT Research Centre.

Results

Participants

The flow of participants through the different stages of the study is presented in Fig. 1. A total of 294 participants had been hospitalized due to a head injury during the 11 year time period between the two surveys (exposed). The remaining 25,662 individuals were not hospitalized for head injury during this period (unexposed). Demographic data for the two groups are presented in Table 1. Prevalence of headache in HUNT2 was similar in the two groups (43.9% versus 41.7%, χ^2 (1) = 0.575, p = 0.45).

Head injuries

Among the 294 individuals with head injuries, 11 experienced two head injuries, adding up to a total of 305 incidents. Taking into account only the first head injury (of those with more than one), 11.9% of the head injuries were minimal, 71.8% were mild, 10.9% were moderate and 5.4% were unclassifiable. There were no severe head injuries. The most common injury mechanism was falling (55.1%), followed by traffic accidents (28.6%) and assault (1.7%).

A CT scan was performed in 56.4% (n = 172), an MRI in 1.0% (n = 3) and a plain X-ray of the head in 3.6% (n = 11) of the cases. The scans revealed traumatic pathology in 16.0% (n = 47). In total, 9.2% (n = 27) of all patients had intracranial pathology. 9.9% (n = 29) had cranial fractures (revealed either by imaging or clinical findings), and 5.1% (n = 15) had both cranial fracture and intracranial pathology.

Headache categories

Among the 25,956 partcipants, 12,830 (49.4%) were headache free in HUNT2 and HUNT3 (stable non-suffering), 6303 (24.3%) suffered from headache in both surveys (stable headache suffering), 4523 (17.4%) reported headache in HUNT2 only (past headache suffering) and 2300 participants (8.9%) had no headache in HUNT2, but reported to suffer from headache in HUNT3 (new headache suffering).

Among the 129 participants with head injury and pre-existing headache, 46 (35.7%) suffered from migraine, 57 (44.2%) from non-migrainous headache and 26 (20.2%) were unclassifiable.

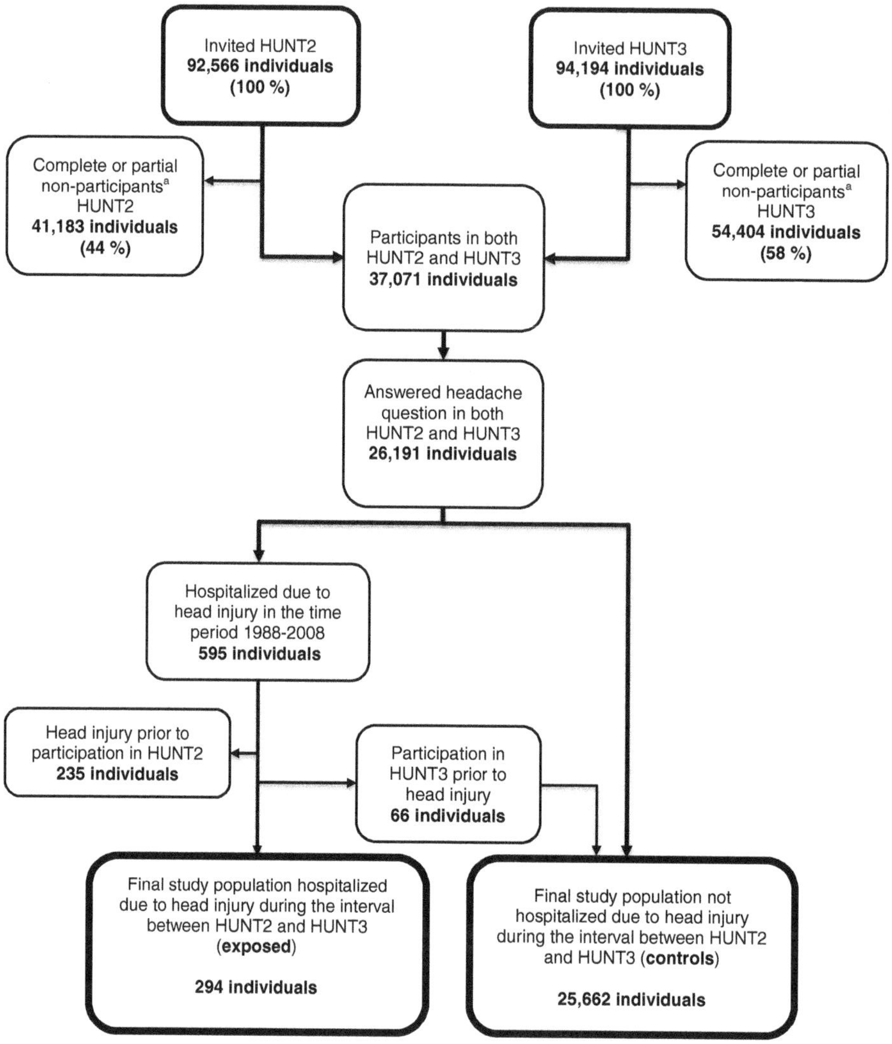

Fig. 1 Flow of participants through the HUNT2 and HUNT3 study and selection of head injury patients. [a]Complete non-participants: Answering no questionnaire. Partial non-participants: Answering part of the questinonnaire, but not the headache screening question. Abbreviations: HUNT = the Nord-Trøndelag Health Study

Individuals with mild head injury were more likely to have new onset of headache (OR 1.74, 95% CI 1.05–2.87) and stable headache suffering (OR 1.70, 95 CI 1.15–2.50) compared to controls (Table 2).

Table 3 demonstrates change in monthly headache frequency between HUNT2 and HUNT3 among participants suffering from headache in both surveys. In the head injury population 15.0% had more frequent headache in HUNT3 than in HUNT 2, in the control population the corresponding proportion was 12.2%.

There was a significant association between exacerbation of headache and head injury (Table 4). There was a nearly doubled odds of exacerbation of headache among those exposed to mild head injury than among the controls (OR 1.93, 95% CI 1.24–3.02) (Table 4). Individuals with head injury were also more likely to have stable headache suffering with unchanged frequency from HUNT2 to HUNT3 than the controls (Table 4). There was no significant relationship between moderate head injury and any of the headache trajectories (Tables 2 and 4).

There were no significant associations between head injury and past headache suffering or improvement of headache status.

No consistent significant interaction was observed between head injury and any of the covariates. The only significant interaction observed was for smoking and only in the case of improvement of headache.

Although no significant interaction was observed between sex and head injury, we did separate analyses for males and females for all headache trajectories. In these separate analyses, significant associations were found only for men (Tables 2 and 4).

Table 1 Demographics and health related variables

	Head injury population	Controls
Variable		
Total number of subjects	294	25,662
Age at participation in HUNT2 (years) (mean ± SD)	48.4 ± 14.7	47.3 ± 13.1
Age at injury (first injury) (years) (mean ± SD)	53.8 ± 15.2	
Age at participation in HUNT3 (years) (mean ± SD)	59.6 ± 14.7	58.5 ± 13.1
Time from head injury (first injury) to HUNT3 (years) (mean ± SD)	4.9 ± 3.2	
Female	137 (46.5)	14,639 (57.0)
Duration of education (HUNT2) (n (%))		
≤ 9 years	82 (27.9)	7535 (29.4)
10–12 years	135 (45.9)	11,663 (45.4)
≥ 13 years	73 (24.8)	6007 (23.4)
HADS score (mean ± SD) (HUNT2)	8.8 ± 5.7	7.4 ± 5.4
HADS score (mean ± SD) (HUNT3)	8.5 ± 6.0	7.3 ± 5.4
BMI (mean ± SD) (HUNT2)	26.2 ± 3.9	26.0 ± 3.6
BMI (mean ± SD) (HUNT3)	27.4 ± 4.3	27.4 ± 4.3
Daily smoking (HUNT2) (n (%))	62 (21.1)	6278 (24.5)
Daily and occasionally smoking (HUNT3) (n (%))	73 (24.8)	5338 (20.8)
Self-reported health poor or less than good (HUNT2) (n (%))	82 (27.9)	5451 (21.2)
Self-reported health poor or less than good (HUNT3) (n (%))	102 (34.7)	6883 (26.8)
Headache sufferer (n (%))		
HUNT2	129 (43.9)	10,697 (41.7)
HUNT3	111 (37.8)	8492 (33.1)
CAGE[a] ≥ 1 (HUNT2) (n (%))	56 (19.0)	3721 (14.5)
CAGE[a] ≥ 1 (HUNT3) (n (%))	58 (19.7)	3834 (14.9)

Abbreviations: *HADS* Hospital Anxiety and Depression Scale, *BMI* Body Mass Index
[a]*CAGE* Modified Norwegian version of the CAGE alcohol-screening instrument

Discussion

This is the first study which presents population based data on headache occurrence after head injury with known pre-injury headache status. Our main finding was that exposure to head injury increased the risk of new onset headache suffering and exacerbation of headache. Also, head injury was positively associated with stable headache suffering, which means that headache was less likely to improve. This confirms findings from several studies with less reliable study designs during the last years [9, 23, 24], but contrast with an earlier population-based study, which did not find an association between previous head injury and headache [12]. However, in that study there was a 22-year interval between the exposure to trauma and inquiry about headache [12].

The data were analyzed with regard to sex differences, since both prevalences of primary headache, as well as injuries to the head, are known to differ between men and women [25, 26]. The available literature concerning any sex-differences for persistent HAIH has been inconsistent [6, 27–29]. We did not find any significant difference between males and females in the effect of a head injury on change in headache status from HUNT2 to HUNT3. In the analyses stratified upon sex, the positive associations from the combined analysis were observed to be significant only among men. This could be an incidental finding.

Earlier studies have shown an inverse dose-response relationship between the severity of head injuries and development of persistent headache [13, 14]. In our analyses the estimated odds for all unfavourable headache trajectories after a mild head injury were higher than the corresponding odds found for moderate head injury. This indicates that although sequelae in general after mild head injuries are milder compared to more severe head injuries, patients with previous mild head injuries may be just as, or even more affected by headache. This seems to confirm the paradoxical finding in earlier studies of a lack of a positive dose-response relationship between head injury severity and HAIH. However, the present study included few moderate head injuries, which gives low power. Furthermore, the classification of head injury severity has differed widely, which makes comparisons between studies difficult [30–32].

Strengths

The major strengths of this study were the large population-based dataset on headache at two time points, combined with extensive objective information on each head injury, retrieved from medical records which eliminated recall bias regarding the head injury and enabled us to classify the head injuries according to severity. We had validated information about the headache status of the participants before the head injury, which enabled us to compare prevalence as well as frequency before and after the time of the head injuries and make comparisons with a non-exposed control group. This has not been possible in earlier studies. The design eliminates recall bias also regarding pre-study headache suffering, which can be a problem in prospective studies, as participants might tend to trivialise headache before the head injury because they understand their headache as a consequence of their head injury. Such possible under-reporting of pre-injury headache could be the reason why several prospective studies report pre-injury headache prevalence far below known headache prevalence in the general population [33–35]. This is especially a problem in studies without control groups. In some studies, using a control group

Table 2 Multivariate regression analyses of the associations between head injury and relative headache status in HUNT3 versus HUNT2 with regard to suffering from headache only

		All		Men	Women
		Adjustment for age and sex	Complete adjustment[a]	Complete adjustment[a]	Complete adjustment[a]
	N	N (OR, 95% CI)	N (OR, 95% CI)	N (OR, 95% CI)	N (OR, 95% CI)
Past headache suffering					
No head injury (reference)	25,662	4474 (ref.)	4474 (ref.)	1603 (ref.)	2871 (ref.)
Any head injury	294	49 (1.21, 0.87–1.69)	49 (1.23, 0.85–1.78)	24 (1.35, 0.82–2.21)	25 (1.06, 0.60–1.86)
Minimal head injury	35	7 (1.15, 0.47–2.80)	7 (0.94, 0.33–2.70)	1 (0.50, 0.06–4.14)	6 (1.17, 0.33–4.18)
Mild head injury	211	36 (1.35, 0.91–2.00)	36 (1.39, 0.89–2.15)	18 (1.53, 0.85–2.75)	18 (1.19, 0.61–2.32)
Moderate head injury	32	5 (1.13, 0.41–3.13)	5 (1.24, 0.43–3.54)	4 (1.41, 0.44–4.49)	1 (0.93, 0.08–10.52)
Stable headache suffering					
No head injury (reference)	25,662	6223 (ref.)	6223 (ref.)	1833 (ref.)	4390 (ref.)
Any head injury	294	80 (1.51, 1.13–2.03)	80 (1.55, 1.12–2.14)	37 (1.65, 1.06–2.56)	43 (1.37, 0.85–2.20)
Minimal head injury	35	10 (1.20, 0.53–2.70)	10 (0.96, 0.38–2.42)	4 (1.22, 0.32–4.60)	6 (0.78, 0.21–2.86)
Mild head injury	211	56 (1.60, 1.12–2.27)	56 (1.70, 1.15–2.50)	27 (1.91, 1.13–3.22)	29 (1.42, 0.80–2.51)
Moderate head injury	32	9 (1.58, 0.66–3.75)	9 (1.45, 0.57–3.70)	4 (0.90, 0.24–3.34)	5 (2.54, 0.45–14.30)
New headache suffering					
No head injury (reference)	25,662	2269 (ref.)	2269 (ref.)	974 (ref.)	1295 (ref.)
Any head injury	294	31 (1.44, 0.96–2.15)	31 (1.37, 0.88–2.15)	21 (1.89, 1.12–3.21)	10 (0.70, 0.29–1.69)
Minimal head injury	35	1 (0.33, 0.04–2.47)	1 (0.38, 0.05–2.90)	1 (0.81, 0.10–6.75)	0 (–)
Mild head injury	211	27 (1.86, 1.20–2.90)	27 (1.74, 1.05–2.87)	17 (2.31, 1.26–4.23)	10 (1.02, 0.41–2.52)
Moderate head injury	32	3 (1.20, 0.34–4.22)	3 (1.30, 0.36–4.65)	3 (1.75 (0.48–6.42)	0 (–)

One analysis was done with head injury as a binary variable (no head injury/any head injury) and a separate analysis was done with head injury in four categories according to head injury severity (no head injury/minimal head injury/mild head injury/moderate head injury). The head injury severity was classified according to the Head Injury Severity Scale (HISS)

Reference category: Stable non-sufferer (absence of headache suffering in both surveys)

Abbreviations: *OR* Odds ratio, *CI* Confidence interval

[a]Analyses are adjusted for age, sex, duration of education, daily smoking, CAGE score ≥ 1 and HADS-score

Table 3 Change in monthly headache frequency between HUNT2 and HUNT3 among participants suffering from headache in both surveys

HUNT2	HUNT3	N (%), head injury population	N (%), controls
Decreased headache frequency[a]		10 (12.5)	939 (15.1)
> 14 days	1–14 days	2 (2.5)	269 (4.3)
7–14 days	< 7 days	8 (10.0)	670 (10.8)
Stable headache frequency[b]		55 (68.8)	4234 (68.0)
< 7 days	< 7 days	46 (57.5)	3833 (61.6)
7–14 days	7–14 days	4 (5.0)	257 (4.1)
> 14 days	> 14 days	5 (6.3)	144 (2.3)
Increased headache frequency[c]		12 (15.0)	757 (12.2)
< 7 days	7–30 days	10 (12.5)	633 (10.2)
7–14 days	> 14 days	2 (2.5)	124 (2.0)
Missing		3 (3.8)	293 (4.7)
Total		80 (100.0)	6223 (100.0)

[a]Less frequent headache (days/month) in HUNT3 compared to HUNT2
[b]Same headache frequency (days/month) in HUNT3 as in HUNT2
[c]More frequent headache (days/month) in HUNT3 compared to HUNT2

with injuries other than head injuries could be an advantage, as one could theorize that physical trauma could cause headache through psychosocial stressors, regardless of which part of the body is injured. However, if the study is epidemiological, the design is population-based and the intention is to investigate whether head injury is a risk factor for development of headache regardless of the underlying mechanism, a community control group is more appropriate [36].

In a previous study, we analysed headache in HUNT3 related to all hospitalized head injuries ($n = 940$) between 1988 and HUNT3 [15]. As in the present study, there was a significant association between head injury and headache. However, in that study we were not able to take headache status before the trauma into account. This was a limitation because in patients with headache complaints a trauma may cause stress which can precipitate an attack of their pre-existing headache. Headache in a trauma setting can be a sign of a serious head injury, and these patients may therefore be referred to a hospital. Hence, one could imagine that pre-existing headache could act as a confounder. However, the present

Table 4 Multivariate regression analyses of the associations between head injury and relative headache status in HUNT3 versus HUNT2 with regard both to suffering from headache as well as to change in headache frequency

		All		Men	Women
		Adjustment for age and sex	Complete adjustment[a]	Complete adjustment[a]	Complete adjustment[a]
	N	N (OR, 95% CI)	N (OR, 95% CI)	N (OR, 95% CI)	N (OR, 95% CI)
Improvement of headache status[1]					
No head injury (reference)	25,662	5413 (ref.)	5413 (ref.)	1852 (ref.)	3561 (ref.)
Any head injury	294	59 (1.22, 0.89–1.68)	59 (1.21, 0.85–1,72)	28 (1.30, 0.81–2.08)	31 (1.06, 0.63–1.80)
Minimal head injury	35	12 (1.62, 0.76–3.44)	12 (1.35, 0.56–3.24)	2 (0.76, 0.15–3.82)	10 (1.65, 0.54–4.98)
Mild head injury	211	40 (1.26, 0.86–1.84)	40 (1.27, 0.83–1.95)	20 (1.39, 0.79–2.47)	20 (1.09, 0.58–2.07)
Moderate head injury	32	6 (1.16, 0.44–3.02	6 (1.23, 0.45–3.31)	5 (1.51, 0.51–4.42)	1 (0.66, 0.06–7.63)
Stable headache suffering and frequency[2]					
No head injury (reference)	25,662	4234 (ref.)	4234 (ref.)	1302 (ref.)	2932 (ref.)
Any head injury	294	55 (1.55, 1.11–2.15)	55 (1.60, 1.12–2.28)	28 (1.86, 1.16–2.99)	27 (1.30, 0.76–2.21)
Minimal head injury	35	5 (0.88, 0.32–2.45)	5 (0.71, 0.23–2.25)	3 (1.37, 0.33–5.68)	2 (0.28, 0.03–2.39)
Mild head injury	211	40 (1.71, 1.15–2.53)	40 (1.83, 1.20–2.79)	20 (2.14, 1.22–3.76)	20 (1.48, 0.79–2.77)
Moderate head injury	32	5 (1.26, 0.44–3.61)	5 (1.06, 0.33–3.40)	3 (0.87, 0.19–4.02)	2 (1.40, 0.18–10.82)
Exacerbation of headache status[3]					
No head injury (reference)	25,662	3026 (ref.)	3026 (ref.)	1181 (ref.)	1845 (ref.)
Any head injury	294	43 (1.55, 1.09–2.21)	43 (1.52, 1.02–2.25)	26 (1.87, 1.14–3.05)	17 (1.08, 0.56–2.08)
Minimal head injury	35	1 (0.24, 0.03–1.83)	1 (0.26, 0.03–2.03)	1 (0.62, 0.07–5.16)	0 (–)
Mild head injury	211	37 (2.00, 1.35–2.98)	37 (1.93, 1.24–3.02)	22 (2.40, 1.37–4.21)	15 (1.37, 0.66–2.85)
Moderate head injury	32	5 (1.56, 0.55–4.41)	5 (1.65, 0.57–4.79)	3 (1.42, 0.39–5.22)	2 (2.09, 0.27–16.16)

One analysis was done with head injury as a binary variable (no head injury/any head injury) and a separate analysis was done with head injury in four categories according to head injury severity (no head injury/minimal head injury/mild head injury/moderate head injury). The head injury severity was classified according to the Head Injury Severity Scale (HISS)

Reference category: Stable non-sufferer (absence of headache suffering in both surveys)

Abbreviations: *OR* Odds ratio, *CI* Confidence interval

[1]Improvement of headache status: Absence of previously reported headache or decrease in its frequency

[2]Stable headache suffering and frequency: Headache suffering in both HUNT2 and HUNT3 with the same frequency in both studies

[3]Exacerbation of headache status: New onset of headache or increased frequency of previously reported headache

[a]Analyses are adjusted for age, sex, duration of education, daily smoking, CAGE score ≥ 1 and HADS-score

study shows that in the head injury group pre-existing headache was not more prevalent than in the control group, while new headache and exacerbation of headache was. We therefore find no reason to suspect the occurrence of such confounding.

Limitations

The study was not designed to determine time of headache onset. Therefore, we cannot specify if the onset of headache was within 7 days after head injury, which is a criterion for classifying a headache as HAIH, according to ICHD-3 beta [10]. However, ICHD-3 beta states that this criterion is somewhat arbitrary and concludes further research is needed into which interval might be more appropriate [10].

The present study included only 32 individuals with a moderate and 35 individuals with a minimal head injury, which gives low power and uncertain results from these groups. Furthermore, generalization of results should be performed with caution, since only 56% of those invited to participate in HUNT2 and 42% of those invited to participate in HUNT3 answered the headache questionnaire.

Patients not examined at a hospital were not included. However, the proportion of patients with head injury being admitted to a hospital after examination by health care providers was larger in the period of data collection than it is today [26, 37]. This can mostly be attributed to increased availability of CT imaging and the implementation of guidelines for initial management of head injury in Norwegian hospitals [38].

Implications for public health

HAIH is one of the most prevalent of secondary headaches worldwide and a potentially preventable one. Everywhere, but especially in low and middle-income countries, head injury is common and most often caused by road traffic injuries, falls and violence [39]. An important step in reducing the incidence of HAIH is therefore head injury preventive strategies [39].

The fact that development of HAIH also, or even especially, occurs after mild head injuries should have implications for the follow-up of patients with mild head injury. In Norway, like many other countries, there are no guidelines for follow-up after mild head injury. We know little about individual factors that predispose to development of persistent HAIH. We therefore suggest that all persons seeking medical advice due to a mild head injury should be encouraged to seek their general practitioner in the case of development of new headache or exacerbation of already existing headache with a duration longer than 3 months. A recent study suggests that a standardized tool might be helpful in the general population of concussion patients to assess for post-traumatic headache [40]. While we await better knowledge of how to best treat HAIH, we suggest using treatment strategies with proven efficacy against the primary headache that it most resembles [41].

Future research

The incidence of mild head injury is high and a close follow-up of all persons experiencing a mild head injury would require a large effort for the health care service. It is therefore especially important to be able to identify persons at risk of developing HAIH and develop clinical guidelines for follow-up after mild head injury. HAIH occurred more frequently in patients with minimal traumatic intracranial haemorrhage after mild TBI than those without in a recent published study [42]. Another study found that persistent HAIH and migraine are associated with differences in brain structure [43]. Both studies suggests that it is possible to find underlying pathophysiology that separates HAIH from the primary headache type it phenotypically resembles. Future research should be aimed at understanding its pathophysiological mechanisms, acquiring knowledge on predictors for development of HAIH and based on this, develop effective preventive measures and treatment options.

Conclusion

Individuals hospitalized due to a mild head injury were more likely to develop new headache suffering or report exacerbation of previously documented headache compared to the surrounding general population. Hence, the present study substantiates HAIH as a true secondary headache entity and not a primary headache misattributed to head injury.

Abbreviations

BMI: Body Mass Index; CAGE: Modified Norwegian version of the CAGE alcohol-screening instrument; CI: Confidence Interval; HADS: Hospital Anxiety and Depression Scale; HAIH: Headache Attributed to Head Injury; HISS: Head Injury Severity Scale; HUNT: the Nord-Trøndelag Health Study; ICD: International Classification of Diseases; ICHD-3 beta: the International Classification of Headache Disorders, beta version of third edition; OR: Odds Ratio

Acknowledgements

The Nord-Trøndelag Health Study (The HUNT Study) is a collaboration between HUNT Research Centre (Faculty of Medicine, Norwegian University of Science and Technology NTNU), Nord-Trøndelag County Council, Central Norway Health Authority and the Norwegian Institute of Public Health.

Funding

This research received no specific grant from any funding agency in the public, commercial, or not-for-profit sectors.

Authors' contributions

LHN, study concept and design, acquisition of data, analysis and interpretation of data, writing of manuscript. KH, analysis and interpretation of data, critical revision of manuscript for intellectual content. AV, study supervision, interpretation of data, critical revision of manuscript for intellectual content. LJS, study concept, interpretation of data, critical revision of manuscript for intellectual content. TF, analysis and interpretation of data, critical revision of manuscript for intellectual content. TP, acquisition of data, critical revision of manuscript for intellectual content. GBG, acquisition of data, critical revision of manuscript for intellectual content. ML, study concept and design, organizing retrieval of data, study supervision, interpretation of data, critical revision of manuscript for intellectual content. All authors read and approved the final manuscript.

Competing interests

The authors declare that they have no competing interests.

Author details

[1]Department of Neuromedicine and Movement Science (INB), Faculty of Medicine and Health Sciences, Norwegian University of Science and Technology, Postbox 8905, 7491 Trondheim, Norway. [2]Department of Neurosurgery, St. Olavs University Hospital, Trondheim, Norway. [3]Norwegian Advisory Unit on Headaches, St. Olavs University Hospital, Trondheim, Norway. [4]Department of Public Health and Nursing, Faculty of Medicine and Health Sciences, Norwegian University of Science and Technology, Trondheim, Norway. [5]Division of Mental Health and Addiction, Oslo University Hospital, Oslo, Norway.

References

1. Abu Bakar N, Tanprawate S, Lambru G, Torkamani M, Jahanshahi M, Matharu M (2016) Quality of life in primary headache disorders: a review. Cephalalgia : an international journal of headache 1:67–91
2. Linde M, Gustavsson A, Stovner LJ, Steiner TJ, Barre J, Katsarava Z et al (2012) The cost of headache disorders in Europe: the Eurolight project. Eur J Neurol (5):703–711
3. Atlas of headache disorders and resources in the world 2011 (2011) A collaborative project of World Health Organization and Lifting The Burden (2011). WHO Press. (ISBN 978 92 4 156421 2. NLM classification: WL 342). www.who.int.
4. Frost RB, Farrer TJ, Primosch M, Hedges DW (2013) Prevalence of traumatic brain injury in the general adult population: a meta-analysis. Neuroepidemiology 40(3):154–159
5. AIR M, Stocchetti N, Bullock R (2008) Moderate and severe traumatic brain injury in adults. The Lancet Neurology 8:728–741
6. Lucas S, Hoffman JM, Bell KR, Dikmen S (2014) A prospective study of prevalence and characterization of headache following mild traumatic brain injury. Cephalalgia: an international journal of headache 2:93–102
7. De Kruijk JR, Leffers P, Menheere PP, Meerhoff S, Rutten J, Twijnstra A (2002) Prediction of post-traumatic complaints after mild traumatic brain injury: early symptoms and biochemical markers. J Neurol Neurosurg Psychiatry (6):727–732
8. Lew HL, Lin PH, Fuh JL, Wang SJ, Clark DJ, Walker WC (2006) Characteristics and treatment of headache after traumatic brain injury: a focused review. Am J Phys Med Rehabil (7):619–627

9. Nampiaparampil DE (2008) Prevalence of chronic pain after traumatic brain injury: a systematic review. JAMA (6):711–719
10. Headache Classification Committee of the International Headache Society (HIS) (2013) The international classification of headache disorders, 3rd edition (beta version). Cephalalgia: an international journal of headache. 9:629–808
11. Couch JR, Lipton RB, Stewart WF, Scher AI (2007) Head or neck injury increases the risk of chronic daily headache: a population-based study. Neurology (11):1169–1177
12. Nestvold K, Stavem K (2007) Headache 22 years after hospitalization for head injury compared with matched community controls. Neuroepidemiology 29(1–2):113–120
13. Theeler B, Lucas S, Riechers RG 2nd, Ruff RL (2013) Post-traumatic headaches in civilians and military personnel: a comparative, clinical review. Headache 53(6):881–900
14. Solomon S (2009) Post-traumatic headache: commentary: an overview. Headache 49(7):1112–1115
15. Hoem Nordhaug L, Vik A, Hagen K, Stovner LJ, Pedersen T, Gravdahl GB et al (2016) Headaches in patients with previous head injuries: a population-based historical cohort study (HUNT). Cephalalgia: an international journal of headache. 11:1009–1019
16. Krokstad S, Langhammer A, Hveem K, Holmen TL, Midthjell K, Stene TR et al (2013) Cohort profile: the HUNT study, Norway. Int J Epidemiol (4):968–977
17. Linde M, Stovner LJ, Zwart JA, Hagen K (2011) Time trends in the prevalence of headache disorders. The Nord-Trondelag health studies (HUNT 2 and HUNT 3). Cephalalgia: an international journal of headache. 5:585–596
18. Hagen K, Zwart JA, Vatten L, Stovner LJ, Bovim G (2000) Head-HUNT: validity and reliability of a headache questionnaire in a large population-based study in Norway. Cephalalgia: an international journal of headache. 4:244–251
19. Hagen K, Zwart JA, Aamodt AH, Nilsen KB, Brathen G, Helde G et al (2010) The validity of questionnaire-based diagnoses: the third Nord-Trondelag health study 2006-2008. J Headache Pain. 11(1):67–73
20. Stein SC, Spettell C (1995) The head injury severity scale (HISS): a practical classification of closed-head injury. Brain Inj 9(5):437–444
21. Mayfield D, McLeod G, Hall P (1974) The CAGE questionnaire: validation of a new alcoholism screening instrument. Am J Psychiatry 10:1121–1123
22. Box GEP, Tidwell PW (1962) Transformation of the independent variables. Technometrics 4:531–550
23. D'Onofrio F, Russo A, Conte F, Casucci G, Tessitore A, Tedeschi G (2014) Post-traumatic headaches: an epidemiological overview. Neurol Sci 35:203–206
24. Hong CK, Joo JY, Shim YS, Sim SY, Kwon MA, Kim YB et al (2017) The course of headache in patients with moderate-to-severe headache due to mild traumatic brain injury: a retrospective cross-sectional study. J Headache Pain 18(1):48
25. Lebedeva ER, Kobzeva NR, Gilev DV, Olesen J (2016) Factors associated with primary headache according to diagnosis, sex, and social group. Headache 56(2):341–356
26. Heskestad B, Baardsen R, Helseth E, Romner B, Waterloo K, Ingebrigtsen T (2009) Incidence of hospital referred head injuries in Norway: a population based survey from the Stavanger region. Scand J Trauma Resusc Emerg Med. 17:6
27. Jensen OK, Nielsen FF (1990) The influence of sex and pre-traumatic headache on the incidence and severity of headache after head injury. Cephalalgia: an international journal of headache. 6:285–293
28. Hoffman JM, Lucas S, Dikmen S, Braden CA, Brown AW, Brunner R et al (2011) Natural history of headache after traumatic brain injury. J Neurotrauma 28(9):1719–1725
29. Xu H, Pi H, Ma L, Su X, Wang J (2016) Incidence of headache after traumatic brain injury in China: a large prospective study. World Neurosurg 88:289–296
30. Evans RW (2010) Persistent post-traumatic headache, postconcussion syndrome, and whiplash injuries: the evidence for a non-traumatic basis with an historical review. Headache (4):716–724
31. Sigurdardottir S, Andelic N, Roe C, Jerstad T, Schanke AK (2009) Post-concussion symptoms after traumatic brain injury at 3 and 12 months post-injury: a prospective study. Brain Inj 6:489–497
32. Couch JR, Bearss C (2001) Chronic daily headache in the posttrauma syndrome: relation to extent of head injury. Headache 41(6):559–564
33. Stacey A, Lucas S, Dikmen S, Temkin N, Bell K, Brown AW et al (2016) Natural history of headache five years after traumatic brain injury. J Neurotrauma 34(8):1558–1564
34. Walker WC, Marwitz JH, Wilk AR, Ketchum JM, Hoffman JM, Brown AW et al (2013) Prediction of headache severity (density and functional impact) after traumatic brain injury: a longitudinal multicenter study. Cephalalgia: an international journal of headache. 12:998–1008
35. Stovner LJ, Schrader H, Mickeviciene D, Surkiene D, Sand T (2009) Headache after concussion. Eur J Neurol 1:112–120
36. Mathias JL, Dennington V Fau - Bowden SC, Bowden Sc Fau – Bigler ED, Bigler ED Community versus orthopaedic controls in traumatic brain injury research: how comparable are they?; Brain Inj. 2013;27(7-8):887-895 1362-301X (Electronic)
37. Heskestad B, Waterloo K, Ingebrigtsen T, Romner B, Harr ME, Helseth E (2012) An observational study of compliance with the Scandinavian guidelines for management of minimal, mild and moderate head injury. Scand J Trauma Resusc Emerg Med 20:32
38. Ingebrigtsen T, Romner B, Kock-Jensen C (2000) Scandinavian guidelines for initial management of minimal, mild, and moderate head injuries. The Scandinavian Neurotrauma committee. J Trauma 4:760–766
39 Hyder AA, Wunderlich CA, Puvanachandra P, Gururaj G, Kobusingye OC (2007) The impact of traumatic brain injuries: a global perspective. NeuroRehabilitation 22:341–353
40. Begasse de Dhaem O, Barr WB, Balcer LJ, Galetta SL, Minen MT (2017) Post-traumatic headache: the use of the sport concussion assessment tool (SCAT-3) as a predictor of post-concussion recovery. J Headache Pain 18(1):60
41. Guidelines for Concussion/mTBI and Persistent Symptoms: Second Edition [Internet]. 2013 [cited 29. november 2017]. Available from: http://onf.org/documents/guidelines-for-concussion-mtbi-persistent-symptoms-second-edition
42. Hong CK, Shim YS, Sim SY, Joo JY, Kwon MA, Kim YB et al (2017) Post-traumatic headache in patients with minimal traumatic intracranial hemorrhage after traumatic brain injury: a retrospective matched case-control study. J Headache Pain. 18(1):64
43. Schwedt TJ, Chong CD, Peplinski J, Ross K, Berisha V (2017) Persistent post-traumatic headache vs. migraine: an MRI study demonstrating differences in brain structure. J Headache Pain 18(1):87

22

Vitamin D deficiency in patients with cluster headache

Jong-Hee Sohn[1], Min-Kyung Chu[2], Kwang-Yeol Park[3], Hong-Yup Ahn[4] and Soo-Jin Cho[5*]

Abstract

Background: Cluster headache is famous for attacks with seasonal and diurnal periodicity. This diurnal and seasonal variation might be related to sunlight and vitamin D metabolism. We investigated the serum vitamin D levels in patients with cluster headache.

Methods: We enrolled patients with cluster headache and age- and sex-matched migraineurs and normal controls. From October 2016 to March 2018, non-fasting serum 25(OH)D concentrations were measured using a chemiluminescent immunoassay. Vitamin D deficiency was defined as a concentration < 20 ng/mL.

Results: The study enrolled 28 patients with cluster headache, 36 migraineurs, and 36 normal controls. In the patients with cluster headache, the serum 25(OH)D concentration averaged 14.0 ± 3.9 ng/mL and 92.8% had vitamin D deficiency. There was no significant difference among the patients with cluster headache, migraineurs, and controls. In the patients with cluster headache, there was no difference in the serum 25(OH)D concentrations between men and women, cluster and remission periods, first and recurrent attack, presence and absence of daily or seasonal periodicity, and 3-month recurrence. In the 14 patients with seasonal periodicity, patients with periodicity of winter to spring had a trend of lower serum 25(OH)D concentrations than those with periodicity of summer to autumn (12.30 ± 1.58 vs. 16.96 ± 4.69 ng/mL, $p = 0.097$).

Conclusions: Vitamin D deficiency is common in patients with cluster headache, but the role of vitamin D deficiency is uncertain, except for its seasonal influence.

Keywords: Vitamin D, Deficiency, Cluster headache, Migraine

Background

Vitamin D is produced in the skin after oral absorption and exposure to sunlight. It is transformed by the liver and kidneys and plays a crucial role in promoting bone and muscle health. Vitamin D deficiency is a global health issue and is associated with inflammation, autonomic function, autoimmune disorders, chronic pain, cancer, and vascular and neurological disorders, in addition to its skeletal roles [1–6].

The estimated prevalence of vitamin D deficiency in North America, Europe and Australia is as high as 20–50% [7–13]. Vitamin D deficiency is more common in Korea (37° N) where the prevalence in male and female adult workers was 69.5 and 83.1%, respectively [14]. The determinants of vitamin D levels are the amount of skin exposure, followed by location, season, personal ultraviolet radiation exposure, vitamin D supplementation, body mass index, and physical activity [15].

A high prevalence of all kinds of headache has been associated with high latitude, suggesting a relationship with vitamin D [16]. However, the inter-relationships of vitamin D deficiency and headache are still uncertain. The studies of vitamin D in primary headache disorders have focused mainly on migraine, although there is no systematic evidence of an association between vitamin D deficiency and migraine [17–19]. There are case reports of migraine patients who improved with vitamin D supplementation [20, 21]. Simvastatin plus vitamin D has been reported to be effective for preventing headache in adults with episodic migraine in randomized clinical trials [22]. Dysfunction of vitamin D-binding protein and polymorphism of the vitamin D receptor gene have been

* Correspondence: dowonc@naver.com
[5]Department of Neurology, Dongtan Sacred Heart Hospital, Hallym University College of Medicine, Keun Jae Bong-gil 7, Hwaseong, Gyeonggi-do 18450, Korea
Full list of author information is available at the end of the article

reported in patients with migraine, while the relationship between the serum vitamin D level and headache frequency in migraine patients is controversial [23–25].

Tension-type headache is the most common primary headache disorder, accounting for most non-migraine headache in population studies. In the Norwegian population, non-migraine type headache was associated with low vitamin D levels with an odds ratio of 1.20 in the lowest quartile compared with the highest quartile group, whereas no significant association was found between migraine and the vitamin D levels [17]. There are also reports that chronic tension-type headache was associated with vitamin D deficiency [26–28].

Cluster headache shows a seasonal predilection, with nocturnal attacks [29–31]. The diurnal and seasonal variation might be related to sunlight and vitamin D metabolism, suggesting a role for vitamin D in cluster headache. There are no published studies of vitamin D in cluster headache, although a poster presentation showed that an anti-inflammatory regimen of vitamin and mineral supplements including vitamin D3 was effective in preventing cluster headaches [32]. Therefore, we investigated the serum vitamin D level in patients with cluster headache and the relationship between vitamin D deficiency and headache parameters compared with migraineurs and healthy controls.

Methods

Subjects

We enrolled patients with cluster headache and age- and sex-matched migraine patients as headache controls and normal controls in a case–control design. This study collected data from patients with cluster headache and migraine treated in the headache clinics of Chuncheon, Dongtan, and Kangnam Sacred Heart Hospitals of Hallym University College of Medicine from October 2016 to March 2018. All participants were between 20 and 65 years of age, and they were examined and classified according to the beta version of the International Classification of Headache Disorders-3 (ICHD-3β) [33] by a board-certified neurologist based on the patient history, a neurological examination, and neuroimaging studies. The control group consisted of volunteers matched for age, gender, and season enrolled. We recruited the control group via advertisements such as posted notices in the hospital. Control participants were required to be headache free (less than 1 headache day per month for an average of 1 year) with no history of primary or secondary headache disorder by the ICHD-3β [31, 33]. Exclusion criteria included subjects who took a vitamin D supplement or medication that influences vitamin D metabolism (e.g., antiepileptic drugs, rifampin, antiretroviral drugs, etc.), severe obesity [body mass index (BMI) > 30], thyroid or parathyroid disease, diabetes, and severe liver or renal disease.

The study protocol and informed consent form were reviewed and approved by the Institutional Review Board of each hospital (2016-439-I). Written informed consent was obtained from all participants before enrolling them in the study.

Demographic data and questionnaire

Demographic data were obtained from all groups, including age, sex, height, weight, place of residence, occupation, level of education, and smoking habit. The data collected on headache patients included frequency of attacks (per month), average headache duration (hours), severity of pain [assessed with a visual analogue scale (VAS) range 0–10], and days per month using abortive medication. The patients with cluster headache completed a detailed semi-structured questionnaire on the headache characteristics, such as autonomic symptoms, diurnal periodicity, time of propensity, and seasonal periodicity. We contacted the patients after at least 3 months and collected data on the recurrence of headache. Eligible patients were interviewed at follow-up outpatient appointments or by telephone. The headache group completed the Headache Impact Test-6 (HIT-6) to measure headache-related impact, Patient Health Questionnare-9 (PHQ-9) to assess depression, Generalized Anxiety Dirorder-7 (GAD-7) to assess anxiety, and Pittsburgh Sleep Quality Index (PSQI) to measure the quality of sleep [34–37].

Measurement and analysis of vitamin D

Non-fasting venous blood samples were collected at the baseline examinations. Serum 25(OH)D concentrations were measured with a chemiluminescent immunoassay using the ARCHITECT i4000 SR (Abbott Diagnostics, IL, USA). The intra- and interassay coefficients of variation of the measurements were 1.7–2.8 and 2.7–4.1%, respectively. The assay was standardized against NIST Standard Reference Material 2972 (NIST, Gaithersburg, ME, USA) and certified by the Centers for Disease Control and Prevention Vitamin D Standardization Program [38]. Vitamin D deficiency was defined as a 25(OH)D < 20 ng/mL, insufficiency as 21–29 ng/mL, and ideal range as 30–50 ng/mL.

The time of the day, month, and year when the vitamin D assessment was performed was recorded [39, 40]. Most experts define vitamin D deficiency as serum 25(OH)D vitamin D levels < 20 ng/mL, although there is no consensus on the optimal serum vitamin D levels [41–44]. A cut-off value of 20 ng/mL was used to divide the samples into "deficient" and "normal" groups in this study [14].

Statistics

Analysis of variance (ANOVA) was used to compare demographic and headache parameters among groups, after confirming the normality of the distribution using the Shapiro-Wilk test. If the normality of the distribution was not confirmed, the Kruskal-Wallis, chi-square test or Fisher's exact test were used to compare data between groups, where appropriate. Serum vitamin D concentrations in subjects with CH, migraine, and controls were compared using analysis of covariance (ANCOVA), with adjustment for potential confounders. The correlations between the serum 25(OH)D concentration and various clinical features were assessed using Pearson's or Spearman correlation coefficient based on the normality of the distribution.

To compare vitamin D concentration according to the headache parameters among the CH group, the Mann-Whitney test was used. ANOVA was used to compare vitamin D concentrations between subgroups in CH patients. Using linear regression analysis, we calculated the odds ratios of vitamin D levels associated with the headache variables. The variables that showed statistical correlations with the vitamin D levels in the univariate analyses, and factors that are known to affect the vitamin D level, were included in the multivariate regression analysis. Linear regression was used to assess the seasonal propensity of serum 25(OH)D concentrations with factors known to affect vitamin D levels (age, male, current smoker, sampling time) [45]. A p-value < 0.05 was considered statistically significant. All analyses were performed using R version 3.5.0 for Windows (R Foundation for Statistical Computing, Vienna, Austria. http://www.r-project.org/) and RStudio version 1.1.442.

Results

Comparison of demographics and vitamin D levels in patients with cluster headache, migraine, and controls

The study enrolled 28 patients with cluster headache, 36 migraineurs, and 36 normal controls. No significant differences were found in the CH and migraine patients compared with the controls in terms of age (38.2, 35.1, and 35.4 years, respectively) or sex (proportion male 85.7, 80.6, and 88.9%, respectively). In addition, there were no differences in BMI, smoking status, sampling season, and sampling time zones (7-10 AM, 11 AM-1 PM, 2-5 PM) among the three groups (Table 1).

The serum 25(OH)D concentrations were 14.0 ± 3.9 ng/mL in the patients with CH, 14.7 ± 5.9 ng/mL in the migraineurs, and 14.6 ± 7.4 ng/mL in the normal controls ($p = 0.884$). After adjustment for potential confounders (sex, age, sampling season, current smoking) by ANCOVA, the serum 25(OH)D concentrations were not different between groups (data not shown, $p = 0.853$). Vitamin D deficiency was present in 92.8% of the patients with CH, 80.6% of the migraineurs, and 83.3% of the normal controls ($p = 0.771$) There were no significant differences in distribution of serum 25(OH)D concentrations between patients with CH, migraine, and controls (Table 1).

Serum 25(OH)D concentrations were higher in those with a sampling season from summer to autumn than those with a sampling season from winter to spring (15.6 ± 5.2 ng/mL vs. 13.3 ± 6.5 ng/mL, $p = 0.003$). No differences

Table 1 Demographic features and vitamin D parameters of the patients with cluster headache, migraineurs, and normal controls

	Cluster Headache ($n = 28$)	Migraine ($n = 36$)	Normal controls ($n = 36$)	p-value
Age, years	38.2 ± 8.5	35.1 ± 8.2	35.4 ± 9.1	0.189
Men (%)	24 (85.7)	29 (80.6)	32 (88.9)	0.607
BMI, kg/m^2	23.3 ± 2.8	23,6 ± 3.7	24.1 ± 3.2	0.583
Smoking habit (%)[a]				0.133
Current	17 (63.0)	15 (41.7)	14 (38.9)	
ex-smoker	3 (11.1)	2 (5.6)	8 (22.2)	
Never	7 (25.9)	19 (52.8)	14 (38.9)	
Pain intensity, VAS	8.5 ± 1.8	6.4 ± 1.7	NA	< 0.001
Vitamin D deficiency (%)	26 (92.8)	29 (80.6)	30 (83.3)	0.771
Distribution of 25(OH)D concentration				0.236
≥ 30 (ng/mL)	0	1 (2.8)	2 (5.6)	
20–29.9 (ng/mL)	2 (7.2)	6 (16.7)	4 (11.1)	
10–19.9 (ng/mL)	23 (82.1)	21 (58.3)	19 (52.8)	
< 10 (ng/mL)	3 (10.7)	8 (22.2)	11 (30.5)	
Sampling seasons				0.349
Winter to spring	15 (53.9)	21 (58.3)	15 (41.7)	
Summer to autumn	13 (46.4)	15 (41.7)	21 (58.3)	

Values are expressed as mean ± standard deviation or number (%)
VAS visual analogue scale
[a]data was not available in one patient with CH

in serum vitamin D concentrations were evident based on the time of blood sample collection when analyzed at one-hour intervals (data not shown). Furthermore, there were no correlations between serum 25(OH)D concentrations and age, BMI, GAD-7 score, or PHQ-9 score, nor were any differences of the level observed between sexes.

Comparison of vitamin D levels in the patients with cluster headache according to clinical factors

In patients with CH, there was no difference in the serum 25(OH)D concentrations between men and women, cluster and remission periods, first and recurrent attack, presence and absence of daily or seasonal periodicity, and 3-month recurrence ($p > 0.05$). In the 14 patients with seasonal periodicity, patients with periodicity of winter to spring had a trend toward lower serum 25(OH)D concentrations than those with periodicity of summer to autumn (12.30 ± 1.58 vs. 16.96 ± 4.69 ng/mL, $p = 0.097$, Table 2).

Vitamin D levels were significantly lower in the subgroup with sampling season between winter to spring relative to other groups. Therefore, we analyzed vitamin D levels in the CH subgroups according to seasonal propensity, and by sample season for the 22 CH patients with recurrence (Table 3). There were significant differences in vitamin D levels between six groups; however, the differences between sampling seasons were not significant. There was no correlation between the vitamin D level and daily frequency, average weeks of cluster period, total bout of cluster period, or HIT-6, GAD-7, or PHQ-9 score.

Table 2 Vitamin D levels according to clinical variables in the patients with cluster headache

	25(OH)D, ng/mL	*p*-value
Sex		0.646
Men ($n = 24$)	13.95 ± 4.08	
Women ($n = 4$)	14.33 ± 2.82	
Recurrence		0.300
First episode ($n = 6$)	14.83 ± 2.42	
Recurrent episode ($n = 22$)	13.78 ± 4.21	
Paired comparison		0.421
Cluster period ($n = 14$)	13.87 ± 3.64	
Remission period ($n = 14$)	14.06 ± 4.56	
Diurnal periodicity		0.728
Present ($n = 16$)	13.69 ± 3.47	
Absent ($n = 12$)	14.41 ± 4.50	
Time of propensity		0.125
Nighttime propensity ($n = 9$)	14.72 ± 3.63	
Daytime propensity ($n = 7$)	11.71 ± 2.63	
Recurrence at 3 months		0.562
present ($n = 2$)	13.00 ± 3.39	
absent ($n = 26$)	14.08 ± 3.97	
Seasonal periodicity		0.188
Present ($n = 14$)	14.63 ± 4.14	
Absent ($n = 8$)	12.29 ± 4.18	
Season of cluster period		0.097
Winter to spring ($n = 7$)	12.30 ± 1.58	
Summer to autumn ($n = 7$)	16.96 ± 4.69	
Sampling season		0.001
Winter to spring ($n = 15$)	11.91 ± 2.63	
Summer to autumn ($n = 13$)	16.41 ± 3.76	

Clinical factors associated with vitamin D levels

The univariate linear analysis showed that sampling from summer to autumn and seasonal propensity for summer to autumn showed significant correlations with the vitamin D level. In the multiple linear regression analysis, however, the significance of seasonal propensity for summer to autumn was lost after adjusting for the sampling season. No changes in significance were observed by the multiple linear regression analysis when controlling for age, current smoking status, and sampling time zone (Additional file 1: Table S1).

Discussion

This study suggested that vitamin D deficiency is very common in patients with cluster headache compared with the prevalence of vitamin D deficiency in Korean adults [14]. However, the significance of vitamin D deficiency is uncertain, except for a subtle seasonal influence.

A few recent observational studies suggested that low serum vitamin D levels were related to some headache disorders, especially migraine and tension-type headache [24, 28, 46, 47]. One study also reported significant relations of lifetime prevalence of both migraine and tension-type headache with latitude [16]. If vitamin D has any association with headache, the prevalence of headache should match the seasonal variation in vitamin D levels. There are data indicating an increased frequency of headache attacks in autumn–winter and the least number of attacks in summer, although there are few studies on the seasonal variation of primary headache disorders, such as migraine and tension-type headache [48–50].

However, the relationship between cluster headache and vitamin D has not been studied previously, although cluster headache has characteristic seasonal rhythmicity. Cluster headache is a primary headache disorder characterized by a unique seasonal and diurnal periodicity. These characteristic features of its periodicity suggest involvement of the hypothalamus, the biological clock [51]. In Korea, seasonal propensity and diurnal periodicity were present in 44.0 and 68.5% of the patients with cluster headache, respectively. Among patients with seasonal propensity and diurnal periodicity, the most frequently cited season and time was spring

Table 3 The 25(OH)D concentration according seasonal propensity and sample seasons in 22 CH patients with recurrence

According to sample seasons	Seasonal propensity		No seasonal propensity ($n = 8$)	p-value
	Winter to spring ($n = 7$)	Summer to autumn ($n = 7$)		
Winter to spring ($n = 12$)	12.28 ± 1.93^{a} ($n = 5$)	13.00 ± 3.39^{c} ($n = 2$)	9.48 ± 1.61^{e} ($n = 5$)	0.001
Summer to autumn ($n = 10$)	12.35 ± 0.07^{b} ($n = 2$)	18.54 ± 4.38^{d} ($n = 5$)	16.97 ± 1.82^{f} ($n = 3$)	

One-way analysis of variance (ANOVA) was done based on normal distribution of vitamin D level among 28 patients with cluster headache. According to post-hoc analysis between 6 groups using Turkey HSD, p-values between a and d was 0.023, p-value between d and e was < 0.001, and p-value between e and f was 0.018. The other comparisons were not significant

CH cluster headache

(37.5%) and night (66.4%), respectively [52]. An inverse relationship between sunshine duration and the monthly incidence of cluster periods was reported in a hospital-based study [53]. A follow-up population-based study found positive correlations between average temperature and sunshine duration with occurrence of cluster periods, and that temperature was associated with precipitating or priming cluster periods [30]. Based on previous results, it is possible that vitamin D and cluster headaches are related. However, our study did not find significant differences in the vitamin D level among cluster headache, migraine, and controls. Although there was no significant difference among groups, the prevalence of vitamin D deficiency was higher in the cluster headache group than in the migraine and control groups. This suggests that vitamin D deficiency is very common in patients with cluster headache compared with the prevalence of vitamin D deficiency in Korean adults [14]. There was also no significant difference in vitamin D levels according to clinical variables in the patients with cluster headache. However, patients with periodicity of winter to spring had a trend of lower serum 25(OH)D concentrations than those with periodicity of summer to autumn in patients with seasonal periodicity. The serum vitamin D level varies with the season, peaking in May to September. The levels tend to be lower from November to March [54–56]. Therefore, we used an arbitrary classification of the sunny season, i.e., summer to autumn, winter to spring.

The vitamin D receptor and 1α-hydroxylase, the enzyme responsible for the formation of the active vitamin, are present in many parts of the central nervous system, including the prefrontal cortex, hippocampus, cingulate gyrus, thalamus, and hypothalamus. The strongest immunohistochemical staining for both the receptor and enzyme was in the hypothalamus [57]. Vitamin D-binding protein was also detected in axonal projections throughout the lateral hypothalamus in the rat [58]. The presence of the vitamin D receptor, 1α-hydroxylase, and vitamin D-binding protein in the hypothalamus suggests a role of vitamin D deficiency in the generation of various primary headache disorders. In addition to the hypothalamus, there is evidence that the pineal gland has a role in the biological regulation of circadian rhythms by producing melatonin [59]. Sunshine has been reported to regulate specific hormonal and neurotransmitter levels, including melatonin [60]. Altered melatonin levels have been documented in cluster headache and the nocturnal serum melatonin level was decreased during cluster periods [61]. Based on the characteristic clinical features and proposed mechanisms of cluster headache, we hypothesized that vitamin D and cluster headache are related. However, our study failed to find any correlations between the serum vitamin D levels and headache characteristics, such as the seasonal and circadian rhythmicity of cluster headache or the association between serum vitamin D levels and recurrence of cluster headache. To determine the associations between vitamin D and the recurrence in cluster headache, a further longitudinal follow-up study of a larger population is required.

Various factors influence serum vitamin D levels, making, it is difficult to speculate on the role of vitamin D in the pathophysiology of cluster headache. Our study could not control for all of the environmental and demographic factors that significantly affect the serum vitamin D levels There was no information on the exposure of the subjects to sunlight, their sun protection habits or the extent of vitamin D supplementation through food, though we did collect information on smoking status, BMI, sampling time, and sampling season, all of which are known to influence vitamin D concentration. We also analyzed the influence of these variables on serum vitamin D levels. There were no significant differences in smoking status and BMI among the three groups. Additionally, current smoking was not a significant determinant of serum vitamin D levels in this study population using multivariate regression analysis. Second, our study had a relatively small sample size due to the rarity of cluster headache. This study suggests that the influence of vitamin D may warrant analysis in a larger cohort of CH patients with seasonal propensity for winter to spring. This study also included mostly men, due to a sex-matched research design, so these findings may not be truly representative of migraine and normal controls, or generalizable to other groups. Third, the outcome variables collected, such as the seasonal propensity, were assessed on self-report by recall and the classification of the sunny season was arbitrary. While we did not obtain fasting serum samples, there were no significant differences in sampling times among the three groups based on the time the blood samples were collected.

Conclusions

In summary, this is the first report to examine serum vitamin D levels in patients with CH compared to those of age-and sex-matched controls controlling for sampling season as well as other clinical variables.. Our preliminary findings suggest that vitamin D deficiency is very common in patients with cluster headache, but the significance of vitamin D deficiency is uncertain, except for the subtle seasonal influence. Further research is needed to determine the role of vitamin D in CH.

Abbreviations

BMI: Body mass index; GAD-7: Generalized Anxiety Dirorder-7; HIT-6: Headache Impact Test-6; ICHD-3β: Beta version of the International Classification of Headache Disorders-3; PHQ-9: Patient Health Questionnare-9; PSQI: Pittsburgh Sleep Quality Index; SE: Standard error; VAS: Visual analogue scale

Acknowledgements

Thanks to my research coordinator, Jung Eun Kwon for sincere cooperation during the procedure.

Funding

This study was supported by Hallym University Research Fund (HURF-2016-54). The role of funding was in the design of the study and collection, analysis, and interpretation of data. No other financial relationships relevant to this publication were disclosed.

Authors' contributions

Conception and design of the experiments: SJC, KYP, JHS, MKC, HYA; Performance of data collection: SJC, JHS, MKC; Data analysis: SJC, KYP, HYA. Writing of the manuscript and final approval: SJC, KYP, JHS, MKC, HYA.

Competing interests

The authors declare that they have no competing interests.

Author details

[1]Department of Neurology, Chuncheon Sacred Heart Hospital, Hallym University College of Medicine, Chuncheon-si, Gangwon-do, Korea. [2]Department of Neurology, Severance Hospital, Yonsei University College of Medicine, Seoul, Korea. [3]Department of Neurology, Chung-Ang University Hospital, Chung-Ang University College of Medicine, Seoul, Korea. [4]Department of Statistics, Dongguk University-Seoul, Seoul, Korea. [5]Department of Neurology, Dongtan Sacred Heart Hospital, Hallym University College of Medicine, Keun Jae Bong-gil 7, Hwaseong, Gyeonggi-do 18450, Korea.

References

1. Gagnon C, Lu ZX, Magliano DJ, Dunstan DW, Shaw JE, Zimmet PZ, Sikaris K, Grantham N, Ebeling PR, Daly RM (2011) Serum 25-hydroxyvitamin D, calcium intake, and risk of type 2 diabetes after 5 years: results from a national, population-based prospective study (the Australian diabetes, obesity and lifestyle study). Diabetes Care 34(5): 1133–1138. https://doi.org/10.2337/dc10-2167
2. Ju SY, Lee YJ, Jeong SN (2013) Serum 25-hydroxyvitamin D levels and the risk of depression: a systematic review and meta-analysis. J Nutr Health Aging 17(5):447–455. https://doi.org/10.1007/s12603-012-0418-0
3. Afzal S, Bojesen SE, Nordestgaard BG (2014) Reduced 25-hydroxyvitamin D and risk of Alzheimer's disease and vascular dementia. Alzheimers Dement 10(3):296–302. https://doi.org/10.1016/j.jalz.2013.05. 17 65
4. Autier P, Boniol M, Pizot C, Mullie P (2014) Vitamin D status and ill health: a systematic review. Lancet Diabetes Endocrinol 2(1):76–89. https://doi.org/10.1016/s2213-8587(13)70165-7
5. Chen WR, Qian YA, Chen YD, Shi Y, Yin d W, Wang H, Zhu P, Liu HW, Sha Y (2014) The effects of low vitamin D on coronary artery disease. Heart Lung Circ 23(4):314–319. https://doi.org/10.1016/j.hlc.2013.08.012
6. Annweiler C, Dursun E, Feron F, Gezen-Ak D, Kalueff AV, Littlejohns T, Llewellyn DJ, Millet P, Scott T, Tucker KL, Yilmazer S, Beauchet O (2015) 'Vitamin D and cognition in older adults': updated international recommendations. J Intern Med 277(1):45–57. https://doi.org/10.1111/joim.12279
7. Gill TK, Hill CL, Shanahan EM, Taylor AW, Appleton SL, Grant JF, Shi Z, Dal Grande E, Price K, Adams RJ (2014) Vitamin D levels in an Australian population. BMC Public Health 14:1001. https://doi.org/10.1186/1471-2458-14-1001
8. Ginde AA, Liu MC, Camargo CA Jr (2009) Demographic differences and trends of vitamin D insufficiency in the US population, 1988-2004. Arch Intern Med 169(6):626–632. https://doi.org/10.1001/archinternmed.2008.604
9. Greene-Finestone LS, Berger C, de Groh M, Hanley DA, Hidiroglou N, Sarafin K, Poliquin S, Krieger J, Richards JB, Goltzman D (2011) 25-Hydroxyvitamin D in Canadian adults: biological, environmental, and behavioral correlates. Osteoporos Int 22(5):1389–1399. https://doi.org/10.1007/s00198-010-1362-7
10. Hypponen E, Power C (2007) Hypovitaminosis D in British adults at age 45 y: nationwide cohort study of dietary and lifestyle predictors. Am J Clin Nutr 85(3):860–868. https://doi.org/10.1093/ajcn/85.3.860
11. Looker AC, Dawson-Hughes B, Calvo MS, Gunter EW, Sahyoun NR (2002) Serum 25-hydroxyvitamin D status of adolescents and adults in two seasonal subpopulations from NHANES III. Bone 30(5):771–777
12. Rockell JE, Skeaff CM, Williams SM, Green TJ (2006) Serum 25-hydroxyvitamin D concentrations of New Zealanders aged 15 years and older. Osteoporos Int 17(9):1382–1389. https://doi.org/10.1007/s00198-006-0118-x
13. Thuesen B, Husemoen L, Fenger M, Jakobsen J, Schwarz P, Toft U, Ovesen L, Jorgensen T, Linneberg A (2012) Determinants of vitamin D status in a general population of Danish adults. Bone 50(3):605–610. https://doi.org/10.1016/j.bone.2011.12.016
14. Jeong H, Hong S, Heo Y, Chun H, Kim D, Park J, Kang MY (2014) Vitamin D status and associated occupational factors in Korean wage workers: data from the 5th Korea national health and nutrition examination survey (KNHANES 2010-2012). Ann Occup Environ Med 26: 28. https://doi.org/10.1186/s40557-014-0028-x
15. Kimlin MG, Lucas RM, Harrison SL, van der Mei I, Armstrong BK, Whiteman DC, Kricker A, Nowak M, Brodie AM, Sun J (2014) The contributions of solar ultraviolet radiation exposure and other determinants to serum 25-hydroxyvitamin D concentrations in Australian adults: the AusD study. Am J Epidemiol 179(7):864–874. https://doi.org/10.1093/aje/kwt446
16. Prakash S, Mehta NC, Dabhi AS, Lakhani O, Khilari M, Shah ND (2010) The prevalence of headache may be related with the latitude: a possible role of vitamin D insufficiency? J Headache Pain 11(4):301–307. https://doi.org/10.1007/s10194-010-0223-2
17. Kjaergaard M, Eggen AE, Mathiesen EB, Jorde R (2012) Association between headache and serum 25-hydroxyvitamin D: the Tromso study: Tromso 6. Headache 52(10):1499–1505. https://doi.org/10.1111/j.1526-4610.2012.02250.x
18. Lippi G, Cervellin G, Mattiuzzi C (2014) No evidence for an association of vitamin D deficiency and migraine: a systematic review of the literature. Biomed Res Int 2014:827635. https://doi.org/10.1155/2014/827635
19. Zandifar A, Masjedi SS, Banihashemi M, Asgari F, Manouchehri N, Ebrahimi H, Haghdoost F, Saadatnia M (2014) Vitamin D status in migraine patients: a case-control study. Biomed Res Int 2014:514782. https://doi.org/10.1155/2014/514782
20. Thys-Jacobs S (1994) Vitamin D and calcium in menstrual migraine. Headache 34(9):544–546
21. Mottaghi T, Askari G, Khorvash F, Maracy MR (2015) Effect of vitamin D supplementation on symptoms and C-reactive protein in migraine patients. J Res Med Sci 20(5):477–482
22. Buettner C, Nir RR, Bertisch SM, Bernstein C, Schain A, Mittleman MA, Burstein R (2015) Simvastatin and vitamin D for migraine prevention: a randomized, controlled trial. Ann Neurol 78(6):970–981. https://doi.org/10.1002/ana.24534

23. Motaghi M, Haghjooy Javanmard S, Haghdoost F, Tajadini M, Saadatnia M, Rafiee L, Zandifar A (2013) Relationship between vitamin D receptor gene polymorphisms and migraine without aura in an Iranian population. Biomed Res Int 2013:351942. https://doi.org/10.1155/2013/351942
24. Mottaghi T, Khorvash F, Askari G, Maracy MR, Ghiasvand R, Maghsoudi Z, Iraj B (2013) The relationship between serum levels of vitamin D and migraine. J Res Med Sci 18(Suppl 1):S66–S70
25. Nagata E, Fujii N, Hosomichi K, Mitsunaga S, Suzuki Y, Mashimo Y, Tsukamoto H, Satoh T, Osawa M, Inoue I, Hata A, Takizawa S (2014) Possible association between dysfunction of vitamin D binding protein (GC globulin) and migraine attacks. PLoS One 9(8):e105319. https://doi.org/10.1371/journal.pone.0105319
26. Prakash S, Makwana P, Rathore C (2016) Vitamin D deficiency mimicking chronic tension-type headache in children. BMJ Case Rep 2. https://doi.org/10.1136/bcr-2015-213833
27. Prakash S, Rathore C, Makwana P, Dave A, Joshi H, Parekh H (2017) Vitamin D deficiency in patients with chronic tension-type headache: a case-control study. Headache 57(7):1096–1108. https://doi.org/10.1111/head.13096
28. Prakash S, Shah ND (2009) Chronic tension-type headache with vitamin D deficiency: casual or causal association? Headache 49(8):1214–1222. https://doi.org/10.1111/j.1526-4610.2009.01483.x
29. Rozen TD, Fishman RS (2012) Cluster headache in the United States of America: demographics, clinical characteristics, triggers, suicidality, and personal burden. Headache 52(1):99–113. https://doi.org/10.1111/j.1526-4610.2011.02028.x
30. Lee YJ, Chen YT, Ou SM, Li SY, Yang AC, Tang CH, Wang SJ (2014) Temperature variation and the incidence of cluster headache periods: a nationwide population study. Cephalalgia 34(9):656–663. https://doi.org/10.1177/0333102413520083
31. Barloese MC (2015) Neurobiology and sleep disorders in cluster headache. J Headache Pain 16:562. https://doi.org/10.1186/s10194-015-0562-0
32. Peter B (2014) A survey of cluster headache (CH) sufferers using vitamin D3 as a CH preventative. Poster presented of the 66th Annual meeting of American Acedemy of Neurology, Philadelphia, April 26–May 03, 2014
33. Headache Classification Committee of the International Headache Society (IHS) (2013) The International Classification of Headache Disorders, 3rd edition (beta version). Cephalalgia 33(9):629–808. https://doi.org/10.1177/0333102413485658
34. Buysse DJ, Reynolds CF, Monk TH, Berman SR, Kupfer DJ (1989) The Pittsburgh sleep quality index: a new instrument for psychiatric practice and research. Psychiatry Res 28(2):193–213
35. Chu MKIH, Ju YS, Yu KH, Ma HI, Kim YJ et al (2009) Validity and reliability assessment of Korean headache impact test-6 (HIT-6). J Korean Neurol Assoc 2009(27):1–6
36. Seo JG, Park SP (2015) Validation of the patient health questionnaire-9 (PHQ-9) and PHQ-2 in patients with migraine. J Headache Pain 16:65. https://doi.org/10.1186/s10194-015-0552-2
37. Seo J-G, Park S-P (2015) Validation of the generalized anxiety disorder-7 (GAD-7) and GAD-2 in patients with migraine. J Headache Pain 16(1):97
38. CDC Vitamin D Standardization-Certification Program (VDSCP)—Total 25hydroxy Vitamin D Certified Procedures (2017) https://www.cdc.gov/labstandards/pdf/hs/CDC_Certified_Vitamin_D_Procedures.pdf. Accessed 8 Dec 2017
39. Holick MF (2017) The vitamin D deficiency pandemic: approaches for diagnosis, treatment and prevention. Rev Endocr Metab Disord 18(2):153–165. https://doi.org/10.1007/s11154-017-9424-1
40. Holick MF, Binkley NC, Bischoff-Ferrari HA, Gordon CM, Hanley DA, Heaney RP, Murad MH, Weaver CM (2011) Evaluation, treatment, and prevention of vitamin D deficiency: an endocrine society clinical practice guideline. J Clin Endocrinol Metab 96(7):1911–1930. https://doi.org/10.1210/jc.2011-0385
41. Thomas MK, Lloyd-Jones DM, Thadhani RI, Shaw AC, Deraska DJ, Kitch BT, Vamvakas EC, Dick IM, Prince RL, Finkelstein JS (1998) Hypovitaminosis D in medical inpatients. N Engl J Med 338(12):777–783. https://doi.org/10.1056/nejm199803193381201
42. Malabanan A, Veronikis IE, Holick MF (1998) Redefining vitamin D insufficiency. Lancet 351(9105):805–806
43. Hollis BW, Wagner CL (2005) Normal serum vitamin D levels. N Engl J Med 352(5):515–516; author reply 515-516. https://doi.org/10.1056/nejm200502033520521
44. Holick MF (2006) High prevalence of vitamin D inadequacy and implications for health. Mayo Clin Proc 81(3):353–373. https://doi.org/10.4065/81.3.353
45. Masood T, Kushwaha RS, Singh R, Sailwal S, Pandey H, Varma A, Singh RK, Cornelissen G (2015) Circadian rhythm of serum 25 OH vitamin D, calcium and phosphorus levels in the treatment and management of type-2 diabetic patients. Drug Discov Therap 9(1):70–74. https://doi.org/10.5582/ddt.2015.01002
46. Prakash S, Kumar M, Belani P, Susvirkar A, Ahuja S (2013) Interrelationships between chronic tension-type headache, musculoskeletal pain, and vitamin D deficiency: is osteomalacia responsible for both headache and musculoskeletal pain? Ann Indian Acad Neurol 16(4):650–658. https://doi.org/10.4103/0972-2327.120487
47. Celikbilek A, Gocmen AY, Zararsiz G, Tanik N, Ak H, Borekci E, Delibas N (2014) Serum levels of vitamin D, vitamin D-binding protein and vitamin D receptor in migraine patients from Central Anatolia region. Int J Clin Pract 68(10):1272–1277. https://doi.org/10.1111/ijcp.12456
48. Soriani S, Fiumana E, Manfredini R, Boari B, Battistella PA, Canetta E, Pedretti S, Borgna-Pignatti C (2006) Circadian and seasonal variation of migraine attacks in children. Headache 46(10):1571–1574. https://doi.org/10.1111/j.1526-4610.2006.00613.x
49. Marrelli A, Marini C, Prencipe M (1988) Seasonal and meteorological factors in primary headaches. Headache 28(2):111–113
50. Cugini P, Romit A, Di Palma L, Giacovazzo M (1990) Common migraine as a weekly and seasonal headache. Chronobiol Int 7(5–6):467–469
51. Pringsheim T (2002) Cluster headache: evidence for a disorder of circadian rhythm and hypothalamic function. Can J Neurol Sci 29(1):33–40
52. Heui-Soo Moon JWP, Kwang-Soo Lee C-SC, Byung-Kun Kim J-MK, Jong-Hee Sohn MKC, Oh K, Cho SJ (2017) Clinical features of cluster headache patients in Korea. J Korean Med Sci 32(3):502–506. https://doi.org/10.3346/jkms.2017.32.3.502
53. Lin KH, Wang PJ, Fuh JL, Lu SR, Chung CT, Tsou HK, Wang SJ (2004) Cluster headache in the Taiwanese - a clinic-based study. Cephalalgia 24(8):631–638. https://doi.org/10.1111/j.1468-2982.2003.00721.x
54. Rapuri PB, Kinyamu HK, Gallagher JC, Haynatzka V (2002) Seasonal changes in calciotropic hormones, bone markers, and bone mineral density in elderly women. J Clin Endocrinol Metab 87(5):2024–2032. https://doi.org/10.1210/jcem.87.5.8475
55. Prince PB, Rapoport AM, Sheftell FD, Tepper SJ, Bigal ME (2004) The effect of weather on headache. Headache 44(6):596–602. https://doi.org/10.1111/j.1526-4610.2004.446008.x
56. Maxwell JD (1994) Seasonal variation in vitamin D. Proc Nutr Soc 53(3):533–543
57. Eyles DW, Smith S, Kinobe R, Hewison M, McGrath JJ (2005) Distribution of the vitamin D receptor and 1 alpha-hydroxylase in human brain. J Chem Neuroanat 29(1):21–30. https://doi.org/10.1016/j.jchemneu.2004.08.006
58. Jirikowski GF, Kaunzner UW, Dief Ael E, Caldwell JD (2009) Distribution of vitamin D binding protein expressing neurons in the rat hypothalamus. Histochem Cell Biol 131(3):365–370. https://doi.org/10.1007/s00418-008-0540-6
59. Peres MF (2005) Melatonin, the pineal gland and their implications for headache disorders. Cephalalgia 25(6):403–411. https://doi.org/10.1111/j.1468-2982.2005.00889.x
60. Golombek DA, Rosenstein RE (2010) Physiology of circadian entrainment. Physiol Rev 90(3):1063–1102. https://doi.org/10.1152/physrev.00009.2009
61. Waldenlind E, Gustafsson SA, Ekbom K, Wetterberg L (1987) Circadian secretion of cortisol and melatonin in cluster headache during active cluster periods and remission. J Neurol Neurosurg Psychiatry 50(2):207–213

23

Pre-treatment with sumatriptan for cilostazol induced headache in healthy volunteers

Katrine Falkenberg[1,2] and Jes Olesen[1,2*]

Abstract

Background: Previous studies indicate that sumatriptan is not effective when second messenger levels are high as after cilostazol provocation. Therefore, we have conducted the present study, where sumatriptan is administrated as pretreatment before cAMP increases due to cilostazol intake. Our hypothesis was that pretreatment with sumatriptan would have a significant effect against cilostazol induced headache in healthy volunteers.

Methods: In a double-blind, randomized, crossover design, 30 healthy volunteers of both sexes received cilostazol 200 mg on two separate days, each day preceded by oral sumatriptan (2 × 50 mg) or placebo. Headache response and accompanying symptoms were registered in a questionnaire by the participants themselves.

Results: Cilostazol induced a mild to moderate headache in all but 3 participants (Range 0–7 on Numerical Rating Scale). There was no significant difference in headache score 2 h ($p = 0.67$) or 4 h ($p = 0.1$) after treatment between the 2 days. Median peak headache score was 1.5 (range 0–5) on the sumatriptan day and 2 (range 0–7) on the placebo day ($p = 0.26$).

Conclusion: Pre-treatment with sumatriptan prevents cilostazol induced headache from developing. However, the placebo group did not develop enough headache to get statistical significant results. The cilostazol pre-treatment model is valuable for experimental headache research and perhaps for testing drugs with another mechanism of action.

Keywords: Headache, Migraine, Pain, Phosphodiesterase type 3, Human migraine model

Background

In recent years, the authors made a dedicated attempt to develop a pragmatic model for testing new anti-migraine drugs. The idea behind the model is to have participants come to the hospital and to be able to induce migraine attacks and treat them. That would enable the drug industry to test their new anti-migraine drug under controlled conditions, inexpensively and in a short period of time. We have tried to develop the model in both healthy volunteers and in patients with migraine without aura (MO) using two different headache inducing substances; Isosorbide-5-mononitrate (5-ISMN, a long lasting NO-donor) and cilostazol (a phosphodiesterase 3- inhibitor).

NO leads to an increase in cGMP in the cell and cilostazol increases cAMP [1, 2]. To validate the model, we tested the effect of sumatriptan on the induced headache. Sumatriptan had no effect on 5-ISMN induced headache [3]. When treating cilostazol induced headache in healthy volunteers with sumatriptan, we saw a trend towards an effect [4] and the trend was stronger when the same study was conducted in MO patients [5]. However, all three studies indicate that sumatriptan is not effective when second messenger levels (cGMP and cAMP), are increased in the system. Therefore, we have conducted the present study, where sumatriptan is administrated as pretreatment before cAMP increases

* Correspondence: jes.olesen@regionh.dk
[1]Danish Headache Center and Department of Neurology, University of Copenhagen, Rigshospitalet Glostrup, Copenhagen, Denmark
[2]Danish Headache Center, Department of Neurology N39, Rigshospitalet Glostrup, University of Copenhagen, Valdemar Hansens vej 5, DK-2600 Glostrup, Denmark

due to cilostazol intake. Our hypothesis was that pre-treatment with sumatriptan would have a significant effect against cilostazol induced headache in healthy volunteers.

Methods

A similar method has been described previously in three studies by the authors [3–5].

Participants

Thirty healthy volunteers (15F/15M) with no history of migraine were included. Inclusion criteria were: healthy subjects of both sexes aged 18–60 years and weighting 45–90 kg.

Exclusion criteria were: any type of headache (except episodic tension-type headache < 1 day per week), serious somatic or psychiatric disease, pregnancy, and intake of daily medication (except oral contraceptives). The participants were informed that cilostazol might induce headache or migraine in some individuals.

Design

We conducted a double-blinded, randomized, balanced, placebo-controlled, cross-over study. The participants received pre-treatment with 50 mg of sumatriptan or placebo 1.5 h prior to oral cilostazol of 200 mg. Together with cilostazol intake, the participants took an additional 50 mg of sumatriptan or placebo. Tmax for both sumatriptan and cilostazol is about 2 h and we thus reach maximum concentration of sumatriptan and cilostazol at the same time. The reason why we also gave sumatriptan 1.5 h prior to cilostazol was to have a high dose of sumatriptan at time of cilostazol intake. Cilostazol dose (200 mg) was chosen based on previous headache-studies.

The central pharmacy of the Capital Region of Copenhagen performed the randomization of the experimental drug in a balanced fashion. The randomization code did not leave the hospital during the study and was not available to the investigators until after termination of the study. We did not break the code until data management took place.

Standard protocol approvals

All participants gave written, informed consent to participate in the study. The study was approved by the Ethics Committee of Copenhagen (H-15011960) and the Danish Data Protection Agency. The study is registered on clinicaltrials.gov (NCT03156920) and was conducted according to the Helsinki II declaration of 1964, as revised in 2008.

All participants were enrolled via the website forsøgsperson.dk [6].

Study procedure

The participants had to be headache free 48 h prior to the study and not to have taken any type of painkillers 12 h before beginning of the study. A pregnancy test was taken at the beginning of each study day on all fertile female participants. All participants had two separate study days at least five days apart. They arrived non-fasting at the clinic between 8:00 a.m. and 12:00 p.m. Full medical history, physical examination, electrocardiography (ECG), vital signs and baseline headache were collected at arrival. All participants received the treatment (placebo or sumatriptan) and waited for 1.5 h before they received cilostazol 200 mg orally together with an additional pill of treatment (the same treatment as the first one). Hereafter the participants were discharged from hospital. In case of severe headache not responding to the experimental treatment, the participants were allowed rescue with nonsteroidal anti-inflammatory drugs (NSAIDs) and paracetamol, but not before two hours after cilostazol. During the study, an emergency phone was always open where participants could call if they experienced severe headaches or discomfort.

Headache parameters

Headache parameters and accompanying symptoms were recorded by the investigator at baseline on a headache questionnaire. Afterward headache intensity, characteristics (unilateral/bilateral, quality and aggravation by physical activity), accompanying symptoms (nausea/vomiting, phono- and photophobia) and side effects were scored on a self-administered questionnaire. The participants had to fill out the questionnaire every 30 min the first 6 h after cilostazol and thereafter every hour until 12 h after cilostazol. The intensity was scored on a Numerical Rating Scale (NRS) from 0 to 10, 1 representing a very mild headache (including feeling of pressing or pulsation), 5 a headache of medium severity and 10 the worst possible headache (10). Missing data were filled in using last observation carried forward.

The following criterion was used for a migraine-like attack induced 0–12 h after administration of cilostazol:

Headache fulfilling criteria C and D for migraine without aura according to the IHS criteria [7].

C. Headache has at least two of the following characteristics:

- Unilateral location
- Pulsating quality
- Moderate or severe pain intensity (moderate to severe pain intensity is considered ≥4 on NRS)
- Aggravation by cough or causing avoidance of routine physical activity

D. During headache at least one of the following:

- Nausea and/or vomiting
- Photophobia and phonophobia.

Statistical analysis

Calculation of sample size was based on the detection of a difference in headache intensity between two experimental days, at 5% significance with 90% power. We estimated that placebo had an effect on 20% and sumatriptan had 60% effect. Standard deviation was estimated based on previous data. The correlation between the 2 days was estimated conservatively at 0.5. We also assumed no carry-over effect. We calculated that at least 18 participants should complete both experimental days. Due to uncertainty regarding these assumptions we decided to include 30 participants. The area under the curve (AUC) for headache score was used as a summary measure for analyzing differences between the groups and was calculated according to the trapezium rule (12). Our primary endpoints were (1) difference in pain intensity difference between sumatriptan and placebo 2 hours after the last treatment, and (2) difference in AUC 0-4 h between the two experimental days. Secondary end-points were difference in median peak headache score, difference in median headache intensity between the two treatments at 4 h, AUC 0-2 h after sumatriptan/placebo and accompanying symptoms as nausea, photo- and photophobia.

Headache intensity scores are presented as medians (range). Differences in AUC for headache scores were tested using the Wilcoxon signed rank test. Difference in pain intensity difference between the sumatriptan day and the placebo day were tested using Mann-Whitney test. The incidence of headache and associated symptoms were analyzed as binary categorical data with McNemar's test. Age and weigh are presented as means. All analyses were performed with SPSS for Windows 11.5 (Chicago, IL, USA), or GraphPad Prism version 7.0. A $p < 0.05$ was considered significant.

Results

Thirty participants (15F, 15 M) with a mean age of 26.5 (19–58 years) and a mean weight on 71.6 kg (48-93 kg), completed the study. Three participants had a first degree relative with migraine (self-reported).

Cilostazol induced a mild to moderate headache (range 1–7 on NRS) in all but three participants. The headache had some migraine features, especially throbbing character and it was aggravated by physical activity (see Table 1 for clinical characteristics of the headache and associated symptoms). Median peak headache score was 1.5 (range 0–5) on the sumatriptan day and 2 (range 0–7) on the placebo day. Median time to peak headache score was 5 h and 4.5 h respectively. Two subjects in each group experienced a migraine-like attack with a mean time of onset of 8.5 h (7 and 10 h) on the sumatriptan day and 4 h (1 and 7 h) on the placebo day.

There was no significant difference in headache score between the 2 days at 2 h after treatment ($p = 0.52$) and thus our primary end-point was negative. Two hours after treatment intake, median headache score was 0 (range 0–3) for the sumatriptan day and 1 (range 0–4) for the placebo day. At 4 h after treatment intake (our secondary end-point) there was no significant difference either ($p = 0.06$). Median headache score 0-12 h after cilostazol for the two treatment groups is illustrated in

Table 1 Clinical characteristics (our secondary end-point) of headache and associated symptoms after cilostazol

	Sumatriptan ($n = 30$)	Placebo ($n = 30$)	P-value*
Number of participants reported headache (range 1–7 on VRS)	27	27	1.00
Median peak headache score (range)	1.5 (0–5)	2 (0–7)	0.26**
No. of participants with			
Throbbing headache	13	15	0.77
Unilateral location	10	8	0.77
Nausea	7	6***	1.00
Aggravation by physical activity	15	17	0.79
Photophobia	7	5	0.72
Phonophobia	4	2	0.61
Rescue medication	0	2	0.48
Migraine-like attack	2	2	1.00

* McNemar's test
** Wilcoxon signed rank test
*** Two subject vomited

Fig. 1 and headache score after treatment is illustrated in Fig. 2.

Our other primary end point, AUC 0-4 h after treatment did not differ between the 2 days ($p = 0.57$). Nor did we see a difference in our secondary end point, difference in peak headache score ($p = 0.26$) see Fig. 3.

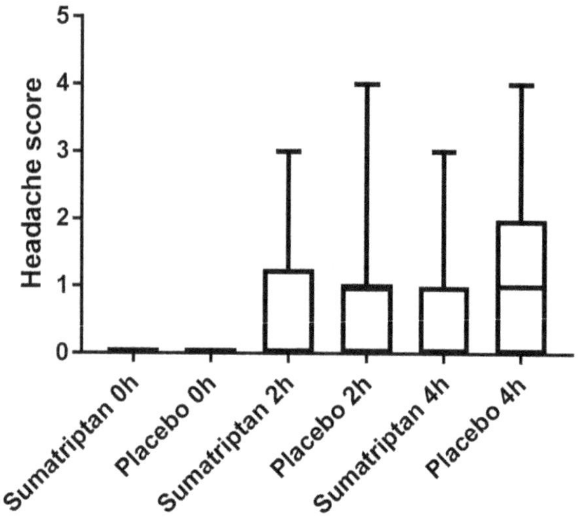

Fig. 2 Headache score after treatment. Headache score 0 h, 2 h and 4 h after treatment with placebo and sumatriptan. There was no difference in headache score at any time-point between the two treatment days

Discussion

Cilostazol induced a mild to moderate headache in 27/30 participants. The median headache score after sumatriptan was 0 and thus sumatriptan may have prevented the headache from developing. However, our end-points were all statistically negative because the placebo group did not develop much headache either (median headache score at 1) (See Fig. 1).

Modifying the model from previous studies

In previous studies, we showed a trend towards an effect of sumatriptan on cilostazol induced headache in both healthy volunteers and in MO patients [2, 3]. The effect was, however, not clear and the model needed modification in order to be valid for future drug testing. Cilostazol induces headache by an increase of cAMP which leads to vasodilatation and sensitization of nerve endings. One possible explanation for the lack of effect of sumatriptan in our previous studies could be that sumatriptan cannot exert its effect when cGMP and cAMP have already accumulated in the cell, which happens after provocation with isosorbide-5-mononitrate and cilostazol respectively [1–3].

Cilostazol inhibits phosphodiesterase 3 and thus prevents cAMP break-down. Therefore, in order for cAMP to be accumulated in the cell due to cilostazol, there must be cAMP in the cell beforehand. Sumatriptan inhibits adenylate cyclase leading to a decreased formation of cAMP in the cell. In the present study we tried to modify the previous model by administering sumatriptan as pretreatment and thus impeding the formation of cAMP before cilostazol provocation. We hypothesized that there would be no cAMP to accumulate in the cell and therefore no headache would occur. Our results suggest that sumatriptan pre-treatment may prevent the headache from developing since median headache score remained 0 until 6 h after sumatriptan. At 6 h the effect of sumatriptan has subsided and the headache score increased to 1, like in the placebo group (see Fig. 1). An explanation why our results all came out statistically negative is that we have a considerably lower headache induction in the present study, compared to previous studies (see elaboration below).

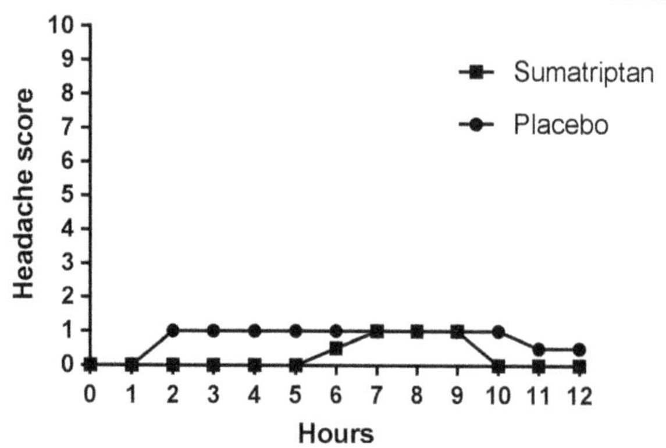

Fig. 1 Headache score 0-12 h after cilostazol. Median headache score 0-12 h after cilostazol. Median headache score was 1 on both days and thus we found no difference between the two treatment days

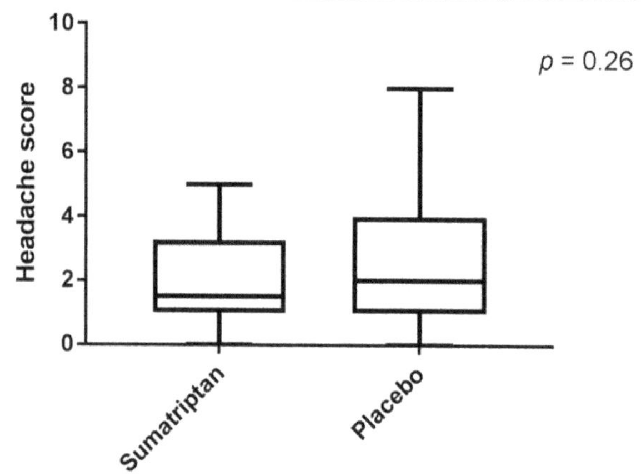

Fig. 3 Peak headache score. Difference in median peak headache score on the two treatment days was not statistical significant

The headache inducing properties of cilostazol in healthy volunteers

It has previously been described that cilostazol induces a headache with migraine characteristics in healthy volunteers and a migraine-like attack in migraine patients [2, 8]. More and more studies are using cilostazol headache models to study the pathophysiology of migraine. Nevertheless, the headache inducing property of cilostazol differs depending on study design.

Our own group has completed 3 such studies: Birk et al. conducted a double-blind randomized placebo-controlled crossover study in which the participant received cilostazol on 1 day and placebo on the other day. The participants were not offered any treatment as part of the study. Cilostazol induced a median peak headache score of 3.5 on NRS.

In a previous study by the present authors, cilostazol induced headache, once established, was treated with sumatriptan and placebo in a double-blind crossover study. Treatment was then given on both study days. Median peak headache score was 2 on the sumatriptan day and 3 on the placebo day. Hence, when the participants receive treatment for the headache (including placebo) we see a milder headache score than if no treatment is offered.

In keeping with that result, the present study where sumatriptan and placebo were given as pretreatment found, median peak headache score of only 1.5 on the sumatriptan day and 2 on the placebo day. When treatment is administered before the headache inducing substance, the placebo effect may thus be even bigger. It is interesting, that the placebo effect seems to be present in experimental headache induction studies to a degree similar to spontaneous migraine attacks.

Can we use the present model for drug testing?

We suggest that the cilostazol pre-treatment model is valuable for experimental headache research and perhaps for novel drug testing, but the model needs some modifications. It could for an example be interesting to conduct the present study on migraine patients, who are known to develop more headache from cilostazol than healthy volunteers.

Conclusion

This study shows that pre-treatment with sumatriptan prevents cilostazol induced headache from developing. However, the placebo group did not develop enough headache to get statistically significant results. We also show by comparison to previous studies that the placebo effect on experimental headache is considerable and should be taken into consideration in future power calculations.

Abbreviations

5-ISMN: Isosorbide-5-mononitrate; AUC: Area under the curve; cAMP: Cyclic adenylate monophosphate; cGMP: Cyclic guanosine monophosphate; ECG: Electrocardiography; IHS: International Headache Society; MO: Migraine without aura; NRS: Numerical rating scale; NSAIDs: Nonsteroidal anti-inflammatory drugs; PDE3: Phosphodiesterase 3; PID: Pain intensity difference

Acknowledgements

This work was supported by Candys Foundation, Grosser L.F. Foghts Foundation, The Hartmann Foundation, Axel Muusfeldt Foundation and Frimodt Heineke Foundation.

Authors' contributions

KF and JO designed the experiment. KF collected and analysed the data. KF and JO wrote the manuscript. All authors read and approved the final manuscript.

Competing interests

The authors declare that they have no competing interests.

References

1. Liu Y, Shakur Y, Yoshitake M et al (2001) Cilostazol (pletal): a dual inhibitor of cyclic nucleotide phosphodiesterase type 3 and adenosine uptake. Cardiovasc Drug Rev 19:369–386
2. Guo S, Olesen J, Ashina M. Phosphodiesterase 3 inhibitor cilostazol induces migraine-like attacks via cyclic AMP increase. Brain. Epub ahead of print 26 August 2014. DOI: https://doi.org/10.1093/brain/awu244
3. Hansen EK, Olesen J (2017) Towards a pragmatic human migraine model for drug testing: 2. Isosorbide-5-mononitrate in healthy individuals. Cephalalgia 37:11–19
4. Hansen EK, Guo S, Ashina M et al (2016) Toward a pragmatic migraine model for drug testing: I. Cilostazol in healthy volunteers. Cephalalgia 36:172–178
5. Falkenberg K, Dunga BÓÁ, Guo S et al (2018) Cilostazol induced migraine does not respond to sumatriptan in a double blind trial. J Headache Pain 19:11
6. National Center for clinical trial registrations. Raske forsøgspersoner søges til migræneforsøg. 2017. www.forsoegsperson.dk. Accessed 28 Aug 2017.
7. (IHS) HCC of the IHS (2013) The international classification of headache disorders, 3rd edition (beta version). Cephalalgia 33:629–808
8. Birk S, Kruuse C, Petersen KA et al (2006) The headache-inducing effect of cilostazol in human volunteers. Cephalalgia 26:1304–1309

24

Headache attributed to aeroplane travel: the first multicentric survey in a paediatric population affected by primary headaches

Debora De Carlo[1†], Irene Toldo[1†], Agnese Maria Tamborino[2], Barbara Bolzonella[1], Maria Giuseppina Ledda[3], Lucia Margari[4], Vincenzo Raieli[5], Margherita Santucci[6], Vittorio Sciruicchio[7], Angelo Vecchio[8], Sergio Zanini[9], Stefano Sartori[1], Michela Gatta[1], Alberto Verrotti[2] and Pier Antonio Battistella[1*]

Abstract

Background: This multicentric survey investigates the prevalence and characteristics of Airplane Headache in children affected by primary headaches.

Methods: Patients with symptoms of Airplane Headache were recruited from nine Italian Pediatric Headache Centres. Each patient was handed a structured questionnaire which met the ICHD-III criteria.

Results: Among 320 children suffering from primary headaches who had flights during their lifetime, 15 (4.7%) had Airplane Headache, with mean age of 12.4 years. Most of the patients were females (80%). The headache was predominantly bilateral (80%) and localized to the frontal area (60%); it was mainly pulsating, and lasted less than 30 min in all cases. Accompanying symptoms were tearing, photophobia, phonophobia in most of the cases (73.3%). More than 30% of patients used medications to treat the attacks, with good results.

Conclusion: Our study shows that Airplane Headache is not a rare disorder in children affected by primary headaches and highlights that its features in children are peculiar and differ from those described in adults. In children Airplane Headache prevails in females, is more often bilateral, has frequently accompanying symptoms and occurs at any time during the flight.

Further studies are needed to confirm the actual frequency of Airplane Headache in the general pediatric population not selected from specialized Headache Centres, with and without other concomitant headache condition, and to better clarify the clinical characteristics, pathophysiology and potential therapies.

Keywords: Headache, Aeroplane travel, Airplane, Primary headaches, Children, Pediatric headache, ICHD-III

Background

Headache disorders in children and adolescents are common disabling problems with a significant impact on the quality of life of both children and parents [1, 2].

Airplane headache (AH) is a relatively rare headache disorder associated only with airplane travel; in particular pain begins during taking off or landing or both [3].

The first adult case of AH was reported in 2004 [4]. Its prevalence is unknown and the underlying pathophysiology is uncertain, although sinonasal barotrauma has been proposed [4–6].

In 2013 Mainardi et al. [7] collected clinical data of 75 patients with symptoms suggestive of AH and proposed provisional diagnostic criteria.

There has been a steadily increase in the number of reported cases in the following years: up to now, 275 adult cases have been described in the literature [7–20] and, recently, two systematic reviews have been published [21, 22]. Most of the known cases of AH are young males. In all cases, symptoms are highly stereotyped. The pain is typically reported as severe and may be described as jabbing, stabbing, or pulsatile in quality. It is usually unilateral and localized to fronto-orbital and

* Correspondence: pierantonio.battistella@unipd.it
†Debora De Carlo and Irene Toldo contributed equally to this work.
[1]Juvenile Headache Centre, University of Padua, via Giustiniani 3, 35128 Padua, Italy
Full list of author information is available at the end of the article

fronto-parietal regions. The headache is short-lived, lasts less than 30 min, and occurs exclusively in relation to airplane travel (most frequently during airplane descent). Accompanying symptoms are usually absent.

So far only 5 cases within the pediatric age group have been described [23–25].

The aim of our study is to investigate the prevalence and characteristics of AH in a large group of children suffering from primary headaches, taking into account *experts' opinion about the pediatric secondary headache diagnostic criteria of ICHD-III beta* [26].

Patients and methods

This study is a multicentric pediatric cohort study. Patients with symptoms suggestive of AH were recruited from 9 Italian Pediatric Headache Centres.

During the study period, all patients were solicited to take part in the study. Following an explanation about the study purposes, each patient was handed a structured questionnaire, aimed at obtaining all the relevant information that could clinically distinguish this peculiar disorder. The questionnaire met the ICHD-III criteria [27].

The inclusion criteria were:

A. At least two episodes of headache fulfilling criterion C.
B. The patient is travelling by aeroplane.
C. Evidence of causation demonstrated by at least two of the following:
1. headache has developed during the aeroplane flight
2. either or both of the following:
   a) headache has worsened in temporal relation to ascent following take-off and/or descent prior to landing of the aeroplane.
   b) headache has spontaneously improved within 30 min after the ascent or descent of the aeroplane is completed.
3. headache is severe, with at least two of the following three characteristics:
   a) unilateral location.
   b) orbitofrontal location.
   c) jabbing or stabbing quality.

D. Not better accounted for by another ICHD-3 diagnosis.
E. Age ≤ 18 years.

The structured questionnaire was composed of 32 questions and included two sections: medical history and details of nature of AH.

A total number of 727 children participated in this survey. The questionnaire was completed by 637 subjects.

Most of the cases were females (364 females, 273 males). The mean age of patients was 11.3 years (range 3.1–18.0).

Results

Age at onset

Among 320 patients who flew during their lifetime, only 15 (4.5%) had AH. Most of the cases were females (12 females, 3 males). The mean age at recruitment was 12.4 years (range 8.2–16.0); the mean age at headache onset was 7.2 years (range 3.1–11.1).

History of coexistent primary headaches

A specific section of the questionnaire focused on the possible coexistence of a primary headache, according to the ICHD-III [27]. In the total study population ($n = 637$), the most commonly associated primary headaches were migraine ($n = 456$; 71.6%) and tension-type headache ($n = 137$; 21.5%). In 29 patients (4.5%) two different coexistent primary headaches could be diagnosed; no patient reported symptoms suggestive of cluster headache (Table 1).

The neurological examination was unremarkable. Basic biochemical and hematologic tests and brain magnetic resonance imaging revealed no abnormalities.

Twelve children (80%) with AH suffered also from migraine. Two patients (13.4%) with AH had also tension-type headache. One patient (6.7%) suffered from new daily persistent headache (Table 2).

Upper respiratory tract disorders

A personal history for allergy was reported by 3 patients (20%), and for sinus infection by 3 patients (20%). No patients had symptoms and/or signs related to inflammatory sinus disorders following an ENT specialist evaluation, performed immediately after the attack.

Clinical features of airplane headache

The clinical characteristics of AH were quite peculiar.

First episode

Seven children (46.7%) presented AH since the first flight experience.

Two patients (13.3%) flew 3–6 times per year, and seven patients (46.7%) flew less than one per year.

Table 1 Classification of headaches in patients

Headache type	N	%
Migraine without aura	368	57.8
Episodic tension-type headache	82	12.9
Migraine with aura	74	11.6
Chronic tension-type headache	55	8.6
Migraine + tension-type headache	29	4.5
Other primary headaches	15	2.3
Chronic migraine	14	2.2
Total	637	100

Table 2 Concurrent primary headaches in AH patients

Headache type	N	%
Migraine with aura	7	46.7
Migraine without aura	5	33.3
Episodic tension-type headache	1	6.7
Chronic tension-type headache	1	6.7
New daily persistent headache	1	6.7
Total	15	100

Consistency of attacks

In 7 children (46.7%) the same type of headache recurred consistently on separate flights; for those patients the pain started exclusively during landing in two, both during take-off and landing in three, during take-off in one and during cruising in one. The attacks occurred in more than 50% of flights only in one child ($n = 1/15$, 6.7%); for this patient the pain started only during take-off. The attacks occurred in less than 50% of flights in 3 patients (20%): exclusively during landing in two and also during cruising in one. In 4 cases (26.7%) the attacks were occasional and unpredictable. One patient reported the occasional occurrence of attacks during cruising only in the case of short-haul flights.

Timing

AH can occur at any time during the flight. More specifically, in three patients (20%) the attacks occurred exclusively during landing; in three patients (20%) AH started only during take-off. Five patient (33.5%) reported headache onset during cruising. In three patients (20%) AH started during both take-off and landing, and in one patient during cruising and landing (Table 3). No patients reported the possible difference in altitude between the arrival and departure airport as potential aggravating or trigger factors.

Duration

The duration was less than 30 min in all patients.

Intensity

The pain intensity was defined as severe by 10 (66.7%), moderate by 3 (20%), and mild by 2 (13.3%) patients.

Table 3 Headache onset with respect to flight timing

	Female n (%)	Male n (%)
Only during landing	3 (20)	0
Only during take-off	1 (6.7)	2 (13.3)
During cruising	4 (26.7)	1 (6.7)
During both landing and take-off	3 (20)	0
During both cruising and landing	1 (6.7)	0
Total	12 (80)	3 (20)

Quality of pain

Quality of headache was most frequently defined as pulsating (8 cases, 53.6%). Other definitions were: pressing in 4 (26.7%), tightening in 3 (20%) patients.

Localization of headache

In the majority of patients (12/15, 80%) the pain was bilateral. In the remaining 3 cases (20%) headache was unilateral; in these cases, the pain constantly recurred on the same side throughout the different attacks in two cases, while in one case (6.7%) the pain occurred on the opposite side in subsequent flights. The pain was more frequently localized to the frontal region (9/15, 60%). In three subjects (20%) the pain spread to the whole head.

Emotional impact

Only three children (20%) were concerned with the fear of suffering from a further attack and therefore were negatively predisposed for future flights. Among these subjects, 2 (13.3%) continued to fly with anxiety and/or worry; one (6.7%) decided to fly only if strictly necessary.

Accompanying symptoms

These were reported by 11 patients (73.3%): tearing, photophobia, phonophobia. No conjunctival injection, nausea, vomiting were reported.

Self-administered manoeuvres

Two patients (13.3%) performed one spontaneous maneuver in order to decrease the intensity of the attacks and to obtain some relief. The self-administered maneuvers were: pressure on the pain site and bracelet. One patient reported a reduction of pain intensity.

Pharmacological treatment

Ten patients (66.7%) did not take any drugs. The remaining 5 patients (3/5 females) used the following medications: acetaminophen (15 mg/kg), ibuprofen (10 mg/kg) and ketoprofen (1.5 mg/kg) were taken within few minutes after the headache onset, with rapid relief (Table 4).

Discussion

The present study was performed on a selected population affected by primary headaches referring to 9 Italian Pediatric Headache Centres and described in details the clinical features of 15 children suffering from brief headache during airplane travel. The clinical features of AH in our pediatric population were quite peculiar and differed from those described in adulthood [7–20].

Even though it is not possible to directly compare these data with those on AH adults recruited from the general population, it seems that AH features significantly differ between the adult and the child population

Table 4 Demographic characteristics and clinical reports of the AH patients

Subject no	Gender	Age (year)	Duration of AH (minutes)	Intensity of pain	Quality of pain	Localization of the headache	Pharmacological treatment
1	F	12.6	30	5	Pressing	Temporal, bilateral	No
2	F	9.7	30	2	Pulsating	Frontal, unilateral	No
3	M	10.5	20	8	Pulsating	Frontal, bilateral	No
4	F	12.8	30	4	Pressing	Frontal, bilateral	No
5	F	8.2	20	9	Pulsating	Frontal, bilateral	Yes, acetaminophen
6	M	11	30	1	Pulsating	Frontal, bilateral	Yes, acetaminophen
7	F	15.5	20	8	Pressing	Frontal, bilateral	No
8	F	11	15	8	Pressing	Diffuse, bilateral	No
9	F	16	25	6	Pulsating	Frontal, bilateral	No
10	F	14	25	8	Tightening	Temporal, bilateral	No
11	F	12	20	9	Pulsating	Diffuse, bilateral	Yes, ketoprofen
12	F	16	30	8	Pulsating	Frontal, bilateral	No
13	F	15	30	9	Pulsating	Frontal, bilateral	No
14	M	9	30	7	Tightening	Diffuse, unilateral	Yes, acetaminophen
15	F	12.5	30	8	Tightening	Occipital, unilateral	Yes, ibuprofen

in terms of several clinical features (intensity, distribution of pain, presence and type of accompanying symptoms, male to female ratio, etc). AH is strictly unilateral in the vast majority of adult cases, its phenotype resembles somehow cluster headache [7]. Moreover, only 20% of the pediatric patients presented a negative predisposition to future flights compared to 80% of the adult patients [7] and no one among the pediatric patients appeared to have restlessness or anxiety during the attack, maybe due to the less intensity of the pain. Children showed less frequently concern for subsequent airplane travel maybe for a reduced memory of the painful experience, for the lower intensity of pain and for a greater curiosity for future airplane travels. Moreover, differently from adults [7], no pediatric patients presented an easily recognizable postictal long-lasting mild headache phase after the AH acute attack.

All our patients suffered from at least one type of primary headache, as they were recruited in specialized pediatric Headache Centres. Only 20% of adults reported in the literature suffered from a concomitant primary headache [5–21]. Interestingly, we have found a relevant association between AH and migraine with aura. Baldacci et al. [10] reported a patient with AH also affected by migraine with aura: this primary headache is more rare compared to migraine without aura and episodic tension-type headache in the pediatric population. Therefore, the association between AH and migraine with aura does not seems to be incidental and deserves further epidemiological studies to better understand the etiopathogenetic mechanisms of this association.

In half of our AH cases, the first attack was concomitant with the first flight and in 46.7% of them occurred during each flight. In adult population the first AH during the first flight occured only in 14% of cases; that is a significant difference. It is likely that in the pediatric population, the headache attack during the flight warns the parents and therefore it is reported more frequently since the first attack.

The sex ratio was different for pediatric AH compared to adults [7–20] and was skewed toward females (80%) in our young patients. In adult population, the AH was unilateral and it was localized to the fronto-orbital area [7–20]. The quality of the headache was often defined as jabbing, stabbing and sharp [7–20]. Signs like tearing, conjunctival injection, nausea, vomiting, photophobia, phonophobia were observed rarely[7–20,] while in our study population some of them (tearing, photophobia, phonophobia) were reported by the majority (73.3%) of patients.

Even though the pain was intense in most cases, only one third used analgesics both in children (33.3%) and in adults (38%) [7–20, 23–25].

Two patients performed one spontaneous maneuver to reduce the pain intensity and to obtain some relief, similar to the maneuvers carried out by patients with migraine, tension-type headache and cluster headache, as previously reported [25].

To the best of our knowledge, so far only 5 pediatric AH patients have been reported in the literature: in 2008 Mainardi et al. [23] described the first pediatric patient with AH; in 2010 Ipekdal et al. [24] described three pediatric AH cases aged between 12 and 14 years; the fifth case was reported in 2015 [25].

In the study of Ipekdal et al. [24], nasal mucosal inflammation, adenoidal and tonsillar hypertrophy and sinusitis were the pathophysiological mechanisms found to be responsible for AH. In all the 3 patients, AH has been solved by treating the underlying disease. In fact, they experienced other airplane travels and reported that they performed headache-free landings without any complication after the treatment.

In our study three children had a past history of sinus infections but none had any clinical evidence of an active sinus disorder during AH attacks.

Comparing the previously reported 5 cases with our series, we found that quality and intensity were similar, while site of pain was previously reported as unilateral [23–25], differently from our cases. A recent research article confirmed that headache caused by airplane travel is not necessarily unilateral, the description of headache may be not specific and the past history of any type of headache should be considered [26].

Given the peculiar clinical features of AH in the pediatric age compared to the adult population, more attention is needed towards this form of secondary headache, for better recognition even without the concomitance of other primary headaches: therefore the next edition of the ICHD should mention this entity also for the pediatric age.

Conclusions

Our study shows that AH is not a rare disorder in children affected by primary headaches and highlights that features of AH in children are peculiar and differ from those described in adults.

The exact mechanism underlying AH remains unclear, but it has been suggested a multifactorial pathogenesis [28].

Further studies are needed in the general pediatric population to confirm the actual frequency of AH; in particular population-based studies might address the issue of analyzing AH incidence, considering a bigger sample not selected in specialized Headache Centres, with and without other concomitant headache condition, with a long-term follow-up evaluation.

Abbreviations

AH: Airplane headache; ENT: Ear, nose and throat; *ICHD-III: International Classification of Headache disorders, 3rd edition*

Acknowledgements

The Authors wish to thank patients and their families for their kind cooperation.

Funding

The authors have no funding to report.

Authors' contributions

DDC: acquisition of data, analysis and interpretation of data, drafting of the manuscript. IT: design and implementation of the research, analysis of the results, drafting and revision of the manuscript. AMT, BB, MGL, LM, VR, MS, VS, AV, SZ: acquisition of clinical data, material support. SS, MG: study supervision and material support. AV, PAB: study concept and design, critical revision of the manuscript for important intellectual content. All authors read and approved the final manuscript.

Competing interests

The authors declare that they have no competing interests.

Author details

[1]Juvenile Headache Centre, University of Padua, via Giustiniani 3, 35128 Padua, Italy. [2]L'Aquila, Department of Pediatrics, San Salvatore Hospital, University of L'Aquila, L'Aquila, Italy. [3]Department of Child and Adolescent Neuropsychiatry, University Hospital of Cagliari, Cagliari, Italy. [4]Child Neuropsychiatry Unit, Department of Neuroscience and Sense Organs, University of "Aldo Moro" Bari, Bari, Italy. [5]Child Neuropsychiatry Unit, Di Cristina Hospital, ARNAS civico, Palermo, Italy. [6]Department of Child Neuropsychiatry, Università degli Studi di Bologna Scuola di Medicina e Chirurgia, Bologna, Italy. [7]Neurologic and Psychiatric Sciences Department, Ist Neurological Clinic, Bari, Italy. [8]Department of Child Neuropsychiatry, Università degli Studi di Palermo, Palermo, Italy. [9]IRCCS "La Nostra Famiglia - E. Medea", Pasian di Prato, Udine, Italy.

References

1. Strine TW, Okoro CA, McGuire LC et al (2006) The associations among childhood headaches, emotional and behavioral difficulties, and health care. Pediatrics 117:1728–1735
2. Brenner M, Oakley C, Lewis D (2008) The evaluation of children and adolescents with headache. Curr Pain Headache Rep 12:361–366
3. Titlić M, Demarin V (2008) Airplane headaches-two new cases and a review of the literature. Acta Med Croatica 62:229–231
4. Atkinson V, Lee L (2004) An unusual case of airplane headache. Headache 44:438–439
5. Berilgen MS, Mungen B (2011) A new type of headache, headache associated with airplane travel: preliminary diagnostic criteria and possible mechanisms of aetiopathogenesis. Cephalalgia 31:1266–1273
6. Mainardi F, Maggioni F, Lisotto C et al (2013) Diagnosis and management of headache attributed to airplane travel. Curr Neurol Neurosci Rep 13:335
7. Mainardi F, Lisotto C, Maggioni F et al (2012) Headache attributed to airplane travel ('airplane headache'): clinical profile based on a large case series. Cephalalgia 32:592–599
8. Berilgen MS, Mungen B (2006) Headache associated with airplane travel: report of six cases. Cephalalgia 26:707–711
9. Evans RW, Purdy RA, Goodman SH (2007) Airplane descent headaches. Headache 47:719–723
10. Mainardi F, Lisotto C, Maggioni F (2007) Headache attributed to airplane travel: three new cases with first report of female occurrence and classifying criteria. J Headache Pain 8(Suppl):12
11. Mainardi F, Lisotto C, Palestini C et al (2007) Headache attributed to airplane travel ('airplane headache'): first Italian case. J Headache Pain 8:196–199
12. Marchioretto F, Mainardi F, Zanchin G (2008) Airplane headache: a neurologist's personal experience. Cephalalgia 28:101
13. Kim HJ, Cho YJ, Cho JY et al (2008) Severe jabbing headache associated with airplane travel. Can J Neurol Sci 35:267–268
14. Coutinho E, Pereira-Monteiro J (2008) 'Bad trips': airplane headache not just in airplanes? Cephalalgia 28:986–987
15. Baldacci F, Lucetti C, Cipriani G et al (2010) Airplane headache' with aura. Cephalalgia 30:624–625
16. Kararizou E, Anagnostou E, Paraskevas GP et al (2011) Headache during airplane travel ("airplane headache"): first case in Greece. J Headache Pain 12:489–491
17. Cherian A, Mathew M, Iype T et al (2013) Headache associated with airplane travel: a rare entity. Neurol India 61:164–166

18. Bui SB, Petersen T, Poulsen JN et al (2016) Headaches attributed to airplane travel: a Danish survey. J Headache Pain 17:50
19. Mainardi F, Maggioni F, Lisotto C, Zanchin G (2015) Should aircrafts never land? Headache attributed to airplane travel: a new series of 140 patients. J Headache Pain 16(suppl1):166
20. Purdy RA (2012) Airplane headache-an entity whose time has come to fly? Cephalalgia 32:587–588
21. Bui SB, Gazerani P (2017) Headache attributed to airplane travel: diagnosis, pathophysiology and treatment – a systematic review. J Headache Pain 18:1–14
22. Nierenburg H, Jackfert K (2018) Headache attributed to airplane travel: a review of literature. Curr Pain Headache Rep 22:48
23. Mainardi F, Broekmann R, Lisotto C, Maggioni F, Mampreso E, Zanchin G (2008) "Airplane headache" may occur in paediatric age: description of the first case. J Headache Pain 9:42
24. Ipekdal H, Karadas O, Erdem G (2010) Airplane headache in pediatric age group: report of three cases. J Headache Pain 11:533–534
25. Rogers K, Rafiq N, Prabhakar P et al (2015) Childhood headache attributed to airplane travel: a case report. J Child Neurol 30:764–766
26. Ozge A, Abu-Arafeh I, Gelfand AA et al (2017) Experts' opinion about the pediatric secondary headache diagnostic criteria of ICHD-III beta. J Headache Pain 18:113
27. Headache Classification Committee of the International Headache Society (IHS) (2018) The international classification of headache disorders, 3rd edition. Cephalalgia 38(1):1–211
28. Bui SBD, Petersen T, Poulsen JN et al (2017) Simulated airplane headache: a proxy towards identification of underlying mechanisms. J Headache Pain 18:1–10

25

Field testing primary stabbing headache criteria according to the 3rd beta edition of International Classification of Headache Disorders

Minwoo Lee[1†], Min Kyung Chu[2†], Juyoung Lee[1], Jinhyuk Yoo[1] and Hong Ki Song[1*]

Abstract

Background: The diagnostic criteria for primary stabbing headache (PSH) in the 3rd beta edition of International Classification of Headache Disorders (ICDH-3 beta) were recently revised. In the ICDH-3 beta, PSH is defined as short-lasting head pain spontaneous occurring as a single stab or series of stabs without autonomic symptoms and involving all head areas (i.e., not limited to the ophthalmic branch region of the trigeminal nerve). The aim of this study was to investigate the validity of the ICHD-3 beta criteria for PSH in a clinic-based setting.

Methods: We prospectively collected data from patients with complaint of headache with stabbing pain without apparent cause at an initial visit to a secondary-care hospital from March 2009 to March 2014. Patients were followed up for 2 weeks to assess changes in clinical characteristics and secondary causes of pain.

Results: Data from 280 patients with headache with stabbing pain without apparent cause were collected, and 245 patients were followed up for 2 weeks. Secondary causes for stabbing headache were observed in 9 patients (herpes zoster in 7 patients and Bell's palsy in 2 patients) after 2 weeks. The remaining 236 patients fulfilled the diagnostic criteria for PSH according to ICHD-3 beta. Only 22 patients met the diagnostic criteria for PSH according to ICHD-2.

Conclusions: All patients with headache with stabbing pain without cranial autonomic symptoms fulfilled the diagnostic criteria for PSH according to ICHD-3 beta at the initial visit. Secondary causes for headache with stabbing pain were revealed in a small proportion (3.7 %) of patients after 2 weeks of follow-up.

Keywords: Primary stabbing headache, Secondary headache, Headache, Criteria, ICHD-3 beta

Background

Stabbing pain in the head that lasts a few seconds is a common type of headache [1–4]. The second edition of the International Classification of Headache Disorders (ICHD-2) proposed diagnostic criteria for this type of headache, which is known as primary stabbing headache (PSH) (code 4.1). These criteria require that head pain occurs exclusively or predominantly in the first division of the trigeminal nerve without apparent cause [5]. Previous studies have shown, however, that PSH can occur outside the trigeminal region, including in the extracephalic regions. The third beta edition of the International Classification of Headache Disorders (ICHD-3 beta), therefore, has revised the diagnostic criteria for PSH (code 4.1) as head pain that occurs spontaneously as a single stab or series of stabs without cranial autonomic symptoms in all head regions [1–4, 6–12].

The diagnostic criteria for PSH according to ICHD-3 beta have not been validated yet. The purpose of this study was 1) to test the validity of the diagnostic criteria for PSH according to ICHD-3 beta; 2) to investigate the clinical characteristics of PSH according to pain location,

* Correspondence: hksong0@hanmail.net
Minwoo Lee and Min Kyung Chu are the first authors of this article.
†Equal contributors
[1]Department of Neurology, Kangdong Sacred Heart Hospital, Hallym University Medical Center, Seongan-ro 150, Gangdong-gu, Seoul 134-701, South Korea
Full list of author information is available at the end of the article

which represents a criterion that changed from ICHD-2 to ICHD-3 beta; and 3) to investigate the clinical characteristics of secondary stabbing headache (SSH) at a follow-up visit among patients diagnosed with PSH at an initial visit.

Methods

Participants

We consecutively recruited patients with short-duration headache without apparent cause who visited the Department of Neurology at Kangdong Sacred Heart Hospital, a secondary-care hospital in Korea, from March 2009 to March 2014. Exclusion criteria included 1) 19 years old or younger; 2) patients with possible causes for stabbing headache; and 3) patients who refused to participate the study. After 5 years of consecutive recruitment, we analyzed data of structured interview and medical records of all the subjects in accordance with the ICHD-3 beta diagnostic criteria of PSH in the present study. This study was approved by the Institutional Review Board of Kangdong Sacred Heart Hospital. Written informed consent was obtained from all participants.

Assessment

A physician (HKS) interviewed all patients using a structured questionnaire and performed the physical examination. The information collected included age; gender; headache duration; location, intensity, frequency, and quality of pain; preceding infection; presence of allodynia; associated symptoms; and recurrence of stabbing headache. Patients were followed up for 2 weeks to investigate response to treatment, change in clinical characteristics, and secondary causes for stabbing headache.

The location of pain was recorded relative to the trigeminal and upper cervical regions. The trigeminal region was subdivided into ophthalmic (V1), maxillary (V2), and mandibular (V3) branches. The upper cervical region was subdivided into the lesser occipital nerve (LON), greater occipital nerve (GON), and greater auricular nerve.

A headache specialist (HKS) treated all patients with PSH. Patients with PSH were treated with gabapentin (300 mg bid), naproxen (275 mg bid), or amitriptyline (5 mg hs) based on the judgement of the specialist. Each patient was categorized as either a responder (cessation of stabbing pain) or non-responder (continuation of stabbing pain) in response to treatment after 2 weeks. After 2 weeks of follow up, we asked our participants to inform us if stabbing headache persisted more than 1 week or occurring other secondary causes of stabbing headache to detect persisting symptoms or late-onset SSH.

Statistics

Data were analyzed using SPSS Statistics for Windows, Version 21 (Armonk, New York, USA). Student's t-tests, chi-square tests, and Mann–Whitney U tests were used for comparison as appropriate. A p-value < 0.05 was considered statistically significant

Results

Subjects

During the study period, a total of 280 patients with stabbing headache were recruited during the initial visit. Of these patients, 243 were prescribed medication for their stabbing headache at the initial visit and 245 were followed for 2 weeks (Fig. 1) *Clinical characteristics at initial visit.*

Of the 280 patients with stabbing headache without apparent cause at the initial visit, 103 were men and 177 were women. The mean age of patients was 51.4 ± 13.3 years. The mean duration from the onset of symptoms to the initial visit was 4.0 ± 3.7 days. The mean visual analog scale (VAS) score for headache intensity was 4.6 ± 1.6. Seventy-four (26.4 %) patients reported mild pain (VAS score 1–3), 165 (58.9 %) reported moderate pain (VAS score 4–6), and 41 (14.6 %) reported severe pain (VAS score 7–10). The duration of a single stab was within 1–2 s in 262 patients (93.6 %) and 3–5 s in 18 patients (6.4 %). No patient reported autonomic symptoms during their headache attacks. There was no predominant pain lateralization (145 on the left, 133 on the right, and 2 on both the left and right). Pain was reported in the LON region in 129 patients, GON region in 80 patients, V1 region of the trigeminal nerve in 27 patients, V2 region in 28 patients, and V3 region in 8 patients. One patient had pain in both the LON and GON, and another patient had pain in both V1 and V2. No patients reported stabbing headache in both the trigeminal and upper cervical regions. A total of 243 patients

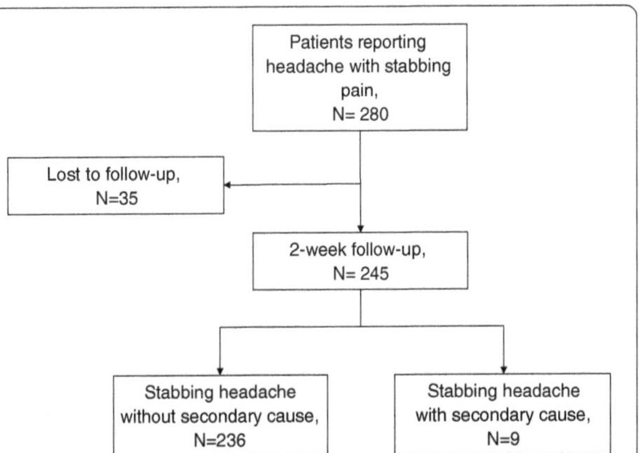

Fig. 1 Flow chart of the number of participants at each stage of the study

(86.8 %) were treated with medication. Fifty-three patients (18.9 %) reported allodynia on the same side of the stabbing headache. Allodynia was reported in 8 patients who reported stabbing headache in the V1 region (Table 1).

Clinical characteristics at follow-up

Of the 245 patients who were followed for 2 weeks after the initial visit, 231 (94.3 %) reported improvements. Mean duration for improvement among the responder group was 3.2 ± 1.9 days. Secondary causes for stabbing headache were observed in 9 patients (3.8 %) (herpes zoster in 7 patients and Bell's palsy in 2 patients); these patients were initially diagnosed with PSH (Table 1). Improvement at follow-up was not significantly different between those who did and did not take medication (189/199 vs. 37/37, respectively; $p = 0.164$). Among 10 PSH patients with persisting stabbing headache at follow-up, no patient additionally visited for their headaches. All 4 SSH patients with persisting stabbing headache at follow-up were diagnosed as having herpes zoster. Three of them improved their stabbing headache after 1 week and the remaining 1 patient improved after 2 weeks.

Validating the ICHD-3 beta criteria for PSH

All 280 patients who participated in the present study fulfilled the diagnostic criteria for PSH at the initial visit. Of the 245 patients who were followed for 2 weeks, 9 (3.2 %) did not meet the criteria for PSH at the second visit due to secondary causes for their stabbing headaches. These patients were diagnosed with SSH. Thus, at follow-up, 236 patients were diagnosed with PSH according to ICHD-3 beta. In contrast, only 28 patients (10.0 %) fulfilled the ICHD-2 criteria for PSH (Fig. 2). The remaining 252 patients were diagnosed with

Table 1 Clinical characteristics of patients with stabbing headache according to ICHD-3 beta criteria at the initial and follow-up visit

	All patients[a] (N = 280)	Primary stabbing headache[b] (N = 236)	Secondary stabbing headache[b] (N = 9)	P-value
Gender				
Male	103 (36.8 %)	89 (37.7 %)	5 (55.5 %)	0.280
Female	177 (63.2 %)	147 (62.3 %)	4 (44.4 %)	
Mean age	51.4 ± 13.3	50.6 ± 13.4	54.6 ± 14.1	0.385
Fixed location		230 (97.5 %)	9 (100 %)	0.628
Pain lateralization				
Unilateral	278 (99.3 %)	234 (99.2 %)	9 (100.0 %)	0.781
Bilateral	2 (0.7 %)	2 (0.8 %)	0 (0.0 %)	
Location of pain				
V1 region	27 (9.6 %)	22 (9.3 %)	1 (11.1 %)	0.857
V2 region	28 (10.0 %)	27 (11.4 %)	1 (11.1 %)	
V3 region	8 (2.9 %)	7 (3.0 %)	0 (0.0 %)	
All trigeminal regions	63 (22.5 %)	55 (23.3 %)	2 (22.2 %)	0.940
Lesser occipital nerve region	129 (46.1 %)	109 (46.2 %)	4 (44.4 %)	
Greater occipital nerve region	80 (28.6 %)	64 (27.1 %)	3 (33.3 %)	
Great auricular nerve	6 (2.1 %)	6 (2.5 %)	0 (0.0 %)	
All upper cervical regions	217 (77.5 %)	181 (76.7 %)	7 (77.8 %)	0.891
Multiple locations	2 (0.7 %)	2 (0.8 %)	0 (0.0 %)	0.782
Visual Analog Scale for pain intensity	4.6 ± 1.6	4.5 ± 1.6	6.8 ± 1.6	<0.001
Onset to hospital visit interval (days)	4.0 ± 3.7	4.0 ± 3.9	5.1 ± 2.4	0.341
Improvement at follow-up visit		226 (95.8 %)	5 (55.5 %)	<0.001
Duration of improvement (days) among responders		3.2 ± 1.9	4.8 ± 1.5	0.060
Preceding infection	21 (7.5 %)	21 (8.9 %)	0 (0.0 %)	0.083
Stressful event	61 (21.8 %)	48 (20.3 %)	4 (7.7 %)	0.083
Allodynia	53 (18.9 %)	45 (19.1 %)	2 (22.1 %)	0.814

[a]Assessed at initial visit
[b]Assessed at follow-up visit
ICHD-3 beta: the third beta edition of the International Classification of Headache Disorders. V1: ophthalmic branch of trigeminal nerve; V2: maxillary branch of trigeminal nerve; V3 mandibular branch of trigeminal nerve

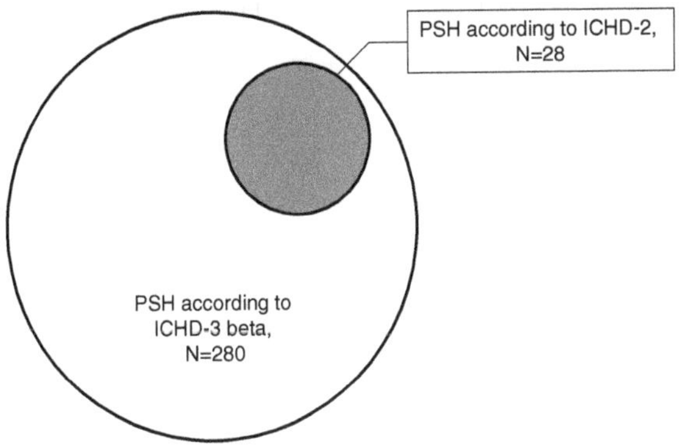

Fig. 2 Distribution of participants diagnosed with primary stabbing headache at the initial visit according to ICHD-3 beta and ICHD-2 criteria. PSH: primary stabbing headache; ICHD-2: the second edition of the international classification of headache disorders; ICHD-3 beta: the third beta edition of the international classification of the headache disorders

trigeminal neuralgia (N = 7, 2.5 %) or unclassified headache (N = 245, 87.5 %) based on ICHD-2 criteria. One patient (4.5 %) who was initially diagnosed with PSH according to ICHD-2 criteria was diagnosed with SSH due to Bell's palsy at follow-up. The proportion of patients with PSH re-diagnosed with SSH at follow-up was not significantly different between ICHD-3 beta and ICHD-2 criteria (9/271 vs. 1/27, $p = 0.919$). No patient was classified as having probable stabbing headache (code 4.7.1) at initial and follow-up visit. The number of patients with PSH re-diagnosed with SSH at follow-up was not significantly different between ICHD-3 and ICHD-2 criteria.

Clinical characteristics of PSH and SSH

We compared demographic and headache characteristics between PSH and SSH. There was no significant difference in gender, age, location of pain, preceding infection, or stressful events between patients with PSH and patients with SSH. VAS for pain was significantly higher in patients with SSH than patients with PSH. Improvement in pain at follow-up was more common in patients with PSH than patients with SSH. The duration of improvement among responders was longer in SSH than PSH (Table 1). However, further follow up of patients with SSH revealed favorable outcome within one month of onset.

Clinical characteristics of PSH involving V1 compared with other regions

Demographic and headache characteristics such as age, gender, VAS for pain, improvement after 2 weeks, duration of improvement among responders, preceding infection, stressful events, and allodynia were not significantly different between patients with PSH who reported V1 region involvement and those who reported involvement of regions other than V1 except stressful event history. Stressful event history was more common among subjects with PSH involving other than V1 region (Table 2).

Clinical characteristics of PSH involving trigeminal area and cervical area

We also compared clinical characteristics at initial visit between PSH involving trigeminal area and cervical area. Stressful event history was significantly higher among PSH subjects involving cervical area than those involving trigeminal area (Table 3).

Discussion

The key findings in the present study are as follows: 1) the diagnostic criteria for PSH in ICHD-3 beta enabled diagnosis of primary headaches with stabbing pain as PSH, most of which were not classified according to ICDH-2 criteria; 2) a small proportion (2.8 %) of new-onset stabbing headaches, which were initially diagnosed as PSH, had secondary causes that were revealed at 2-week follow-up; 3) pain intensity was more severe and pain improvement was slower among patients with SSH than that in patients with PSH.

This is the first study to field test the ICHD-3 beta diagnostic criteria for PSH. In the present study, all 280 subjects with short-lasting stabbing headache without apparent cause and without autonomic symptoms at the initial visit fulfilled the diagnostic criteria for PSH according to ICHD-3 beta. In contrast, only 9.6 % of patients met the criteria for PSH according to ICHD-2. This finding suggests that most primary stabbing headaches without cranial autonomic symptoms fulfill the diagnostic criteria for PHS.

One important change in the diagnostic criteria for PSH in ICHD-3 beta from ICHD-2 was the definition of pain location. The diagnostic criteria for PSH in ICHD-3 beta included all head regions, whereas criteria in ICHD-2 included the V1 region only [12]. To investigate the clinical characteristics of PSH according to pain location, we compared patients with PSH involving the V1 region to patients with PSH involving non-V1 regions. Age, gender, pain intensity, improvement of pain, duration of improvement among responders, preceding infection, stressful events, and allodynia were not significantly different according to pain location. These findings suggest that all clinical characteristics of PSH except pain location are similar between ICHD-3 beta and ICHD-2.

Another change in ICHD-3 beta criteria from ICHD-2 criteria was the definition of accompanying symptoms.

Table 2 Clinical characteristics of primary stabbing headache by ICHD-3 beta criteria at initial visit according to the pain location between V1 and other than V1

	V1 region[a] N = 28	Other than V1 region[b] N = 252	P-value
Gender			
Male	13 (46.4 %)	90 (35.7 %)	0.265
Female	15 (53.6 %)	162 (64.3 %)	
Age	50.5 ± 13.4	51.5 ± 13.3	0.912
Visual analog scale for pain intensity	4.4 ± 1.3	4.7 ± 1.6	0.160
Improvement at follow-up[c]	22 (100.0 %)	204 (95.3 %)	0.301
Mean duration of improvement (days) among responders	4.1 ± 3.1	3.5 ± 2.7	0.135
Preceding infection	4 (14.2 %)	17 (6.7 %)	0.151
Stressful event history	2 (7.1 %)	59 (23.4 %)	0.048
Allodynia	8 (28.5 %)	45 (17.8 %)	0.170

[a]One patient had stabbing headache in both the V1 and V2 regions
[b]V2, V3, lesser occipital nerve, greater occipital nerve, great auricular nerve, and multiple dermatomes. One patient with multiple dermatomes, including V1, were included
[c]22 out of 28 patients with pain at V1 region and 216 out of 252 patients with pain at other than V1 regions were followed at 2 weeks after initial visit, respectively
ICHD-3 beta: the third beta edition of the International Classification of Headache Disorders. V1: ophthalmic branch of trigeminal nerve; V2: maxillary branch of trigeminal nerve; V3 mandibular branch of trigeminal nerve

Diagnostic criteria for PHS in ICHD-2 included as a criterion that no accompanying symptoms were present [5]. According to ICHD-2, PSH was excluded as a diagnosis if stabbing headache without apparent cause was accompanied by symptoms such as nausea, vomiting, photophobia, or phonophobia [1, 5]. In ICHD-3 beta, this criterion was revised to a lack of "cranial autonomic symptoms" [12]. However, we did not investigate accompanying symptoms except allodynia, and no patient reported cranial autonomic symptoms in the present study. This change in the definition of accompanying symptoms in ICHD-3 beta may have excluded fewer primary headaches with stabbing pain as PSH than ICHD-2.

PSH has been considered responsive to indomethacin [13–16]. Responsiveness to indomethacin was described in the "*Comments*" of ICHD-1 and ICHD-2 [5, 17]. However, responsiveness to indomethacin was removed from ICHD-3 beta [12]. In the present study, no patient was treated with indomethacin, and most patients with PSH improved at follow-up. Mean duration for improvement was 3.2 days among responders. In addition, improvement at follow-up was not significantly different between patients who did and did not take medication.

Table 3 Clinical characteristics of primary stabbing headache by ICHD-3 beta criteria at initial visit according to the pain location between trigeminal and cervical areas

	Trigeminal area[a] N = 55	Cervical area[b] N = 225	P-value
Gender			
Male	23 (41.8 %)	80 (35.5 %)	0.388
Female	32 (58.9 %)	145 (64.5 %)	
Age	49.5 ± 13.4	51.8 ± 13.2	0.968
Visual analog scale for pain intensity	4.4 ± 1.6	4.7 ± 1.6	0.787
Improvement at follow-up	43 (97.8 %)	188 (97.9 %)	0.937
Mean duration of improvement (days) among responders[c]	3.8 ± 3.2	3.4 ± 2.7	0.145
Preceding infection	5 (10.9 %)	16 (7.1 %)	0.617
Stressful event history	6 (6.8 %)	55 (24.4 %)	0.029
Allodynia	14 (25.4 %)	39 (17.3 %)	0.168

[a]V1, V2 and V3 dermatomes
[b]Lesser occipital nerve, greater occipital nerve, great auricular nerve, and multiple dermatomes. One patient with multiple dermatomes, including V1 region, were included
[c]44 out of 55 patients with pain at trigeminal area and 192 out of 225 patients with pain at cervical area were followed at 2 weeks after initial visit, respectively
ICHD-3 beta: the third beta edition of the International Classification of Headache Disorders

These findings suggest that most patients with PSH have a good prognosis; specific responsiveness to indomethacin was difficult to conclude.

Our study, which followed patients who were initially diagnosed with PSH, revealed that a small but significant proportion of patients were found to have SSH at follow-up. Previous studies have reported secondary causes for stabbing headache, including Bell's palsy, herpes zoster, cerebral infarction, transient ischemic attack, post-infection, thalamic hemorrhage, autoimmune diseases, pituitary tumor, Chiari Malformation Type 1, C1-C2 subluxation, meningioma, and multiple sclerosis [2, 6, 15, 18–24]. We compared clinical characteristics of PSH and SSH and found no significant differences except in pain intensity. This finding suggests that the risk for SSH is higher for a PSH-diagnosed stabbing headache with severe pain intensity. The risk for SSH was not significantly different between ICHD-3 beta and ICHD-2 criteria in the present study.

Bell's palsy and herpes zoster have been reported as common causes of secondary stabbing headache [6, 24]. Retroauricular stabbing pain in Bell's palsy often presents 2–3 days before the onset of facial weakness [25, 26]. Herpes zoster is usually accompanied by short-lasting stabbing pain in the involved sites. Pain in herpes zoster often presents 4–5 days before the presentation of skin lesions [26]. Most stabbing headaches are reported to be improved within 2 weeks [1, 2]. Given these findings, we followed patients with PSH for 2 weeks. However, stabbing headache persisted in some patients, and some SSH may have been classified as PSH in the present study.

Our study has several limitations. First, we did not perform nerve block or examine tenderness in the occipital area to diagnosis occipital neuralgia (ON). According to ICHD-3 beta, ON pain is associated with tenderness over the affected nerve branch or trigger points at the emergence of the greater occipital nerve or C2 distribution [12]. Temporary relief of the pain by local anesthetic block is also required. ON in the GON and LON areas may have been diagnosed as PSH in the present study. Second, not all patients were treated, and treatment medication was not the same across patients. In the present study, a headache specialist decided which treatment to administer to each patient based on his judgement. The rate and duration of improvement was similar between patients who did and did not receive treatment. This finding is consistent with previous studies in which PSH is reported to be an easily treatable headache disorder [1, 2]. Third, we did not investigate prior history of migraine or other primary headache disorders. Though rather speculative, previous studies reported that 21 - 38 % of patients with primary stabbing headache had history of migraine [2, 16].

The strengths of this study are its large sample size, 2-week follow-up to investigate changes in clinical characteristics and secondary causes, comparisons of diagnostic criteria between ICHD-3 beta and ICHD-2, and headache diagnosis by a headache specialist, which may avoid inter-examiner bias. Future work will include a longer duration of follow-up and exclusion of ON via an examination of tenderness and performance of a nerve block.

Conclusion

In summary, the diagnostic criteria for PSH according to ICHD-3 beta are valid and enable the diagnosis of most primary headaches with stabbing pain, which were not classified according to ICDH-2. A small proportion of participants with PSH according to ICHD-3 beta criteria at the initial visit were re-diagnosed with SSH at 2-week follow-up owing to secondary causes. This information may provide a better understanding of PSH and it diagnostic criteria according to ICHD-3 beta.

Abbreviations

GON: greater occipital nerve; ICHD-2: International Classification of Headache Disorders, 2nd edition; ICHD-3 beta: International Classification of Headache Disorders, 3rd edition (beta version); LON: lesser occipital nerve; ON: occipital neuralgia; PSH: primary stabbing headache; SSH: secondary stabbing headache.

Competing interests

The authors declare that they have no conflicts of interest in the research described in "Field testing primary stabbing headache criteria according to the 3rd beta edition of International Classification of Headache Disorders: a clinic-based study".

Authors' contributions

MWL conceived and designed the study, analysed data, and wrote the manuscript. MKC designed the study, analysed data and wrote manuscript. JL and JY collected data of this study. HKS conceived and designed the study, collected and analysed data, and wrote the manuscript. All authors read and approved the final manuscript.

Acknowledgements

The authors would like to thank Gallup Korea for providing technical support for the Korean Headache Survey.

Author details

[1]Department of Neurology, Kangdong Sacred Heart Hospital, Hallym University Medical Center, Seongan-ro 150, Gangdong-gu, Seoul 134-701, South Korea. [2]Department of Neurology, Kangnam Sacred Heart Hospital, Hallym University, Seoul, South Korea.

References

1. Fuh JL, Kuo KH, Wang SJ (2007) Primary stabbing headache in a headache clinic. Cephalalgia 27(9):1005–1009

2. Shin JH, Song HK, Lee JH, Kim WK, Chu MK (2007) Paroxysmal stabbing headache in the multiple dermatomes of the head and neck: a variant of primary stabbing headache or occipital neuralgia? Cephalalgia 27(10):1101–1108
3. Sjaastad O, Pettersen H, Bakketeig LS (2001) The Vågå study; epidemiology of headache I: the prevalence of ultrashort paroxysms. Cephalalgia 21(3):207–215
4. Sjaastad O, Pettersen H, Bakketeig LS (2002) The Vågå study of headache epidemiology II. Jabs: clinical manifestations. Acta Neurol Scand 105(1):25–31
5. Headache Classification Subcommittee of the International Headache Society (IHS) (2004) The International Classification of Headache Disorders. Cephalalgia 24(suppl 1):8–160
6. Martins IP, Parreira E, Costa I (1995) Extratrigeminal ice-pick status. Headache 35(2):107–110
7. Piovesan EJ, Kowacs PA, Lange MC, Pacheco C, Piovesan LR, Werneck LC (2001) Prevalence and semiologic aspects of the idiopathic stabbing headache in a migraine population. Arq Neuropsiquiatr 59(2-A):201–205
8. Raskin NH, Schwartz RK (1980) Icepick-like pain. Neurology 30(2):203–205
9. Selekler HM, Budak F (2004) Idiopathic stabbing headache and experimental ice cream headache (short-lived headaches). Eur Neurol 51(1):6–9
10. Selekler MH, Komsuoglu SS (2004) Extracephalic stabbing pain temporally related to cephalic ones. Headache 44(7):719–721
11. Sjaastad O, Pettersen H, Bakketeig LS (2003) Extracephalic jabs/idiopathic stabs. Vågå study of headache epidemiology. Cephalalgia 23(1):50–54
12. Headache Classification Committee of the International Headache Society (2013) The international classification of headache disorders, 3rd edition (beta version). Cephalalgia 33(9):629–808
13. Dodick DW (2004) Indomethacin-responsive headache syndromes. Curr Pain Headache Rep 8(1):19–26
14. Mathew NT (1981) Indomethacin responsive headache syndromes. Headache 21(4):147–150
15. Rozen TD (2004) Short-lasting headache syndromes and treatment options. Curr Pain Headache Rep 8(4):268–273
16. Guerrero AL, Herrero S, Penas ML, Cortijo E, Rojo E, Mulero P, Fernandez R (2011) Incidence and influence on referral of primary stabbing headache in an outpatient headache clinic. J Headache Pain 12(3):311–313
17. Headache Classification Committee of the International Headache Society (1988) Classification and diagnostic criteria for headache disorders, cranial neuralgias and facial pain. Cephalalgia 8(Suppl 7):1–96
18. Levy MJ, Matharu MS, Meeran K, Powell M, Goadsby PJ (2005) The clinical characteristics of headache in patients with pituitary tumours. Brain 128(Pt 8):1921–1930
19. Piovesan EJ, Zukerman E, Kowacs PA, Werneck LC (2002) COX-2 inhibitor for the treatment of idiopathic stabbing headache secondary to cerebrovascular diseases. Cephalalgia 22(3):197–200
20. Ergün U, Özer G, Sekercan S, Artan E, Kudiaki C, Üçler S, Coskun Ö, Inan L (2009) Headaches in the different phases of relapsing-remitting multiple sclerosis: a tendency for stabbing headaches during relapses. Neurologist 15(4):212–216
21. Mascellino AM, Lay CL, Newman LC (2001) Stabbing headache as the presenting manifestation of intracranial meningioma: a report of two patients. Headache 41(6):599–601
22. Rampello L, Malaguarnera M, Rampello L, Nicoletti G, Battaglia G (2012) Stabbing headache in patients with autoimmune disorders. Clin Neurol Neurosurg 114(6):751–753
23. Robbins MS (2011) Transient stabbing headache from an acute thalamic hemorrhage. J Headache Pain 12(3):373–375
24. Lewis GW (1958) Zoster sine herpete. Br Med J 2(5093):418–421
25. Lee G, Lee D, Seok J, Yoo J (2011) Clinical analysis of Bell's palsy in One university hospital. J Korean Neurol Assoc 29(4):285–290
26. Roper A, Brown R (2005) Adams and Victor's Principles of Neurology, 8th edn. McGraw-Hill, Columbus

Chronic cluster headache and the pituitary gland

Annelien De Pue[1*], Bart Lutin[2] and Koen Paemeleire[1]

Abstract

Background: Cluster headache is classified as a primary headache by definition not caused by an underlying pathology. However, symptomatic cases of otherwise typical cluster headache have been reported.

Case presentation: A 47-year-old male suffered from primary chronic cluster headache (CCH, ICHD-3 beta criteria fulfilled) since the age of 35 years. A magnetic resonance imaging (MRI) study of the brain in 2006 came back normal. He tried several prophylactic treatments but was never longer than 1 month without attacks. He was under chronic treatment with verapamil with only a limited effect on the attack frequency. Subcutaneous sumatriptan 6 mg injections were very effective in aborting attacks. By February 2014 the patient developed a continuous interictal pain ipsilateral to the right-sided cluster headache attacks. An indomethacin test (up to 225 mg/day orally) was negative. Because of the change in headache pattern we performed a new brain MRI, which showed a cystic structure in the pituitary gland. The differential diagnosis was between a Rathke cleft cyst and a cystic adenoma. Pituitary function tests showed an elevated serum prolactin level. A dopamine agonist (cabergoline) was started and the headache subsided completely. Potential pathophysiological mechanisms of pituitary tumor-associated headache are discussed.

Conclusion: Neuroimaging should be considered in all patients with CCH, especially those with an atypical presentation or evolution. Response to acute treatment does not exclude a secondary form of cluster headache. There may be shared pathophysiological mechanisms of primary and secondary cluster headache.

Keywords: Cluster headache, Pituitary gland, Secondary headache

Background

Cluster headache (CH) is classified as a primary headache by definition not caused by an underlying pathology. However, numerous symptomatic cases of otherwise typical CH have been reported. We want to report a case of a man with typical chronic cluster headache (CCH) and a pituitary lesion only found on repeat MRI. Potential mechanisms underlying this association are discussed. We hope this will be useful to other clinicians taking care of patients suffering from this devastating condition [1].

Case presentation

A 47 year-old man was diagnosed with CH at the age of 35. A 1,5 Tesla MRI of the brain in another hospital was reportedly normal. The patient came under our care in 2011. The headache attacks and pattern were compatible with a primary CCH diagnosis according to the criteria of the International Headache Society (ICHD-3 beta, 3.1.2) [2]. The patient described attacks of strictly right-sided orbitotemporal headache associated with ipsilateral tearing and nasal congestion. The attacks lasted from 20 to 60 min, with a frequency up to 4 attacks per day, often including one attack at night. The most consistent trigger was alcohol intake. Subcutaneous sumatriptan 6 mg injections were very effective in aborting attacks, inhaled high-flow oxygen was not. Despite different prophylactic treatments (verapamil up to 480 mg/day, lithium up to 800 mg/day, topiramate up to 400 mg/day) the patient was never longer than 1 month without attacks. By February 2014 the patient developed a continuous interictal pain ipsilateral to the right-sided CH attacks. At that point in time he was under chronic treatment with verapamil (maximal tolerated dose of 560 mg/day) for 6 months with only a mild effect on attack frequency. An indomethacin test (up to 225 mg/day orally) was negative. Because of the change in headache pattern we decided

* Correspondence: annelien.depue@Ugent.be
[1]Department of Neurology, Ghent University Hospital, De Pintelaan 185, B-9000 Ghent, Belgium
Full list of author information is available at the end of the article

to perform a new brain MRI, which showed a cystic structure in the pituitary gland (Fig. 1). The differential diagnosis was between a Rathke's cleft cyst or a cystic adenoma. Pituitary function tests (PFTs) came back normal, except for an elevated prolactin level (68.4 μg/L, normal values 4–17 μg/L) and a low free testosterone level (4.44 ng/dL, normal values 6–25 ng/dL). This could be due to verapamil-induced hyperprolactinemia or a prolactinoma. There was no galactorrhea, gynaecomastia, or erectile dysfunction (but he acknowledged a low libido), and visual fields were full. The patient was not willing to stop the treatment with verapamil as he feared an increase in cluster attack frequency. The patient was referred to an endocrinologist, who started carbergoline, a dopamine agonist, at a dose of 0,25 mg twice a week. Within a few weeks after the start of the cabergoline treatment the CH attacks subsided completely and verapamil could be successfully stopped. The serum prolactin and testosterone levels normalized. A repeat MRI in October 2015 demonstrated a 30 % reduction in size of the cystic pituitary lesion. At present the patient has been on carbergoline treatment for 1,5 year and the cluster headaches haven't returned ever since and prolactin levels remained within normal range. Interestingly, the patient reports to experience a new type of unilateral frontotemporal headache attacks since about 6 months. These attacks are milder and shortlasting (seconds), and the pain is rather stabbing. There are no associated cranial autonomic symptoms. These attacks are not disabling and the patient does not need treatment for them. We have labeled these probable short-lasting unilateral neuralgiform headache attacks (ICHDI-3 beta, 3.5.3) within the given context.

Discussion

Secondary cluster headache

The lesion in the pituitary and the headaches could just be a co-occurrence. However the temporal relationship between the initiation of carbergoline treatment and disappearance of the cluster headache attacks suggests a potential causal relationship with the pituitary lesion and (worsening of) the headache condition. This adds to numerous recent reports of secondary cluster-like headache (CLH). By definition before concluding to a primary headache potential causative disorders should be excluded to rule out a secondary CLH. Edvardsson reviewed 63 cases of symptomatic CH associated with vascular problems (44 %), tumours (40 %) or inflammation/infection (11 %) [3]. Of the 63 cases 48 % fulfilled the criteria for CH. A larger cohort of 156 cases of CLH showed a similar distribution of causative disorders [4]. On first observation, 50 % of CLH perfectly mimicked CH at presentation [5]. Furthermore, the response to typical CH medications does not exclude a secondary form. Red flags could be older age at onset, abnormal-duration/frequency/localization, change in clinical characteristics or response to treatment, or an abnormal neurological/general examination [4, 5]. These findings suggest that neuroimaging should be considered in all patients with CH, even typical cases. The ICHDIII beta criteria for secondary headache disorders require evidence of causation, which includes that 'headache has significantly worsened in parallel with worsening of the presumed causative disorder' and 'headache has significantly improved (or disappeared) in parallel with improvement of the presumed causative disorder'. In our patient neuro-imaging was done early in his headache trajectory and results came back normal. However, in

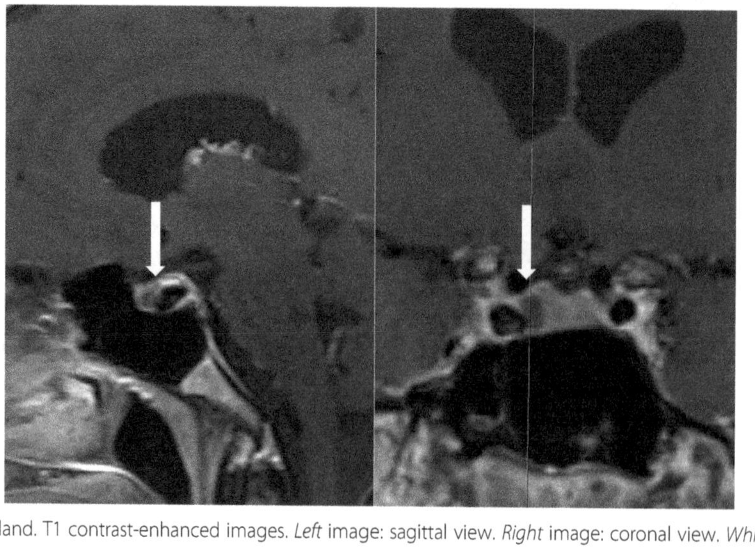

Fig. 1 MRI of the pituitary gland. T1 contrast-enhanced images. *Left* image: sagittal view. *Right* image: coronal view. *White* arrow indicates cystic structure in the pituitary

retrospect we noted that the spatial resolution of the initial MRI of the brain at the level of the pituitary gland was too low to exclude that the cystic structure (Fig. 1) was already present. Even though interictal headache in cluster headache is not an uncommon phenomenon [6], it was the change in headache history in our patient that sparked repeat neuro-imaging.

Pathophysiology

The pathophysiology of secondary CLH associated with pituitary disorders is not well-known. A few hypotheses are considered and summarized in Fig. 2. The long-held theory that CH was the related to a cerebrovascular problem radically changed in the late nineties with CH attacks being recoined as neurovascular in origin and with an important role for the hypothalamic-pituitary axis in the generation of these attacks. Functional imaging studies (fMRI, PET), neuro-endocrine changes (melatonin, cortisol, testosterone, ...) and the circadian/circannual rhythmicity all point to an alteration in the hypothalamus [7–10]. Also lithium, which is one of the known preventative treatment options for CH, is heterogeneously distributed in the brain and seems to accumulate in the hypothalamus and pituitary gland [11, 12]. The pain during cluster headache attacks is attributed to activation of the trigeminovascular system and cranial autonomic symptoms are generated via the trigeminal-autonomic reflex [13–15].

A structural lesion in the hypothalamic-pituitary axis could lead to an autonomic imbalance resulting in an attack-wise presentation of complaints. Others have suggested that the headache due to a lesion in the pituitary is a result of dura mater stretch or invasion of the cavernous sinus. Indeed, the cavernous sinus lateral to the sella turcica contains the ophthalmic and maxillary branches of the trigeminal nerve as well as the internal carotid artery, which are structures that can generate pain. However, in a systematic study of headache in patients with pituitary tumors, no correlation between pituitary volume and headache or between headache and cavernous sinus invasion was found [16]. Pituitary tumor-associated headache may have a biochemical-neuroendocrine basis rather than a structural one [16]. Finally, there is some evidence for the role of "nociceptive peptides" [17]. The presence of calcitonin gene related peptide (CGRP) or substance P in pituitary tumors does not seem to be associated with headache [15]. Other candidate peptides are vasoactive intestinal peptide (VIP), pituitary adenylate cyclase-activating protein and neuropeptide Y.

Pituitary function tests, prolactin and dopamine agonist

A few additional questions are provoked by this case. Is the raised serum prolactin level due to the lesion in the pituitary or induced by the high dose of verapamil? Is the effect of cabergoline proving that the lesion is a prolactinoma and the cause of the headache? Is the positive effect of carbergoline due to the normalization of serum prolactin? Is there a need for screening with PFT's in CH?

There are physiologic, pituitary and systemic (including medications, such as verapamil) causes of hyperprolactinemia [18]. Pituitary causes include prolactin-secreting pituitary adenoma or disconnection hyperprolactinemia due to a lesion that compresses the pituitary stalk [18]. L-type calcium channel blockers, such as verapamil, are known to cause a doubling of serum prolactin levels [19]. Since the patient was reluctant to stop verapamil because of fear increased CH attack frequency, we could not distinguish between both mechanisms prior to initiation of cabergoline treatment. Cabergoline is a long acting D2 dopamine receptor agonist that inhibits prolactin secretion. There

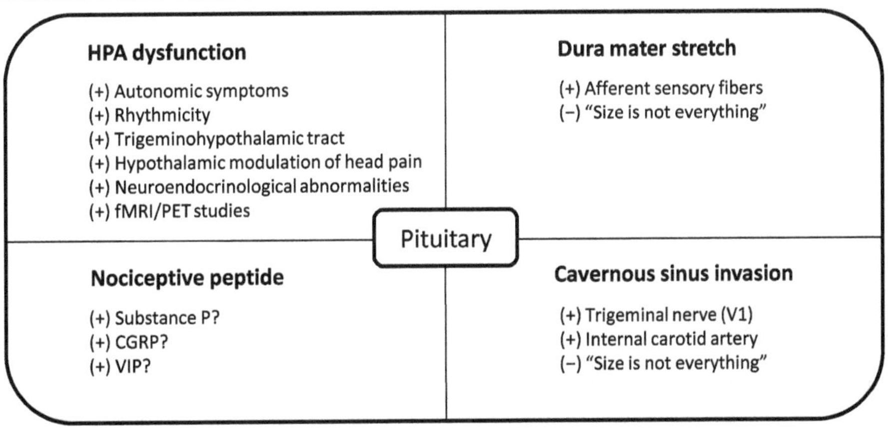

Fig. 2 Potential pathophysiological links with the pituitary gland in cluster headache. (+) arguments pro (-) arguments con. "Size is not everything" is a reference to an article of Levy et al. [16]. V1 is the ophthalmic branch of the trigeminal nerve. HPA = hypothalamic-pituitary axis. The figure is further explained in the text under the heading "pathophysiology"

are reported cases of microprolactinomas manifesting with headache that resolved after administration of a dopamine agonist [20, 21], but there are also reports stating the opposite [22]. The effect of cabergoline on headache doesn't seem to be associated with the normalization of serum prolactin [20]. Potential mechanisms include alterations to the pain-modulating dopaminergic system and carbergoline, an ergot derivative, also possesses significant affinity for certain subtypes of serotonergic and adrenergic receptors. A normal MRI of the brain does not exclude a microadenoma [23], and PFT's should therefore be considered in (refractory) patients with CCH or other (TAC).

Conclusion

Neuroimaging should be considered in all patients with CCH, especially those with an atypical presentation or evolution. When performing brain imaging it seems important to pay extra attention to the pituitary/parasellar region. Response to acute treatment does not exclude a secondary form of CH. PFTs should be considered in patients suffering from (refractory) CCH or other TACs. Cabergoline may have a dramatic effect on CH in patients with coexistent hyperprolactinemia.

Consent

The patient gave written informed consent to have his case published.

Abbreviations

CCH: chronic cluster headache; CGRP: calcitonin gene-related peptide; CH: cluster headache; CLH: cluster-like headache; ICHD-3 beta: The International Classification of Headache Disorders Third Edition, beta version; mg: milligram; MRI: magnetic resonance imaging; ng/dl: nanogram per deciliter; PFT: pituitary function tests; TAC: trigeminal autonomic cephalalgias; TCC: trigeminocervical complex; VIP: vasoactive intestinal peptide; µg/l: microgram per liter.

Competing interests

The authors declare that they have no competing interests.

Author's contributions

ADP drafted the manuscript and made Fig. 2. BL provided the MRI images. KP had substantial contribution to the manuscript and its content. All authors read and approved the final manuscript.

Author details

[1]Department of Neurology, Ghent University Hospital, De Pintelaan 185, B-9000 Ghent, Belgium. [2]Department of Radiology, Ghent University Hospital, Ghent, Belgium.

References

1. Marteletti P, Mitsikostas D-D (2015) Cluster headache: a quasi-rare disorder needing reappraisal. J Headache Pain 16:59
2. Headache Classification Committee of the International Headache Society (IHS) (2013) The International classification of headache disorders, 3rd Edition (beta version). Cephalalgia 33(9):629–808
3. Edvardsson B (2014) Symptomatic cluster headache: a review of 63 cases. Springer Plus 3:64
4. Mainardi F, Trucco M, Maggioni F et al. (2010) Cluster-like headache. A comprehensive reappraisal. Cephalalgia 30:399–412
5. Wilbrink LA, Ferrari MD, Kruit MC et al. (2009) Neuro-imaging in trigeminal autonomic cephalgias : when, how, and of what? Curr Opinion Neurol 22(3):247–253
6. Marmura MJ, Pello SJ, Young WB (2010) Interictal pain in cluster headache. Cephalalgia 30(12):1531–1534
7. May A, Bahra A, Buchel C et al. (1998) Hypothalamic activation in cluster headache attacks. Lancet 351:275–278
8. Sprenger T, Boecker H, Tolle TR et al. (2004) Specific hypothalamic activation during a spontaneous cluster headache attack. Neurology 62:516–517
9. Morelli N, Pesaresi I, Cafforio G et al. (2008) Functional magnetic resonance imaging in episodic cluster headache. J Headache Pain 10:11–14
10. Leone M, Bussone G (1993) A review of hormonal findings in cluster headache. Evidence for hypothalamic involvement. Cephalalgia 13:309–317
11. Edelfors S, Gothgen I (1971) Distribution of electrolytes within the brain in lithium treated rats. Acta Pharmacol Toxicol 29(4):11, abstract
12. Pfeifer WD, Davis LC, van der Velde CD (1976) Lithium accumulation in some endocrine tissues. Acta Biol Med Ger 35(11):1519–23
13. May A (2005) Cluster headache: pathogenesis, diagnosis, and management. Lancet Neurol 366:843–855
14. Goadsby PJ (2002) Pathophysiology of cluster headache: a trigeminal autonomic cephalgia. Lancet Neurol 1:251–257
15. Nesbitt AD, Goadsby PJ (2012) Cluster headache. BMJ 344:37–42
16. Levy MJ, Jäger R, Powell M et al. (2004) Pituitary volume and headache - size is not everything. Arch Neurol 61:721–725
17. Levy MJ, Classey JD, Maneesri S, Meeran K, Powell M, Goadsby PJ (2004) The association between calcitonin gene-related peptide (CGRP), substance P and headache in pituitary tumours. Pituitary 7(2):67–71
18. Tritos NA, Klibanski A (2015) Hyperprolactinemia. JAMA 314(16):1742–3
19. Kelley SR, Kamal TJ, Molitch ME (1996) Mechanism of verapamil calcium channel blockade-induced hyperprolactinemia. Am J Physiol 270(1 Pt 1):E96–100
20. Kallestrup MM, Kasch H, Österby T et al. (2014) Prolactinoma-associated headache and dopamine agonist treatment. Cephalalgia 34(7):493–502
21. Gabrielli M, Gasbarrini A, Fiore G et al. (2002) Resolution of migraine with aura after successful treatment of a pituitary microadenoma. Cephalalgia 22:149–150
22. Levy M, Matharu MS, Goadsby PJ (2003) Prolactinomas, dopamine agonist and headache: two case reports. Eur J Neurol 10:169–174
23. Hauache OM, Rocha AJ, Maia AC et al. (2002) Screening for macroprolactinaemia and pituitary imaging studies. Clin Endocrinol (Osf) 57(3):327–331

27

Medication overuse headache in Europe and Latin America: general demographic and clinical characteristics, referral pathways and national distribution of painkillers in a descriptive, multinational, multicenter study

Ninett Louise Find[1,2], Rossana Terlizzi[2,3], Signe Bruun Munksgaard[2], Lars Bendtsen[2], Cristina Tassorelli[4], Giuseppe Nappi[4], Zaza Katsarava[5], Miguel Lainez[6], Maria Teresa Goicochea[7], Beatriz Shand[8], Ricardo Fadic[8], Santiago Spadafora[9], Marco Pagani[10], Rigmor Jensen[2*] and COMOESTAS Consortium

Abstract

Background: Medication overuse headache (MOH) is a very disabling and costly disorder due to indirect costs, medication and healthcare utilization. The aim of the study was to describe general demographic and clinical characteristics of MOH, along with the national referral pathways and national painkillers distribution in several European and Latin American (LA) Countries.

Methods: This descriptive cross-sectional observational study included 669 patients with MOH referred to headache-centers in Europe and LA as a part of the COMOESTAS project. Information about acute medication and healthcare utilization were collected by extensive questionnaires, supplemented with structured patient interviews.

Results: Triptans were overused by 31 % European patients and by 6 % in LA ($p < 0.001$), whereas ergotamines were overused by 4 % in Europe and 72 % in LA ($p < 0.001$). Simple analgesics were overused by 54 % in Europe and by 33 % in LA ($p < 0.001$), while combination-analgesics were more equally overused (24 % in Europe and 29 % in LA). More European patients (57 %) compared with LA patients (27 %) visited general practitioners ($p < 0.001$), and 83 % of European patients compared to 38 % in LA consulted headache specialists ($p < 0.001$). A total of 20 % in Europe and 30 % in LA visited emergency rooms ($p = 0.007$).

Conclusion: There are marked variations between LA and Europe in healthcare pathways and in acute medication overuse regarding patients with MOH. This should be considered when planning prevention campaigns against MOH.

Keywords: Medication overuse headache, Healthcare utilization, Overuse of acute medication, International variation

* Correspondence: rigmor.jensen@regionh.dk
[2]Danish Headache Center, Neurological Department, Glostrup Hospital, Glostrup, Denmark
Full list of author information is available at the end of the article

Background

Medication overuse headache (MOH) is a globally prevalent and disabling chronic disorder, affecting up to 2 % of populations [1–6]. In Europe, MOH is a fast growing economic burden for society, due to reduced productivity at work, absenteeism from work, cost of medication, and healthcare-resource utilization [5].

Epidemiological studies performed on general populations in western countries report a high degree of healthcare use among patients suffering from chronic headache, often complicated by MOH, especially in the primary sector [2, 6, 7]. In addition, a smaller French study found a high number of contacts to the emergency room (ER) among patients with chronic headache with and without medication overuse [8].

However, healthcare systems differ considerably among nations in regards to organization, referral pathways and financing of healthcare costs. This may contribute to international variations in healthcare utilization among patients with MOH.

Similarly, cultural, economic and political differences may contribute to an international variation in the use of acute medications [3, 6, 7, 9, 10]. A Spanish epidemiological study reported simple analgesics as the most consumed type of drug, followed by ergotamines, among patients with chronic daily headache (CDH) and acute medication overuse [3]. Scandinavian studies report the same tendency towards a high preference for simple analgesics, accompanied by combination-analgesics [7, 10]. It has been described that patients with MOH in USA have a higher use of opioids and barbiturates compared with other nations [6, 9].

The literature regarding healthcare utilization and pattern of medication overuse among patients with MOH in Latin America (LA) is sparse, which also has been mentioned by Allena et al. [11]. A better characterization of this population may assist and direct prevention campaigns and relevant therapy of MOH. Recently, a paper of the COMOESTAS project concerning clinical and demographical characteristics of LA patients with MOH has been published [12].

The current study characterizes and compares the general demographic and clinical characteristics of MOH, the referral pathways and the pattern of acute medication distribution and overuse between European and LA patients suffering from MOH referred to headache centers, in a multinational, multicenter setup.

Methods

Study design

The present study is a descriptive, cross-sectional, observational part of the COMOESTAS project. The main objective of the COMOESTAS project was to compare MOH-relapse rates six months after a structured, multidisciplinary detoxification program between MOH patients using a newly developed, electronic headache-diary system or a paper headache diary, and the main results are in progress for publication [13]. The highly positive effect of the treatment program on disability, depression and anxiety has recently been published [14].

Study population

Patients referred to six national headache centers or clinics in Germany (University Hospital, Essen), Denmark (Danish Headache Center, Copenhagen), Italy (C. Mondino National Neurological Institute, Pavia), Spain (University Clinical Hospital, Valencia), Argentina (Foundation for Combating Neurological Diseases of Childhood, Buenos Aires) and Chile (Pontificia Universidad Católica de Chile, Santiago) were included consecutively from August 2008 to February 2009.

Patients were included if they were diagnosed with MOH according to the revised ICHD-II MOH-criteria [15], and capable of filling in paper and/or electronic diaries. The MOH diagnosis was based on 2 months previous history and at least 1 month with headache diary, in total 3 months overuse. Exclusion criteria were a current diagnosis of co-existent, significant and complicating medical or psychiatric illnesses; significant overuse of 'pure' opioids (patients overusing combination drugs containing opioids were allowed), benzodiazepines and barbiturates; overuse of alcohol and other drugs of addiction; current treatment with migraine-prophylactic drugs, inefficacy of previous, adequate detoxification programs; pregnancy or breastfeeding; or inability to reliably provide medical history.

At inclusion in the program, baseline characteristics were collected using extensive questionnaires supplemented with structured patient interviews. Information about primary headache diagnoses referred to the time before medication overuse and was based on the ICHD-II criteria. Both MOH and primary headache diagnosis were also revised retrospectively according to ICHD-III [16].

Questionnaire of referral pathway, financing of healthcare costs, pathways and subsidization of acute medication

In order to obtain relevant background information on the organization of national healthcare systems, all headache centers were asked how patients were referred to a headache specialist, and if referral was needed for ER. In addition, we gathered information on how headache-related healthcare costs were covered.

Also, background information about medication subsidization and pathways (over-the-counter (OTC) drugs versus prescription-requiring analgesics) was obtained.

Healthcare utilization and acute medication overuse

Data concerning healthcare utilization and acute medication overuse were collected by extensive questionnaires supplemented with structured interviews at the time of inclusion in the program. Firstly, we focused on the proportion of patients having healthcare consultations (General practitioner (GP), headache specialist consultations, and ER visits) and instrumental investigations (EEG, MR- and CT-scans and X-rays) in the year preceding therapy. Headache specialist consultations mainly included visits at neurologists and in a few cases neuro-surgeons.

Secondly, this study focused on acute medication overuse at the time of MOH-diagnosis. This was reported as proportion of patients with specific drug-overuse: Triptans, ergotamines, simple analgesics, opioids, combination-analgesics (analgesics combined with codeine, caffeine and/or antiemetics) or poly-overuse (combination of acute analgesics without overuse of a single drug-type). A patient was diagnosed with more than one MOH subtype if more than one type of drug was overused simultaneously. In addition, proportions of patients with specific drug-overuse were reported in groups separated according to primary headache diagnosis (migraine, tension type headache (TTH) or migraine plus TTH).

All results are shown for the total population, grouped by European and LA headache centers, and sub-grouped by national headache centers.

Statistics

Statistical Package for Social Sciences (SPSS) version 20 was used for statistics. Data were either shown as proportions or as mean and SD in brackets. Chi-square Fischer's exact tests were used for 2×2 tables and Pearson's chi-square tests were used for 2×3 tables in order to compare proportions between Europe and LA, while Student's independent t-tests were used to compare means. A value of $p < 0.050$ was considered as significant. All p-values were two-tailed.

Ethical issues

Local ethics committees from all headache centers approved the study (the local ethical committee at Essen University Hospital, local ethical committee at Pavia University, local ethical committee at Valencia University Clinical Hospital, Research Ethics Committee at the Medical School of Pontificia Universidad Católica de Chile and the Ethics Committee and Biomedical Research at FLENI in Argentina). In Denmark, such studies are exempted from the approval process, as the study did not foresee any new pharmacological treatment or interventions and was hence approved without application. All included patients gave informed consent before taking part.

Results

Study population

A total of 1362 patients with potential MOH were screened in the 6 centers. Of these, 669 were enrolled in the study (Fig. 1).

The majority were 30–55 years old (67.7 %), females (79.4 %), and with onset of primary headache in their teens (64.4 %) (Table 1). The age, gender difference and age at onset of primary headache were very similar in all headache centers, and there was no significant difference between Europe and LA. Baseline characteristics including the proportions of primary headache diagnosis, marital status, educational level and headache frequency are shown in Table 1.

Noteworthy, there were some significant differences in the proportion of primary headache diagnosis, although in general, most of patients had previous migraine or a combination of migraine and TTH, and only a minority had TTH as primary headache diagnosis (Table 1).

Referral pathway and financing of healthcare costs

To be referred to a headache specialist in Denmark and Spain, patients need (Table 2) referral by their GP who function as gatekeeper. In Italy, patients need to be referred to a specialist by their GP, or can self-refer on private basis. In Germany, Argentina and Chile, patients could contact headache specialists directly by self-referral. There was free access for ER in all countries (Table 2).

In the European countries, the governments finance headache specialist consultations in full, except in Italy, where a partial contribution is requested from the patients. In LA, the costs of headache specialist consultations are covered by private healthcare assurances or out of own pocket. Financing of costs of instrumental investigations is presented in Table 2.

Headache-related healthcare utilization

Only 26.5 % of the LA patients had GP consultations for their headache in the year preceding inclusion in the study, compared with 56.7 % of the European patients ($p < 0.001$) (Fig. 2). It should be mentioned that only 6.8 % of the Italian patient group were screened through preliminary GP visits, which is far lower than the proportion of patients from LA (Fig. 3). In contrast, 77.1 % of the German patients had GP consultations, and of those, 35.4 % visited the GP more than 6 times per year, corresponding to a visit more than every second month (see Additional file 1: Table S1).

The vast majority of European patients (82.7 %), especially the Italian group (95.7 %), had seen a headache specialist prior to admission to the headache center, while this was only the case for 37.6 % of the LA patients ($p < 0.001$) (Figs. 2 and 3).

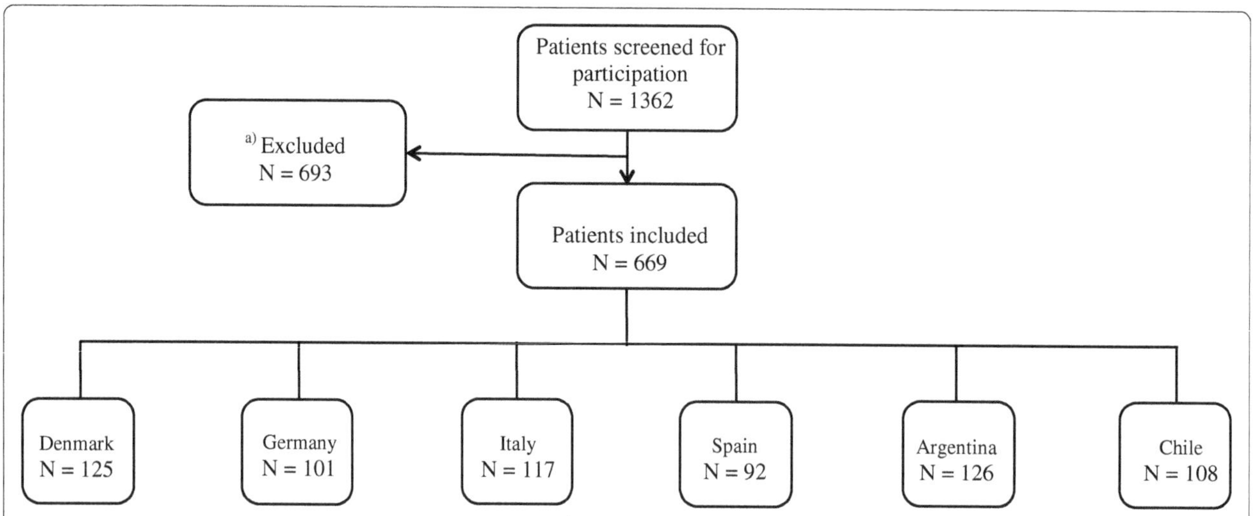

Fig. 1 Study population. The flowchart illustrates the population. [a]Patients ($N = 444$) were excluded for 3 main reasons: previous detoxifications (mostly in the European Centers), wrong referral diagnosis (mostly in the LA Centers) and refusal to participate (equal distribution between EU and LA areas). Furthermore, 191 patients did not fullfill the criteria after filling out headache diary or did not have an internet spot available at home or nearby. Finally, 58 patients were excluded because they did not show up to the following visit or dataset was incomplete. Of the included patients, 435 came from Europe and 234 came from Latin America

In LA, 29.9 % of the patients had headache-related ER visits, compared to 20.4 % of the European patients (p = 0.007) (Fig. 2). The proportions of patients with ER visits varied considerably among all centers, e.g., in Spain, 50.6 % of the patients visited the ER, in contrast to only 6.0 % of the Italian patient group and 20.6 % of the Argentinian patient group (Fig. 3).

The frequencies of headache-related instrumental investigations are presented in Table 1. There was no significant difference between Europe and LA.

Characterization of medication overuse patterns

While ergotamines were the most frequently overused analgesics among patients from LA (72.2 %), they were only overused by 3.7 % of the European patients with MOH ($p < 0.001$) (Fig. 4). In contrast, triptans were overused by 30.8 % of European patients with MOH and only by 5.6 % of LA patients ($p < 0.001$). The same pattern for ergotamines and triptans was seen when separating patients according to primary headache diagnosis (Table 3). Among the European patient groups, the Spanish had the lowest percentage of triptan overusers (13.0 %) and the highest percentage of ergotamine overusers (7.6 %) (Fig. 5). In contrast, Italy had the highest rate of triptan overusers among the European patients (41.9 %) (Fig. 5).

Simple analgesics were overused in all patient groups, corresponding to 46.9 % in the study population, and 15.4 % were daily users (Additional file 2: Table S2). In LA, 33.3 % of the patients overused simple analgesics (Fig. 4). However, significantly more patients from Europe (54.3 %) overused simple analgesics ($p < 0.001$), and noteworthy it was the case for 80.4 % of the Spanish group.

Combination-analgesics were often overused in Chile (59.3 %), Denmark (37.6 %), Germany (22.8 %) and Italy (21.4 %), while they were only overused by a minority of MOH patients in Spain (8.7 %) and Argentina (3.2 %) (Fig. 5). No significant difference in terms of overuse of combination-analgesics was observed between Europe and LA ($P = 0.14$), except among the group of patients with previous migraine (Table 3). In general, only a small proportion was diagnosed with an opioid-overuse (1.5 %) or poly-overuse (2.2 %). There was no significant difference in duration of medication overuse between Europe and LA ($P = 0.13$) (Additional file 2: Table S2). For the total population 59.8 % had a medication overuse for 1–5 years, and 23 % for more than 5 years.

The policy about whether a particular analgesic requires prescription is different among all the countries, as in the case with medication subsidization (summarized in Table 4).

Most patients in the study population only had a single MOH diagnosis (75.6 %), while 23 % had two MOH diagnoses and 1.5 % had three kind of medication overuse (Additional file 3: Table S3).

Discussion

The findings in this study demonstrate a marked variability between Europe and LA regarding general and clinical characteristics of patients as well as the organization of healthcare systems, and headache-related healthcare utilization, medication-overuse and medications availability.

Table 1 Baseline Characteristics

		Denmark	Germany	Italy	Spain	Argentina	Chile	Europe	Latin America	*p*-value	Total
N		125	101	117	92	126	108	435	234		669
Age, years	<30	13.6	26.7	18.8	15.2	31.2	20.4	18.4	26.1		21.1
	30–55	71.2	63.4	72.6	70.7	58.4	70.4	69.7	63.7	0.058	67.7
	>55	15.2	9.9	8.5	14.1	10.4	9.3	12.0	9.8		11.2
Gender, female		77.6	74.3	82.1	80.4	80.2	81.5	78.6	80.8	0.55	79.4
High educational level[a]		87.2	40.4	71.8	49.5	80.2	67.6	64.4	74.4	0.009*	67.9
Marital status, married		70.4	52.0	58.1	68.1	50.8	55.6	62.4	53.0	0.021*	59.1
Primary headache diagnosis	Migraine[b]	30.4	80.2	82.9	46.7	72.2	79.6	59.5	75.6		65.2
	TTH[b]	26.4	2.0	0.9	16.3	5.6	1.9	11.7	3.8	<0.001*	9.0
	Migraine and TTH[b]	43.2	17.8	16.2	37.0	22.2	18.5	28.7	20.5		25.9
Age of onset of primary headache, years		23.4 (13.0)	18.1 (9.2)	14.1 (6.0)	18.9 (9.9)	16.2 (6.2)	19.7 (10.1)	18.8 (10.5)	17.8 (8.4)	0.22	18.4 (9.8)
Headache frequency, days/month[c]		25.8 (5.5)	25.1 (5.6)	23.3 (6.0)	23.6 (5.0)	22.1 (6.4)	23.0 (5.7)	24.5 (5.7)	22.5 (6.1)	<0.001*	23.8 (5.9)
Duration of overuse in years	<1	13.6	21.8	11.1	16.3	19.0	22.2	15.4	20.5		17.2
	1–5	67.2	54.5	58.1	57.6	61.9	57.4	59.8	59.8	0.13	59.8
	>5	19.2	22.4	30.8	26.1	19.0	20.4	24.8	19.7		23.0
EEG[d]		7.3	31.8	0.9	4.7	8.0	2.8	10.0	5.6	0.055	8.4
Scans (CT and MR)[d]		29.3	42.3	20.5	36.4	40.0	21.3	31.0	31.3	0.93	31.1
X-rays[d]		5.7	21.2	2.6	14.1	12.8	0.9	9.8	7.3	0.32	8.9

Age, gender, educational level, marital status, primary headache type: Proportion of patients in percent. Age of onset of primary headache and headache frequency: Mean (SD). Duration of overuse: Percent of patients categorized into three intervals. EEG, Scans and X-rays: Percent of patients, who had these instrumental investigations performed in the year preceding therapy

TTH tension type headache, *EEG* electro encephalogram, *CT* computer tomography scan, *MR* magnetic resonance scan

[a]High educational level = High/technical school or university degree

[b]Migraine = Migraine with aura, migraine without aura and chronic migraine. TTH = episodic and chronic forms

[c]Headache frequencies refer to the time of inclusion in the study and thereby to the MOH diagnosis

[d]*N* = 643

$^{*}p < 0.05$. p-values correspond to comparison between Europe and Latin America

The patient groups showed significant differences in the distribution of primary headache diagnoses between Europe and LA countries. Considering the significantly higher level of education for LA patients and the fact that they have to pay out of their own pocket in order to receive the attention of a headache specialist, it is possible that the observed difference may be related to a different social class of subjects with higher income, more frequently single and tend to be younger. Of course cultural or real epidemiological differences cannot be ruled out.

The inhomogeneous distribution of primary headache diagnoses may theoretically have affected the proportions of the types of overused analgesics, since e.g., triptans and ergotamines are recommended for treatment for migraine only. However, when separating the groups according to primary headache diagnosis, we almost found the same results as in the whole group with a few exceptions as mentioned.

Only a minority of the patients reported pure TTH as primary headache. This could be due to less disability compared to patients with concomitant migraine, contributing to fewer referrals to headache centers. According to previously published Scandinavian studies concerning MOH, approximately 20–30 % percent suffered from pure TTH as primary diagnosis [17, 18], which is comparable to the findings in the Danish and Spanish group in this study.

Prior studies have characterized the use of healthcare in the general population [7, 10, 19], and our patients with MOH presented a multifold higher rate of access to headache specialists. This reflects that our study population was much more affected by headache, and emphasizes the unmet need for focused prevention and management strategies.

The fact that far more European patients had consultations with GPs and headache specialists compared with LA patients - while the latter more frequently

Table 2 Referral pathway and financing of healthcare costs for patients

	Denmark	Germany	Italy	Spain	Argentina	Chile
Referral pathways						
Referral needed for headache specialist consultation	Yes	No	Yes or self-refer on private basis	Yes	No	No
Who are able to refer the patients to a headache specialist?	GP[a] Other specialists ER[a] Other doctors	–	GP	GP Other specialists ER	–	–
Referral needed for emergency room visits	No	No	No	No	No	No
Financing of healthcare costs for patients						
Free Access	GP Headache Specialist ER EEG, MR-, CT-scan and X-rays	GP Headache Specialist ER EEG, MR-, CT-scan and X-rays	GP Headache Specialist[b] ER[c] EEG[b], MR-[d], CT-scan[d] and X-rays[e]	GP Headache Specialist ER EEG, MR-, CT-scan and X-rays	–	GP – ER MR-, CT-scan and X-rays
Private healthcare assurance	–	–	–	–	GP Headache Specialist ER EEG, MR-, CT-scan and X-rays	GP Headache Specialist ER EEG, MR-, CT-scan and X-rays
Out of own pocket	–	–	– Headache Specialist[b] ER[c] EEG[b], MR-[d], CT-scan[d] and X-rays[d]	–	– Headache Specialist – –	GP Headache Specialist ER EEG, MR-, CT-scan and X-rays

GP general practitioner, *ER* emergency room, *EEG* electro encephalogram, *CT* computer tomography scan, *MR* magnetic resonance scan
[a]Referral after a relevant therapy course performed by a general neurologist
[b]Patients < 6 years or > 65 years are exempted for covering the healthcare costs. Without exemption contribution is required according to income
[c]Free access if appropriate request (real emergency)
[d]Patients < 6 years or > 65 years are exempted for covering the healthcare costs. Without exemption contribution is required depending on income
Free access = government covers the costs

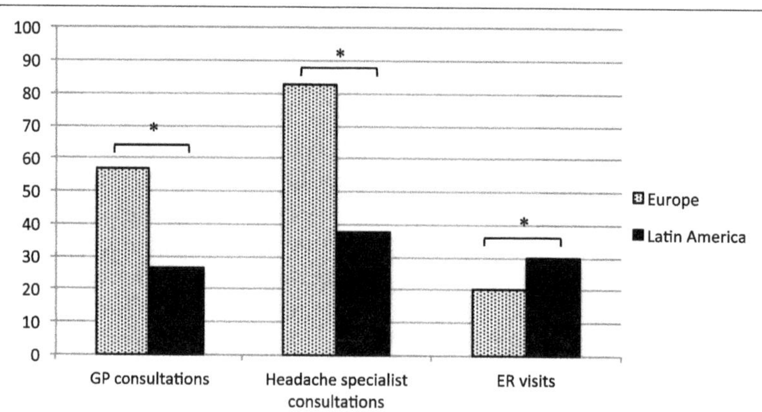

Fig. 2 Headache-related healthcare consultations among patients with medication overuse headache in Europe and Latin America. The bar chart compares the proportion of patients (in percent) from Europe and Latin America with general practitioner (GP) consultations, headache specialist consultations and emergency room (ER) visits in the year preceding inclusion of the study. *$p < 0.05$

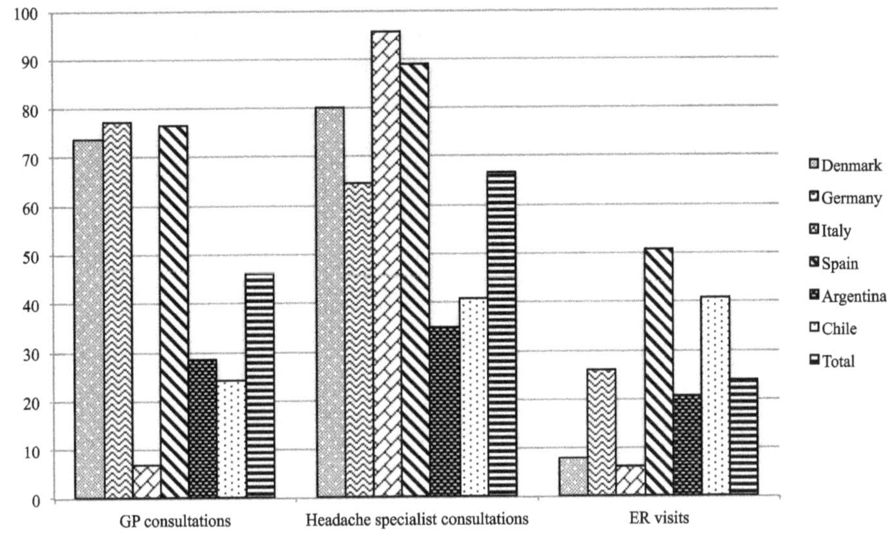

Fig. 3 Healthcare consultations among patients with medication overuse headache. The bar chart presents the proportion of patients (in percent) from each headache clinic with general practitioner (GP) consultations, headache specialist consultations and emergency room (ER) visits in the year preceding inclusion of the study

access ER - may be due to different organization of the healthcare systems. Headache centers were non-existing in Chile (the first one was activated within the initiatives of the COMOESTAS Project 2008–2010) and only one headache center was available in Buenos Aires, a city with several millions of inhabitants. It must be noted that another possible reason for less GP and headache specialist contacts in LA could be less focus in society on headache as a disorder requiring therapy. We have observed a high frequency of EEG examinations in Germany in contrast to the existing guidelines [20] and practice in other countries. In general, EEG is not recommended for the diagnosis of headache but national practice may still vary.

In general, it seems that the healthcare system is not used in the appropriate manner, because a considerable proportion of MOH patients, both from Europe and LA, seek help at the ER, which does not seem as the optimal setting for managing a chronic condition. Furthermore, when considering the very high use of GP visits in some European countries, it could be important to clarify whether some European patients used the healthcare system at too high extent, thus contributing to an unnecessarily increased economic burden for society. In

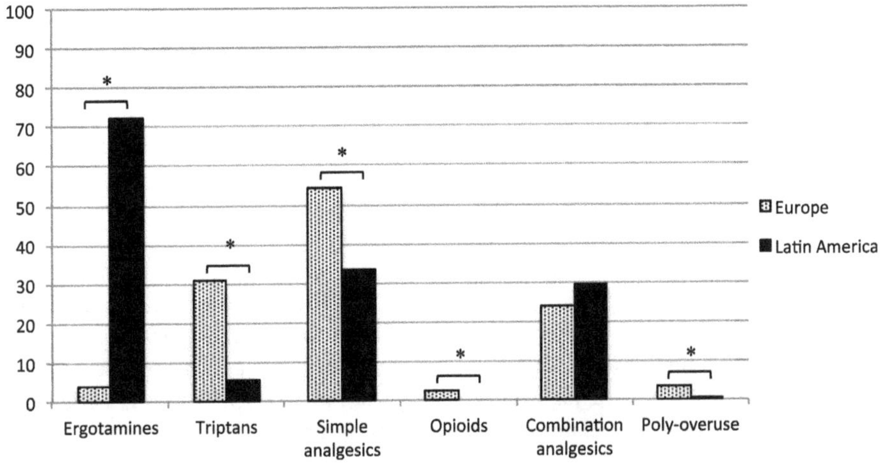

Fig. 4 Type of overused analgesics in Europe and Latin America. The bar chart compares the proportion of patients (in percent) in Europe and Latin America with specific drug-overuse. A single patient can be diagnosed with more than one type of overuse. $^{*}p < 0.05$

Table 3 MOH sub-diagnosis in relation to primary headache diagnosis

Primary headache diagnosis	Acute analgesics	Denmark	Germany	Italy	Spain	Argentina	Chile	Europe	Latin America	*P*-value	Total
N		38	81	97	43	91	86	259	177		436
Migraine	Ergotamines	5.3	1.2	4.1	2.3	81.3	62.8	3.1	72.3	<0.001*	31.2
	Triptans	55.3	37.0	47.4	16.3	4.4	8.1	40.2	6.2	<0.001*	26.4
	Simple analgesics	26.3	60.5	29.9	79.1	26.4	34.9	47.1	30.5	0.001*	40.4
	Opioids	5.3	6.2	0.0	0.0	0.0	0.0	2.7	0.0	0.045	1.6
	Combination-analgesics	18.4	21.0	21.6	4.7	3.3	62.8	18.1	32.2	0.001*	23.9
	Poly-overuse	5.3	2.5	3.1	4.7	0.0	1.2	3.5	0.6	0.54	2.3
N		33	2	1	15	7	2	51	9		60
TTH	Ergotamines	0.0	0.0	0.0	6.7	100.0	100.0	2.0	100.0	<0.001*	16.7
	Triptans	0.0	0.0	0.0	6.7	0.0	0.0	2.0	0.0	1.00	1.7
	Simple analgesics	81.8	50.0	100.0	86.7	42.9	0.0	82.4	33.3	0.005	75.0
	Opioids	3.0	0.0	0.0	0.0	0.0	0.0	2.0	0.0	1.00	1.7
	Combination-analgesics	36.4	100.0	0.0	13.3	0.0	50.0	31.4	11.1	0.42	28.3
	Poly-overuse	3.0	0.0	0.0	0.0	0.0	0.0	2.0	0.0	1.00	1.7
N		54	18	19	34	28	20	125	48		173
Migraine and TTH	Ergotamines	3.7	0.0	0.0	14.7	14.3	40.0	5.6	66.7	<0.001*	22.5
	Triptans	33.3	22.2	15.8	11.8	3.6	5.0	23.2	4.2	0.003*	17.9
	Simple analgesics	38.9	66.7	63.2	79.4	35.7	55.0	57.6	43.8	0.13	53.8
	Opioids	3.7	0.0	0.0	0.0	0.0	0.0	1.6	0.0	1.00	1.2
	Combination-analgesics	51.9	22.2	21.1	11.8	3.6	45.0	32.0	20.8	0.19	28.9
	Poly-overuse	1.9	0.0	10.5	2.9	0.0	0.0	3.2	0.0	0.58	2.3

Percentage of patients with specific MOH sub-diagnosis related to primary headache diagnosis. Number of each group are included in the table. Migraine includes forms with aura, without aura and chronic forms. TTH (Tension Type Headache) includes episodic and chronic forms. *p*-values correspond to comparison between Europe and Latin America. $^{*}p < 0.05$

this case, a more focused effort to recognize and treat patients with MOH may contribute to fewer, but more relevant healthcare contacts.

It can be difficult to compare the use or ER accesses across different health care systems, since primary care systems and emergency systems may be fundamentally different. In this study there was free access in all countries. The findings concerning medication overuse in Europe are in line with results reported in previous studies from European countries [3, 7, 10]. In the present study, simple analgesics were overused in 80 % of the MOH patients from Spain, which is in agreement with the findings of a previous Spanish study, where simple analgesics also were the most overused drugs [3]. The results from the Danish patient group, showing highest preference for simple analgesics, followed by combination-analgesics, were supported by two previous Scandinavian studies [7, 10]. Also in the case of the ergotamine overuse in LA, our findings are reinforced by a recently published review that reports a high prevalence of ergotamine-overuse in LA, and a relatively high prevalence of triptan-overuse in Europe [21].

Ergotamines are highly potent drugs for treating migraine. In LA, ergotamines are sold as OTC analgesics at low prices in contrast to Europe where ergotamines require prescription. This may explain the widespread use in LA. In the eighties and nineties, overuse of ergotamines was a major problem in Europe, and a German study from 2002 reported that 13 % of the patients with MOH overused ergotamines [22]. The availability and, for some countries, the subsidization of triptans in Europe explain the marked decrease in ergotamine overuse and the associated increase in triptan overuse. The distribution policy of triptans, based on prescriptions, obviously did not succeed in deterring overuse. The ergotamine-triptan switch observed in Europe has also been reported in the United States [23], thus suggesting that replacement of ergotamines by triptans is likely to occur in the future in LA. It should be mentioned, that even though prescription was required for ergotamines in Spain, many patients managed to obtain ergotamines without. This could explain why patients from the Spanish group had the highest European proportion of ergotamine-overuse.

This study also reported other differences in the medication overuse pattern among the European countries. Italian patients tended to use more triptans than other European patients, which may be explained by the fact

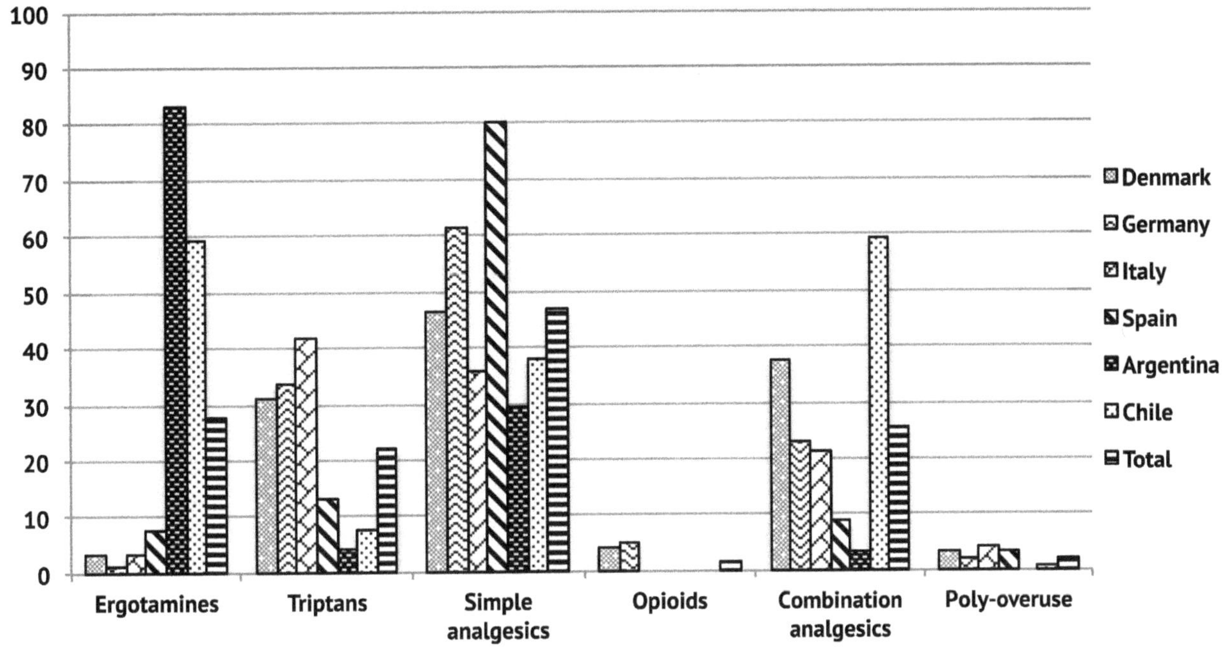

Fig. 5 Type of overused analgesics. The bar chart compares the proportion of patients (in percent) from each headache clinic with specific drug-overuse. A single patient can be diagnosed with more than one type of overuse

that triptans are the only analgesics with subsidization in Italy. Next to simple analgesics, triptans were the most often overused acute medication in Germany, even though there was no subsidization to triptans. Nevertheless, some triptans, e.g., naratriptan, are available as OTC analgesics. In Denmark, most simple analgesics and combination-analgesics are OTC analgesics, which probably made them the most often overused analgesics. The same phenomenon was observed in the German patient group. In Spain, the far most common overused analgesics were simple analgesics, which are available as OTC and subsidized.

In Argentina, simple analgesics are OTC analgesics, as in Denmark, Spain and Germany, and may also in this case contribute to overuse in almost one-third of the Argentinian patients. In Chile, combination-analgesics were overused almost as often as ergotamines. Both kinds of analgesics are sold as inexpensive OTC drugs.

Even though this study describes huge international variations in particular patterns of medication overuse, the underlying factors encouraging medication overuse seem to be the same in all countries: high availability and low prices. This is supported by previously published Asian studies, which reported a high prevalence of OTC analgesic overuse too [24–26]. Thereby, high availability and low costs of acute medication are global challenges for preventing MOH. When having the knowledge about which analgesics that are most commonly overused, specifically targeted clinical and political initiatives can be more easily initiated, e.g., smaller packages of analgesics and focused prevention campaigns spreading out information about the nature of MOH, thereby changing patients' behavior.

Methodological considerations

To our knowledge, no previous study has described and compared general demographic and clinical characteristics of MOH, along with the referral pathways and national painkillers distribution in several European and LA Countries. We did this multicenter, multinational setup in a large MOH population, which is a major strength of this study. The present study is unique as it describes patients accessing headache centers and specialized care, carefully classified by means of prospective diaries. The fact that the study was conducted on patients attending specialized center of course represents a selection bias making this study less applicable to patients in the primary sector and therefore prevents generalization of the results.

It is noteworthy that in the original study design MOH patients overusing barbiturates or pure opioid overuse were excluded, as well as patients with benzodiazepine overuse [13, 14]. This makes the study less applicable for specific groups of patients with high use of barbiturates, opioids and benzodiazepines. It should also be mentioned that patients with significant comorbid psychiatric illnesses were excluded. However, this study

Table 4 Medication pathways and subsidization

	Denmark	Germany	Italy	Spain	Argentina	Chile
OTC analgesics[a]	–	–	–	–	Ergotamines	Ergotamines[k]
	–	Triptans[d]		–	–	Triptans[l]
	Simple analgesics[b]	Simple analgesics[e]		Simple analgesics[g]	Simple analgesics	Simple analgesics
	–	–		–	–	–
	Combination-analgesics[c]	Combination-analgesics[f]		Combination-analgesics	–	Combination-analgesics[m]
Prescription needed	Ergotamines	Ergotamines	Ergotamines	Ergotamines[h]	–	–
	Triptans	Triptans[d]	Triptans	Triptans	Triptans	–
	Simple analgesics[b]	Simple analgesics[e]	Simple analgesics	–	–	–
	Opioids	–	Opioids	Opioids	Opioids	Opioids
	Combination-analgesics[c]	Combination-analgesics[f]	Combination-analgesics	–	Combination-analgesics	–
Analgesics with subsidization	Ergotamines	–	–	Ergotamines	–	–
	Triptans		Triptans	Triptans	Triptans[j]	
	–		–	Simple analgesics	Simple analgesics	
	Opioids		–	Opioids	Opioids	
	–		–	Combination-analgesics[i]	Combination-analgesics	
Analgesics without subsidization	–	Ergotamines	Ergotamines	–	Ergotamines	Ergotamines[k]
	–	Triptans	–	–	–	Triptans[l]
	Simple analgesics[b]	Simple analgesics	Simple analgesics	–	–	Simple analgesics
	–	Opioids	Opioids	–	–	Opioids
	Combination-analgesics[c]	Combination-analgesics	Combination-analgesics	Combination-analgesics[i]	–	Combination-analgesics[m]

[a]Over-the-counter analgesics
[b]Most simple analgesics are OTC. Prescription is only required for large packages or higher doses. Only prescribed simple analgesics are subsidized
[c]Combination-analgesics containing opioids, phenazone and ergotamine require prescription with a few exceptions. Only ergo-caffeine are subsidized
[d]Most triptans require prescription. Few triptans, e.g., Naratriptan, are OTC
[e]Most simple analgesics are OTC, except Ibuprofen 600 mg
[f]Combination-analgesics containing caffeine do not require prescription, while those containing opioids do
[g]Simple analgesics are OTC. However, prescription is used at least in 60 %
[h]Ergotamines require prescription. Nevertheless, many patients manage to acquire it without
[i]Some compounds are subsidized
[j]Triptans are only subsidized partially
[k]Ergotamines are inexpensive and easily available. All kind of ergotamins are combined with either caffeine, acetoaminophen or NSAIDS
[l]Triptans are expensive and available only at pharmacies
[m]Combination-analgesics are inexpensive. There are no combinations with codeine. Most common combination-analgesics contain caffeine, dipirone, chlorphenamine and ergotamine

is applicable to patients with less complex psychiatric disorders and less severe MOH cases, representative for a significant part of the clinical MOH population in primary and specialized care. However, it may be difficult to compare use of emergency across health care systems due to different organizations of the link between the primary care sectors and the emergency systems. In some countries, there may be differences in how emergency rooms and emergency departments are organized. This study does not distinct between that.

The patients were included in 2008 and 2009. Some changes concerning acute medication overuse and healthcare utilization may have occurred since then. The present data remain however important as, to the best of our knowledge, no other study has provided relevant information on this topic in the subsequent years. It could be interesting to repeat the study for comparing with our results.

Conclusion

MOH definitely represent a serious cross-continental issue, although demographic and clinical variability may exist, along with differences in referral patterns, use of healthcare resources and overuse of acute medications overuse in the 2 continents.

A clear message from our data is this: drugs are overused when they are easily accessible and at low price. A focused effort to recognize and treat patients with MOH may contribute to fewer, but more targeted healthcare contacts. Furthermore, clinical and political initiatives for awareness and prevention campaigns based on information of MOH can be better facilitated and targeted when having the knowledge about which types of analgesics that are more likely to become overused by headache sufferers in a particular part of the world.

Additional files

Additional file 1: Table S1. Headache-related healthcare system utilization. Number of consultations per year are categorizes into 4 groups, and shown as percentage of the student population. [1]Missing data on 3 patients from Germany and 5 patients from Spain, respectively. (PDF 55 kb)

Additional file 2: Table S2. Medication overuse headache sub-diagnosis and duration of medication overuse. The table characterizes the medication overuse headache (MOH) sub-diagnosis. Results are shown as percent of patients with a specific MOH sub-diagnosis. Numbers in brackets presents the proportion of the patient population that used a specific analgesics 30 days/month. *p*-values correspond to comparison of MOH sub-diagnosis between Europe and Latin America. $^*p < 0.05$. [1]A patient can have more than one MOH sub-diagnosis. [2]Intake of combination of acute medication ≥ 15 days/month without overuse of a single drug. (PDF 67 kb)

Additional file 3: Table S3. Multiple medication overuse headache sub-diagnoses and specific combination of medication overuse. The table characterizes the proportion of patients with multiple medication overuse headache (MOH) sub-diagnoses and the specific medication overuse profile. The data are shown as percentages. (PDF 66 kb)

Abbreviations
CDH: chronic daily headache; COMOESTAS: Continuous Monitoring of Medication Overuse headache in Europe and Latin America; ER: emergency room; GP: general practitioner; LA: Latin America; MOH: medication overuse headache; OTC: over the counter drugs; TTH: tension type headache.

Competing interests
The authors declare that they have no competing insterests.

Authors' contributions
NLF has participated in acquiring data, analyzed data and drafted the manuscript. RT has reviewed the manuscript. SBM, LB, CT and RJ has participated in designing the study, acquiring and analyzed data, and critically reviewed the manuscript. GN, ZK, ML, MTG, RF, SS and MP participated in designing the study, acquired and analyzed data, and reviewed the manuscript. The members of the COMOESTAS Consortium contributed to patients' enrollment and/or data collection. All authors have given final approval of this version.

Acknowledgement
This work was supported by the COMOESTAS Project – EC contract number 215366 (COMOESTAS) FP7 – Thematic priority ICT.

COMOESTAS Consortium
M. Allena, G. Sances, G. Sandrini and F. Blandini (Headache Science Center, C. Mondino National Neurological Institute, Dept. of Brain and Behavioral Sciences, University of Pavia, Italy). M. Rapsch (Department of Neurology, University Hospital of Essen, Germany). B. Lopez (Foundation of the Valencian Community, University Clinical Hospital, Spain). D. Cerquetti (Foundation for Combating Neurological Diseases of Childhood, Argentina). B. Shand (Pontificia Universidad Católica de Chile, Chile). M. Osa (Universidad Isalud, Argentina).

Author details
[1]Faculty of Health Science, University of Copenhagen, Copenhagen, Denmark. [2]Danish Headache Center, Neurological Department, Glostrup Hospital, Glostrup, Denmark. [3]Department of Biomedical and NeuroMotor Sciences (DIBINEM), Alma Mater Studiorum, Bologna University, Ospedale Bellaria, Bologna, Italy. [4]Headache Science Center, C. Mondino National Neurological Institute C. Mondino Foundation, Dept. of Brain and Behavioral Sciences, University of Pavia, Pavia, Italy. [5]Department of Neurology, University Hospital of Essen, Essen, Germany. [6]Foundation of the Valencian Community, University Clinical Hospital, Barcelona, Spain. [7]Foundation for Combating Neurological Diseases of Childhood, Buenos Aires, Argentina. [8]Pontificia Universidad Católica de Chile, Santiago, Chile. [9]Universidad Isalud, Buenos Aires, Argentina. [10]Bioengineering and Medical Informatics Consortium, Pavia, Italy.

References
1. Westergaard ML, Glümer C, Hansen EH, Jensen RH (2014) Prevalence of chronic headache with and without medication overuse: Associations with socioeconomic position and physical and mental health status. Pain 155(10):2005–13
2. Lantéri-Minet M, Auray J-P, El Hasnaoui A et al (2003) Prevalence and description of chronic daily headache in the general population in France. Pain 102:143–9
3. Colás R, Muñoz P, Temprano R, Gómez C, Pascual J et al (2004) Chronic daily headache with analgesic overuse: epidemiology and impact on quality of life. Neurology 62(8):1338–42
4. Evers S, Marziniak M (2010) Clinical features, pathophysiology, and treatment of medication-overuse headache. Lancet Neurol 9:391–401
5. Linde M, Gustavsson A (2012) The cost of headache disorders in Europe: the Eurolight project. Eur J Neurol 19:703–e43
6. Scher AI, Lipton RB, Stewart WF, Bigal M (2010) Patterns of medication use by chronic and episodic headache sufferers in the general population: results from the frequent headache epidemiology study. Cephalalgia 30:321–8
7. Kristoffersen ES, Grande RB, Aaseth K et al (2012) Management of primary chronic headache in the general population: the Akershus study of chronic headache. J Headache Pain 13(2):113–20
8. Maizels M (2002) Health Resource Utilization of the Emergency Department Headache "Repeater.". Headache 42:747–753
9. Bigal ME, Lipton RB (2009) Overuse of acute migraine medications and migraine chronification. Curr Pain Headache Rep 13:301–7
10. Jonsson P, Linde M, Hensing G, Hedenrud T (2012) Sociodemographic differences in medication use, health-care contacts and sickness absence among individuals with medication-overuse headache. J Headache Pain 13:281–90
11. Allena M, Katsarava Z, Nappi G (2009) From drug-induced headache to medication overuse headache. A short epidemiological review, with a focus on Latin American countries. J Headache Pain 10:71–76
12. Shand B, Goicochea MT, Valenzuela R et al (2015) Clinical and demographical characteristics of patients with medication overuse headache in Argentina and Chile: analysis of the Latin American Section of COMOESTAS Project. J Headache Pain 16:83
13. Tassorelli C, Jensen R, Allena M (2014) A consensus protocol for the management of medication-overuse headache: Evaluation in a multicentric, multinational study. Cephalalgia 34:645–655
14. Bendtsen L, Munksgaard S, Tassorelli C et al (2013) Disability, anxiety and depression associated with medication-overuse headache can be considerably reduced by detoxification and prophylactic treatment. Results from a multicentre, multinational study (COMOESTAS project). Cephalalgia 0:1–8
15. Olesen J, Bousser M-G, Diener H-C et al (2006) New appendix criteria open for a broader concept of chronic migraine. Cephalalgia 26:742–6. doi:10.1111/j.1468-2982.2006.01172.x
16. Road C (2013) The International Classification of Headache Disorders, 3rd edition (beta version). Cephalalgia 26:742–6
17. Munksgaard SB, Bendtsen L, Jensen RH (2012) Detoxification of medication-overuse headache by a multidisciplinary treatment programme is highly effective: a comparison of two consecutive treatment methods in an open-label design. Cephalalgia 32:834–44
18. Hagen K, Albretsen C, Vilming ST et al (2009) Management of medication overuse headache : 1-year randomized multicentre open-label trial. Cephalalgia 29:221–232

19. Lyngberg AC, Rasmussen BK, Jørgensen T, Jensen R (2005) Has the prevalence of migraine and tension-type headache changed over a 12-year period? A Danish population survey. Eur J Epidemiol 20:243–9
20. Sandrini G, Friberg L, Coppola G et al (2011) Neurophysiological tests and neuroimaging procedures in non-acute headache (2nd edition). Eur J Neurol 18:373–81
21. Kristoffersen ES, Lundqvist C (2014) Medication-overuse headache: a review. J Pain Res 7:367–78
22. Limmroth V, Katsarava Z, Fritsche G et al (2002) Features of medication overuse headache following overuse of different acute headache drugs. Neurology 59:1011–4
23. Meskunas CA, Tepper SJ, Rapoport AM et al (2006) Medications associated with probable medication overuse headache reported in a tertiary care headache center over a 15-year period. Headache 46:766–72
24. Dong Z, Chen X, Steiner TJ et al (2014) Medication-overuse headache in China: Clinical profile, and an evaluation of the ICHD-3 beta diagnostic criteria. Cephalalgia. doi:10.1177/0333102414552533
25. Imai N, Kitamura E, Konishi T et al (2007) Clinical features of probable medication-overuse headache: a retrospective study in Japan. Cephalalgia 27:1020–3
26. Ravishankar K (2008) Medication overuse headache in India. Cephalalgia 28: 1223–6

Assessment of headache characteristics in a general adolescent population: a comparison between retrospective interviews and prospective diary recordings

Anne-Berit Krogh[1,2*], Bo Larsson[3], Øyvind Salvesen[4] and Mattias Linde[1,5]

Abstract

Background: Reliable information on headache characteristics, including frequency and intensity, headache-associated impairment, and use of analgesic medications, may depend on the assessment method used. This study analyzed the correlations between headache characteristics determined in structured interviews and those determined in prospective diary recordings kept by adolescents in the general population.

Methods: In this cross-sectional school-based study, a representative sample of 488 adolescents aged 12–18 years were interviewed about headaches experienced during the previous year. Headache diaries for a three-week period were kept by 393 participants: 244 girls (62 %) and 149 (38 %) boys.

Results: Most adolescents (88 %) who reported headaches during their interview also recorded headaches in their diary. In contrast, 51 % of those who reported being headache-free during the last year recorded headaches in their diary. In the interviews, frequent headaches (at least 50 % of days during the last year) were reported by 2.9 % of participants, while 25.5 % reported this headache frequency in their diary. Overall, the ratings of headache frequency were significantly higher in diaries than in interviews ($p < 0.001$). Significant but low correlations were observed between intensity levels reported retrospectively and prospectively (rho = 0.28; $p < 0.001$) and between average scores of headache-related impairment reported retrospectively and prospectively (rho = 0.35; $p < 0.001$). The use of medications by those who reported one or more current headache disorder during their interview was significantly lower in prospective recordings than in the retrospective interview estimates ($p < 0.001$).

Conclusions: There is inconsistency in the estimates of headache characteristics between retrospective reports and diary recordings. A comprehensive picture of headache complaints among adolescents may be better obtained through a combination of prospective diary recordings and interviews by school health and clinical services.

Keywords: Headache, Epidemiology, Diary, Interview, Questionnaire, Adolescents

Background

Headache disorders are among the most common health problems in adolescents [1]. These include primary headaches, with tension-type headache (TTH) and migraine being the most common, and secondary headache disorders [2, 3]. Headache disorders in school children often lead to reduced quality of life and poorer psychosocial function in schoolwork, leisure activities, and social relations [4, 5], as well as to psychological problems, such as depression and anxiety [6, 7]. Studies monitoring the severity of headache disorders and the response to treatment usually include the frequency of attacks as their main outcome criterion. Outcomes of previous studies suggest that prospective recordings in diaries may provide a more reliable and comprehensive picture of headache occurrence in young people than retrospective assessments based on questionnaires and interviews [8–10].

* Correspondence: Anne-Berit.Krogh@ntnu.no
[1]Department of Neuroscience, Faculty of Medicine, Norwegian University of Science and Technology, N-7489 Trondheim, Norway
[2]Faculty of Health and Social Science, Norwegian University of Science and Technology, Trondheim, Norway
Full list of author information is available at the end of the article

Most previous clinical studies comparing retrospective and prospective data used sample sizes ranging from 52 to 214 participants [11–15]. Community-based surveys have also yielded somewhat inconsistent results. For example, a Dutch study with children and adolescents aged 9–16 years found that questionnaires overestimated headache intensity and duration when compared with diary recordings, whereas the estimates were equal for headache frequency [8]. A recent Swedish school-based study with adolescents aged 12–18 years reported that questionnaires overestimated headache intensity and underestimated headache frequency and duration when compared with diary recordings [7]. These earlier studies did not include all types of headache. For example, the Dutch study only included school children who reported a headache frequency of at least once a week [8], and the Swedish study excluded adolescents who considered their headaches to be disease-related (approximately one-third of those screened) [7].

The relative paucity of community surveys comparing retrospectively-obtained information and prospective diary recordings of headache characteristics among adolescents suggests further comparisons are needed. Therefore, the present study investigated the agreement between these two sources of information in determining the frequency and intensity of headaches, headache-associated impairment, and the use of medications to treat headache among a sample of adolescents in the general population. In addition, this study analyzed the sensitivity, specificity, and positive and negative predictive values of agreement between retrospectively-reported headaches experienced at least every other day, frequent medication, and prospective information recorded in headache diaries.

Methods

Sample selection and recruitment

All secondary and high schools in the county of South-Trøndelag in Norway were surveyed, with 899 eligible students invited to participate using stratified cluster sampling. Randomization was stratified by school location (see below) and age/grade: grade 8 (ages 12–13 years), grade 10 (ages 14–15 years), and grade 12 (ages 16–18 years). The sample distribution corresponded to the distribution of the county's population: 59 % of students were from urban areas, 28 % were from the inland/mountain region, and 13 % were from coastal municipalities.

At the time of the study, there were 74 secondary and high schools in South-Trøndelag, 13 of which were invited to participate. As there were large differences in school sizes, with more students attending schools in urban than in rural areas, more rural schools were included to obtain the required number of participants. Of the 13 invited schools, four were located in urban areas and nine in rural (inland/mountain or coastal) areas. Seven of the initially invited schools declined to participate and were replaced by seven other schools. The four participating urban schools included two secondary schools (participants in grades 8 and 10) and two high schools (participants in grade 12). The nine participating rural schools included four secondary schools and one high school from the coastal region, and three secondary schools and one high school from the inland/mountain region. Details of the recruitment procedure have been described elsewhere [16, 17].

Data collection

This study was conducted in two phases. Initially, each adolescent participated in a face-to-face, structured interview with a single interviewer (first author). All interviews were conducted in a suitable room at the participating schools during a regular school day, with interviews lasting 20 minutes on average. A questionnaire was completed during each interview. Immediately afterward, participants were asked to keep a prospective headache diary for a three-week period. Two data collection procedures were used for diaries, one based on paper recordings and the other internet-based [17]. Data were collected from March 2012 to February 2013.

Questionnaire

The questionnaire used in the interviews was developed for school-based studies of headaches in Sweden [9, 18] and translated into Norwegian. As an opening question, each participant was asked whether he/she had experienced a headache during the previous year. Adolescents who answered "Yes" were asked to report their usual headache frequency as "<1 day/month," "1–3 days/month," "1–3 days/week," or "Every other day or more often." Participants were also asked if they had experienced more than one type of headache during the previous year. Those who answered "Yes" were asked about the characteristics of and symptoms associated with each headache type. Specifically, participants were asked to report the frequency, intensity (three-point scale: 1 = mild, 2 = moderate, 3 = severe), and duration of episodes, as well as accompanying symptoms.

Participants were asked to complete the Pediatric Migraine Disability Assessment (PedMIDAS). This scale was developed to assess disability in children and adolescents with chronic pain, including headache, and has been used in clinical studies and epidemiological surveys [19–21]. The PedMIDAS consists of six questions addressing the number of days totally or partially lost owing to headache in the last three months across three domains (school, home, and social activities). A total score was calculated for each participant by summing the number of days reported for each item for all headaches [20].

Participants were asked if they had experienced headaches (of any type) for at least 15 days per month during the previous three months. They were also asked about the frequency analgesic medications were used, with response options being "Never," "1–9 days/month," and "10 days/month or more often." Adolescents who used medication were asked the names of those medications. Special consideration was made during the interview to avoid alerting participants to the concept of medication overuse headache (MOH), to avoid influencing their reports of medication use during the next phase of the study.

Headaches were classified as episodic migraine with or without aura, chronic migraine, probable migraine, episodic TTH, infrequent TTH or frequent TTH, chronic TTH, or MOH, according to the International Classification of Headache Disorders (ICHD-3 beta) [22]. Probable TTH was combined with definite TTH. MOH was defined as having any headache (including the most bothersome headache) for more than half of the days during the previous three months and treating it with medication on at least 10 days per month. A headache that did not meet any of the ICHD-3 beta criteria was labeled "unclassifiable."

The headache diaries included two intensity items: (1) "How intense was your worst headache today?", and (2) "How intense was your headache on average during the day?" Both items were rated on a 0–10 numerical rating scale (NRS), with 0 = No pain and 10 = Worst imaginable/unbearable pain. Other items included: "How did you function in your daily activities today?" (rated on a 0–3 scale: 0 = No difficulties, 1 = Minor difficulties, 2 = Medium difficulties, and 3 = Major difficulties); and "Did you take any acute medications to treat headache today?" (No/Yes).

A similar paper-based diary (0–5 scale) was originally developed for adults with headaches [23] but has been widely used in intervention studies with adolescents experiencing frequent headaches [24]. Participants who filled out their diary via the internet and who had not logged on before 9 PM each day were sent reminders through a short text message service (SMS). Those who used a paper-based diary were reminded once a week.

Categorization of headache frequency and medication use

Having a headache was defined as an NRS score of ≥1. For comparisons between questionnaire data, raw scores of headache frequency obtained from the diaries were categorized into three levels: ≤10 %, 11–49 %, and ≥50 % of the days. The corresponding levels and cutoff points in the questionnaire were: <3 days a month (≤10 %), 1–3 days a month or 1–3 days a week (11–49 %), and at least every other day (≥50 %).

The raw scores for medication use in the diary recordings were categorized as "Never," "Use medications but not very frequently" (at least once but less than 33.3 % of the days in diary recordings), and "Use medications frequently" (33.3 % or more of the recorded days).

Statistical analysis

Descriptive statistics with means, standard deviations (SD), and percentages with 95 % confidence intervals (CI) were computed. The sensitivity, specificity, positive predictive value (PPV), and negative predictive value (NPV) of interview information for having any headache, headaches ≥50 % of the days, and very frequent medication during the previous year were calculated relative to diary determinations of the same parameters. Kappa statistics with 95 % CI were used to assess the agreement between diary and interview data. Spearman's rank correlation coefficient (rho) was used to estimate relationships between ordinal variables. Independent t-tests and analysis of variance were used to estimate differences between group means. Differences between groups were analyzed with the McNemar–Bowker test of cell proportion symmetry. Statistical significance was set at a two-tailed p-value less than 0.05. All statistical analyses were performed with SPSS Statistics for Windows version 22 (IBM SPSS Statistics for Windows, Version 22.0. Armonk, NY: IBM Corp.).

Ethics

The research protocol was approved by the Norwegian Ethical Committee for Medical Research. Informed consent was obtained from each participant and documented in accordance with Ethical Committee requirements. Parental consent was obtained for participants younger than 16 years old.

Results

Study sample

The flow of participants through the different stages of the study is presented in Fig. 1.

Of the 488 adolescents aged 12–18 years who were interviewed, 276 (57 %) were girls and 212 (43 %) were boys. No participants were disqualified because of lack of internet access. Of the participating adolescents, 393 (81 %) returned diaries: 244 (62 %) girls and 149 (38 %) boys, with an average age of 15.1 ± 1.7 years. Of those who filled out diaries, 214 (54 %) used paper-based and 179 (46 %) used internet-based diaries. Paper-based diaries covered an average of 15.9 ± 8.9 days and internet diaries an average of 12.9 ± 6.9 days over the three-week period.

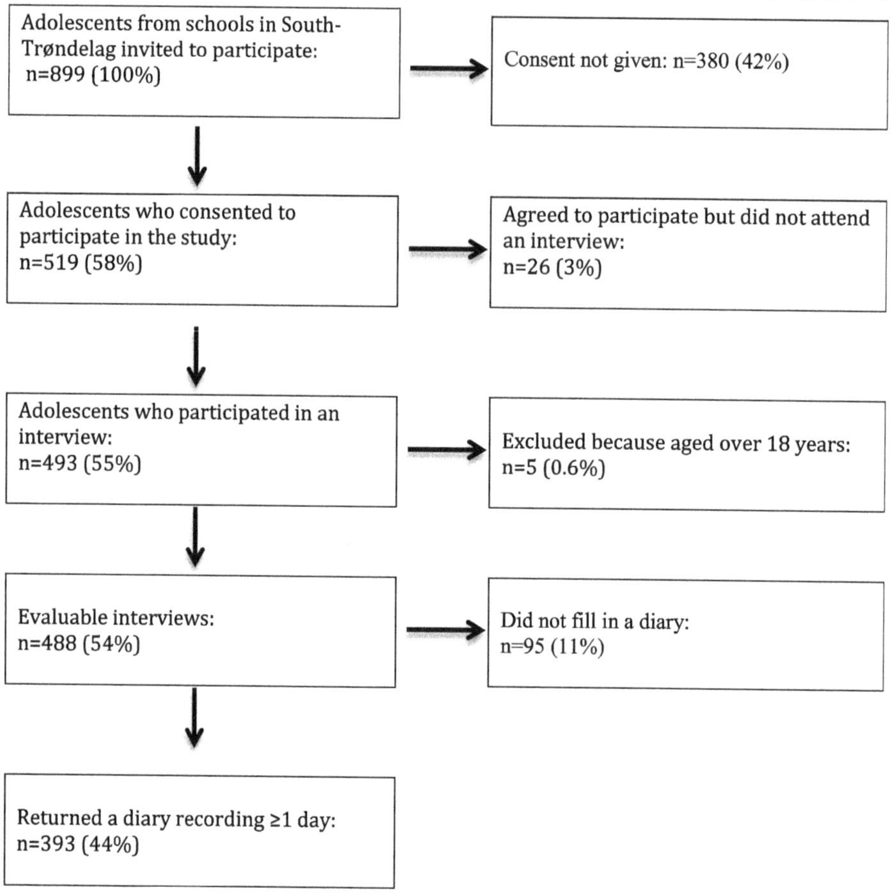

Fig. 1 Flow of participants through the study

Having headaches

Of the 393 participants who completed the interview and diary, 346 (88 %) retrospectively reported headaches in their interviews. Of these, 310 (90 %) reported only one type of headache, and 36 (10 %) reported more than one type. In total, 206 (53 %) were classified as TTH, 130 (33 %) as migraine or probable migraine, one (0.3 %) as MOH, and 11 (3 %) as unclassifiable. Of those who reported more than one type of headache, 31 (86 %) reported TTH as the second headache type and five had migraine or probable migraine.

Of the 346 participants who reported they had experienced headaches during the previous year, 304 (88 %) also documented headache occurrence in their diary. In contrast, of those who did not report a current headache disorder in their interview, 51 % recorded headaches in their diary (Table 1). Comparisons of headache frequency levels reported in interviews with the recorded

Table 1 Sensitivity, specificity, and predictive values of retrospective headache reports (last one year) vs. three-week prospective diary recordings

		Diary			
		Headache	No headache	Total	
Interview	Headache	304	42	346	PPV[a]:304/346 = 88 %
	No headache	23	24	47	NPV[b]:24/47 = 51 %
	Total	327	66	393	
		Sensitivity: 304/327 = 93 %	Specificity: 24/66 = 36 %		

Kappa: 0.33 (95 % CI: 0.20–0.45). McNemar–Bowker test of cell proportion symmetry: $p = 0.019$
[a]Positive predictive value
[b]Negative predictive value
Only participants who filled in the diary for ≥1 day are included in the table

days of headaches in diaries showed fair agreement, with a Kappa value of 0.33 (95 % CI: 0.20–0.45).

Headache frequency

Overall, the ratings of headache frequency were significantly higher in the diaries than in the interviews ($p < 0.001$). Although 81 % of participants retrospectively reported one type of active headache disorder during their interview and estimated the frequency as ≤10 % of days, only 27 % recorded such levels in their diary (Table 2). In interviews, the number of participants reporting headaches as occurring ≤10 % of the days was significantly higher than in diaries ($p < 0.001$). In contrast, diary reports of headaches on 11–49 % and ≥50 % of the days were significantly ($p < 0.001$) higher than in interviews. There was only a slight agreement between interview and diary reports of having headaches on at least 50 % of days and one or more headache disorders (Kappa 0.14, 95 % CI: 0.05–0.23; Table 3). Seventy four percent of participants who retrospectively reported having headaches on fewer than 50 % of days per month recorded such headaches in their diary (Table 3).

Headache intensity

During interviews, 30 (13.8 %) participants reported mild intensity, 132 (60.6 %) moderate intensity, and 56 (25.7 %) reported severe intensity. The mean ± SD NRS intensity score recorded in the diaries was 1.9 ± 0.83. For those who reported that they had headaches the previous year in their interview and also recorded at least one headache in their diary, there was a significant but low Spearman correlation between questionnaire intensity levels and mean diary NRS intensity scores (rho = 0.28, $p < 0.001$). Participants who reported headaches during the previous year had significantly higher average (t(199) = −6,39, $p < 0.001$) and worst (t(202) = −8.96, $p < 0.001$) intensity levels in their diary than those who did not.

Impairment

During the interviews, 207 (95 %) participants had a PedMIDAS score lower than 11 (the limit for a definition of mild disability) and only 11 (5 %) had higher scores. In the diaries, 29 (13.3 %) participants recorded no difficulties during the three-week period, 89 (40.8 %) reported minor difficulties, 71 (32.6 %) reported medium difficulties, and 29 (13.3 %) reported major difficulties. Total mean interview PedMIDAS scores showed significant Spearman correlations with average (rho = 0.36, $p < 0.001$) and maximum (rho = 0.25, $p < 0.001$) impairment scores in the diaries.

Table 2 Headache frequency reported by adolescents retrospectively (last one year) and during three-week prospective diary recordings

Headache frequency (proportion of days)	Interview ($n = 310$)	Diary ($n = 310$)	Overall	Post hoc test
	n (%)	n (%)	*p*-value	*p*-value[a]
≤10 %	252 (81.3)	84 (27.1)	<0.001	<0.001
11–49 %	49 (15.8)	147 (47.4)		<0.001
≥50 %	9 (2.9)	79 (25.5)		<0.001

Only participants who reported having had one type of headache last year in their interview and filled in the diary for ≥1 day are included in the table
[a]McNemar–Bowker test of cell proportion symmetry

Table 3 Sensitivity, specificity, and predictive values of headache for ≥50 % of days: retrospective reports (last one year) vs. three-week prospective diary recordings

		Diary			
		Headache ≥50 % days	Headache <50 % days	Total	
Interview	Headache ≥50 % days	10	1	11	PPV[a]: 10/11 = 91 %
	Headache <50 % days	86	249	335	NPV[b]: 249/335 = 74 %
	Total	96	250	346	
		Sensitivity: 10/96 = 10 %	Specificity: 249/250 = 99 %		

Kappa: 0.14 (95 % CI: 0.05–0.23). McNemar–Bowker test of cell proportion symmetry: $p < 0.001$
[a]Positive predictive value
[b]Negative predictive value
Only participants who reported having had a headache (at least one type) in the last year in their interview and who had filled in a diary for ≥1 day are included in the table

Medication use

Of participants who reported one or more current headache disorder during their interview, the frequency of medication use reported in diaries was significantly lower than that reported in interviews ($p < 0.001$) (Table 4). "No use of medication" was significantly more common in diary recordings ($p < 0.001$), whereas "Medication use but not very frequently" was significantly less common in diaries ($p < 0.001$). There was no agreement between information obtained in interviews and in diary recordings for very frequent medication use (Kappa −0.01, 95 % CI: −0.22–0.00). Of the 346 participants who reported headaches in their interview, only three (0.9 %) also reported very frequent medication use, whereas none of these participants documented very frequent medication use in their diary. In contrast, none of those (2.3 %) who recorded they used medication very frequently in their diary reported very frequent medication in their interview.

Medication type

In total, 329 participants used acute headache medication, and 171 (52.0 %) reported using only one class of drug: 154 (90.1 %) used paracetamol alone, 18 (10.5 %) used a nonsteroidal anti-inflammatory drug (NSAID),

Table 4 Frequency of medication use reported by adolescents: interviews (last one year) vs. three-week prospective diary recordings

Medication frequency	Interview ($n = 346$)	Diary ($n = 346$)	Overall	Post hoc
	n (%)	n (%)	*p*-value	*p*-value[a]
Never	82 (23.7)	198 (57.2)	<0.001	<0.001
Use but not very frequently	261 (75.4)	140 (40.5)		<0.001
Very frequently	3 (0.9)	8 (2.3)		0.23

Use but not very frequently: taking medication on 1 to <33.3 % of all recording days. Very frequent: taking medication on ≥33.3 % of all recording days
Only participants who reported having had headache (at least one type) during the last year in their interview and filled in the diary for ≥1 day are included in the table
[a]McNemar–Bowker test of cell proportion symmetry

and two (1.2 %) used triptans. Of the 155 participants who used combinations of two classes of acute drugs, 152 (98.1 %) used paracetamol and a NSAID, and three (1.9 %) were treated with paracetamol and codeine. Three participants used a combination of three classes of acute drugs: two used paracetamol, a NSAID, and codeine, and one used paracetamol, a NSAID, and triptans. Only three participants (0.3 %) were on prescriptive prophylactic drug treatment.

Discussion

This general population-based study of 393 school-aged adolescents investigated the agreement and relationships between retrospective interviews and prospectively recorded diaries over a three-week period to assess headache characteristics, impairment, and medication use. Overall, the findings showed low correlations and agreement between the two data sources for estimates of headache frequency and intensity, impairment, and medication use. The PPV was high, with most adolescents who reported headache during their interview also documenting a headache in subsequent diary recordings. However, the NPV was over 50 %, suggesting that diary data may identify more individuals with headaches than information obtained during a conventional interview. In the present study, more than half of those who did not report any headaches during their interview recorded a headache during the diary period, although these headaches were of low intensity. In a smaller school-based Swedish study with children and adolescents conducted in 2003, about one-third of those who did not report any headache in a questionnaire recorded headache in their three-week diary; these headaches were primarily of low intensity, a finding consistent with the results of the present study.

While the occurrence of low frequency headaches was higher in the interviews than in diary recordings, the occurrence of high frequency headaches was lower in interviews than in diaries. Similar comparisons have been made in four general population-based studies [7–9, 13]. The results of two of these studies, one Dutch [8] and one Finnish [13], are consistent with our findings [9], with the frequency of headache episodes showing good agreement between interview and prospective diary information.

Interestingly, our findings of a higher prevalence of headaches occurring every day or almost every day in diaries than in interviews resulted in a PPV of 91 %. Many participants who did not report such headache levels in interviews reported them in diaries. An NPV of 74 % indicated a high probability that very high headache frequencies will be captured in diaries, despite individuals stating in interviews that they do not have headaches. Further, a specificity of 99 % indicated there were few false positives. This finding has clear implications for the assessment of frequent and very frequent headaches among adolescents in schools and other health care settings.

Our finding of a low but significant correlation between headache intensity reported in interviews and prospective diary recordings is consistent with the results of a recent Swedish study with school children and adolescents [7]. In that study, headache intensity was higher in questionnaires than in diary recordings. Again, the discrepancy in these findings emphasizes the need for both retrospective interview data and prospective diary information.

Severe disability levels due to headache were rare, as shown in both interview and diary reports, and is consistent with findings for adolescents in the general German population [21]. The impairment levels observed in the present study contrasted strongly with those reported on the PedMIDAS for chronic pain, including headaches, in selected samples of adolescents referred to a tertiary clinic [19, 20]. The PedMIDAS categories were originally developed and validated in a clinical sample of children with migraine [19]. Children with chronic headaches scored much higher than children with non-chronic headaches, and higher than the adolescents in the present sample [8]. Thus, impairment levels in a clinical sample were less sensitive in assessing adolescents with very frequent or severe headaches.

Many adolescents who retrospectively reported use of analgesic medications did not confirm this in their diaries. However, this might have been due to the rather limited three-week recording period. Alternatively, the three-week diary period might have been sufficient to capture very frequent use of analgesic medications. Interestingly, none of the adolescents who reported these levels in interviews also documented them in diaries. The eight adolescents who reported very frequent use of analgesics in their diaries did not report this in their interviews.

This study had several limitations. Data in the diaries were not complete, owing to non-adherence to study protocols. This suggests the need for analyses to be based on the percentage of days completed [17]. This might have biased our estimates regarding the proportions of days with headache, because participants may have been more compliant with their diaries on days with than without a headache. Another limitation was our use of different scales for headache intensity and headache impairment in the interviews and diaries, preventing a determination of levels of agreement. The diary recordings were restricted to three weeks, a time period short enough to be subject to external influences of time factors in the school setting (e.g., variations in the burden of academic work and stress load). The limited recording period might have biased our assessments of retrospective reports of headaches experienced during the previous year compared with a somewhat different but adjacent recording period of three weeks. However, the limited recording period chosen for this study was intended to optimize user adherence among adolescents attending regular schools. Such a time period is also thought to be optimal for recordings of frequent headaches [7, 25–27].

A strength of the present study was its inclusion of a relatively large sample representative of adolescents in the general population, enabling us to extrapolate our results to the general community. Another strength was the lack of delay between completion of the interviews and initiation of diary recordings. The study was conducted over a one-year period (two semesters) and was not restricted to a specific school time or activity. This means that recall bias for the last year potentially caused by particularly restful or stressful periods, such as recently having had a vacation or school examinations, were evenly balanced. Our study also included headaches occurring every day or almost every day, and of the chronic tension type, MOH, or chronic migraine [22]. Our definition of medication use on at least one-third of the days was specifically investigated, because of its clinical use as a definition of MOH.

Conclusions

There was low agreement and correlation of headache characteristics, impairment, and medication use between retrospective questionnaires and prospective diary information. This suggests that a diary given to an adolescent with headaches may provide information complementary to that obtained during a clinical interview. These findings suggest the usefulness of keeping diaries for children and adolescents with recurrent headaches in school health care systems and clinical services.

The findings also suggest a need for additional general population-based studies, addressing agreements between retrospective and prospective reports when assessing various characteristics of head pain, disability, and medication use. Further work is needed to determine the optimal recording timeframe for diary recordings, as adherence rates may decrease over time, thus reducing the validity of estimates. Various types of reminders may also enhance participation rates in similar community-based surveys.

Abbreviations

ICHD-3 beta: the third International Classification of Headache Disorders (2013), a beta version; MOH: Medication overuse headache; NPV: Negative predictive value; NSAID: Non-steroidal anti-inflammatory drug; PedMIDAS: Pediatric Migraine Disability Assessment; PPV: Positive predictive value; TTH: Tension-type headache.

Competing interests

The authors declare that they have no competing interests.

Author contributions

Study concept and design: BL, ML. Acquisition of data: ABK. Statistical analysis: ØS. Writing of the manuscript: ABK, ML, BL, ØS. Critical revision of the manuscript for important intellectual content: ML, BL. Final approval of the version to be submitted: ABK, ML, BL, ØS.

Acknowledgments

The authors express their gratitude to participating students and the directors and staff of participating schools for their cooperation and contribution to this study. The authors would also like to thank Dean Per Borgersen and students, Per Stian Hoff, Malene Dae, and Ida Rosèn, at the Faculty of Informatics and e-Learning at the University College of South-Trøndelag, Norway, for their cooperation in developing and maintaining the procedures and program for the internet diary.

Author details

[1]Department of Neuroscience, Faculty of Medicine, Norwegian University of Science and Technology, N-7489 Trondheim, Norway. [2]Faculty of Health and Social Science, Norwegian University of Science and Technology, Trondheim, Norway. [3]Regional Centre for Child and Youth Mental Health and Child Welfare, Central Norway, Norwegian University of Science and Technology, Trondheim, Norway. [4]Unit for Applied Clinical Research, Faculty of Medicine, Norwegian University of Science and Technology, Trondheim, Norway. [5]Norwegian Advisory Unit on Headaches, St. Olav's University Hospital, Trondheim, Norway.

References

1. Berg Kelly K, Ehrvér M, Erneholm T, Gundevall C, Wennerberg L (1991) Self-reported health status and use of medical care by 3,500 adolescents in western Sweden. Acta Paediatr Scand 80:837–843
2. Laurell K, Larsson B, Eeg-Olofsson O (2004) Prevalence of headache in Swedish schoolchildren, with a focus on tension-type headache. Cephalalgia 24:380–388
3. Anttila P, Metsähonkala L, Sillanpää M (2006) Long-term trends in the incidence of headache in Finnish schoolchildren. Pediatrics 117:1197–1201
4. Karwautz A, Wöber C, Lang T, Bïck A, Wagner-Ennsgraber C, Vesely C, Kienbacher C, Wöber-Bingöl C (1999) Psychosocial factors in children and adolescents with migraine and tension-type headache: a controlled study and review of the litterature. Cephalalgia 19:32–43
5. Kernick D, Reinhold D, JI C (2009) Impact of headache on young people in a school population. Br J Gen Pract 59(566):678–81
6. Larsson B (2009) Migrän och spänningshuvudvärk hos barn och tonåringar. (Migraine and tension-type headache among children and adolescents). Studentlitteratur, Lund
7. Larsson B, Fichtel A (2014) Headache prevalence and characteristics among adolescents in the general population: a comparison between retrospect questionnaire and prospective paper diary data. J Headache Pain 15:1–10. doi:10.1186/1129-2377-15-80

8. van den Brink M, Bandell-Hoekstra EN, Abu-Saad HH (2001) The occurrence of recall bias in pediatric headache: a comparison of questionnaire and diary data. Headache 41:11–20
9. Laurell K, Larsson B, Eeg-Olofsson O (2003) Headache in schoolchildren: agreement between different sources of information. Cephalalgia 23:420–428
10. Lundqvist C, Clench-Aas J, Hofoss D, Bartonova A (2006) Self-reported headache in schoolchildren: parents underestimate their children's headaches. Acta Paediatr 95:940–946. doi:10.1080/08035250600678810
11. Richardson G, McGrath P, Cunningham S, Humphreys P (1983) Validity of the headache diary for children. Headache 23:184–187
12. Labbé EE, Williamsson DA, Southard DR (1985) Reliability and validity of children's reports of migraine headache symptoms. J Psychopathol Behav Assess 7:375–383
13. Metsähonkala L, Sillanpää M, Tuominen J (1997) Headache diary in the diagnosis of childhood migraine. Headache 37:240–244
14. Lewandowski AS, Palermo TM, Kirchner LH, Drotar D (2009) Comparing diary and retrospective reports of pain and activity restriction in children and adolescents with chronic pain conditions. Clin J Pain 25:299–306
15. Heyer GL, Perkins SQ, Rose SC, Aylward SC, Lee JM (2014) Comparing patient and parent recall of 90-day and 30-day migraine disability using elements of the PedMIDAS and an Internet headache diary. Cephalalgia 34(4):298–306
16. Krogh A-B, Larsson B, Linde M (2015) Prevalence and disability of headache among Norwegian adolescents: a cross-sectional school-based study. Cephalalgia 35(13):1181–91
17. Krogh A-B, Larsson B, Salvesen Ø, Linde M (2015) A comparision between prospective Internet-based and paper diary recordings of headache among adolescents in the general population. Cephalalgia Online First Service June:1–11
18. Laurell K, Larsson B, Eeg-Olofsson O (2005) Headache in schoolchildren: Association with other pain, family history and psychosocial factors. Pain 119(119):150–158
19. Hershey AD, Powers SW, Vockell AL, LeCates SL, Segers A, Kabbouche MA (2004) Development of a patient-based grading scale for PedMIDAS. Cephalalgia 24:844–849. doi:10.1111/j.1468-2982.2004.00757.x
20. Hershey AD, Powers SW, Vockell AL, LeCates S, Kabbouche MA, Maynard MK (2001) PedMIDAS: development of a questionnaire to assess disability of migraines in children. Neurology 57:2034–2039
21. Kroner-Herwig B, Heinrich M, Vath N (2010) The assessment of disability in children and adolescents with headache: adopting PedMIDAS in an epidemiological study. Eur J Pain 14:951–958. doi:10.1016/j.ejpain.2010.02.010
22. Headache Classification Committee of the International Headache Society (2013) The International Classification of Headache Disorders, 3rd edition (beta version). Cephalalgia 33:629–808. doi:10.1177/0333102413485658
23. Blanchard EB, Andrasik F (1985) The headache diary. Management of headaches: a psychological approach. Chapter 5. Pergamon Press, New York
24. Larsson B, Carlsson J, Fichtel Å, Melin I (2005) Relaxation treatment of recurrent headache among adolescents: results from a school-based replication series. Headache 45:692–704
25. Osterhaus SO, Passchier J (1992) The optimal length of headache recording in juvenile migraine patients. Cephalalgia 12:297–299
26. Larsson B, Fichtel A (2012) Headache prevalence and characteristics among school children as assessed by prospective paper diary recordings. J Headache Pain 13:129–136. doi:10.1007/s10194-011-0410-9
27. Andrasik F, Lipchik GL, McCrory DC, Wittrock DA (2005) Outcome measurement in behavioral headache research: headache parameters and psychosocial outcomes. Headache 45:429–437. doi:10.1111/j.1526-4610.2005.05094.x

Permissions

All chapters in this book were first published in TJHP, by Springer; hereby published with permission under the Creative Commons Attribution License or equivalent. Every chapter published in this book has been scrutinized by our experts. Their significance has been extensively debated. The topics covered herein carry significant findings which will fuel the growth of the discipline. They may even be implemented as practical applications or may be referred to as a beginning point for another development.

The contributors of this book come from diverse backgrounds, making this book a truly international effort. This book will bring forth new frontiers with its revolutionizing research information and detailed analysis of the nascent developments around the world.

We would like to thank all the contributing authors for lending their expertise to make the book truly unique. They have played a crucial role in the development of this book. Without their invaluable contributions this book wouldn't have been possible. They have made vital efforts to compile up to date information on the varied aspects of this subject to make this book a valuable addition to the collection of many professionals and students.

This book was conceptualized with the vision of imparting up-to-date information and advanced data in this field. To ensure the same, a matchless editorial board was set up. Every individual on the board went through rigorous rounds of assessment to prove their worth. After which they invested a large part of their time researching and compiling the most relevant data for our readers.

The editorial board has been involved in producing this book since its inception. They have spent rigorous hours researching and exploring the diverse topics which have resulted in the successful publishing of this book. They have passed on their knowledge of decades through this book. To expedite this challenging task, the publisher supported the team at every step. A small team of assistant editors was also appointed to further simplify the editing procedure and attain best results for the readers.

Apart from the editorial board, the designing team has also invested a significant amount of their time in understanding the subject and creating the most relevant covers. They scrutinized every image to scout for the most suitable representation of the subject and create an appropriate cover for the book.

The publishing team has been an ardent support to the editorial, designing and production team. Their endless efforts to recruit the best for this project, has resulted in the accomplishment of this book. They are a veteran in the field of academics and their pool of knowledge is as vast as their experience in printing. Their expertise and guidance has proved useful at every step. Their uncompromising quality standards have made this book an exceptional effort. Their encouragement from time to time has been an inspiration for everyone.

The publisher and the editorial board hope that this book will prove to be a valuable piece of knowledge for researchers, students, practitioners and scholars across the globe.

List of Contributors

Kedar Manandhar and Ajay Risal
Department of Neuroscience, Norwegian University of Science and Technology, Edvard Griegs Gate, Trondheim, NO 7489, Norway
Dhulikhel Hospital, Kathmandu University Hospital, Kavre, Dhulikhel, Nepal

Timothy J. Steiner
Division of Brain Sciences, Imperial College London, London, UK
Department of Neuroscience, Norwegian University of Science and Technology, Edvard Griegs Gate, Trondheim, NO 7489, Norway

Martina Curto
Department of Psychiatry, Harvard Medical School, Boston, MA, USA
Department of Molecular Medicine, Sant'Andrea Medical Center, Sapienza University of Rome, Via di Grottarossa 1035-1039, Rome 00189, Italy
Regional referral headache center, Sant'Andrea Hospital, Rome, Italy

Francesca Perugino
Department of Molecular Medicine, Sant'Andrea Medical Center, Sapienza University of Rome, Via di Grottarossa 1035-1039, Rome 00189, Italy

Maurizio Simmaco, Luana Lionetto and Matilde Capi
Advanced Molecular Diagnostics, IDI-IRCCS, Rome, Italy

Paolo Martelletti
Regional referral headache center, Sant'Andrea Hospital, Rome, Italy
Department of Molecular Medicine, Sant'Andrea Medical Center, Sapienza University of Rome, Via di Grottarossa 1035-1039, Rome 00189, Italy

Francesco Fazio
IRCCS Neuromed, Pozzilli, Italy

Andrea Negro
Department of Molecular Medicine, Sant'Andrea Medical Center, Sapienza University of Rome, Via di Grottarossa 1035-1039, Rome 00189, Italy
Advanced Molecular Diagnostics, IDI-IRCCS, Rome, Italy

Maria Adele Giamberardino
Headache Center and Geriatrics Clinic, Department of Medicine and Science of Aging, "G. D'Annunzio" University, Chieti, Italy

Ferdinando Nicoletti
IRCCS Neuromed, Pozzilli, Italy Department of Physiology and Pharmacology, Sapienza University of Rome, Rome, Italy

Sebastian Bao Dinh Bui, Torben Petersen, Jeppe Nørgaard Poulsen and Parisa Gazerani
Department of Health science and Technology, Faculty of Medicine, Aalborg University, Aalborg, Denmark

Are Holen
Pain Unit, St Olavs University Hospital, Trondheim, Norway
Department of Neuroscience, Norwegian University of Science and Technology, Nevrosenteret Øst, St Olavs Hospital, 7006 Trondheim, Norway

Ching-I Hung and Chia-Yih Liu
Department of Psychiatry, Chang Gung Memorial Hospital, Linkou, Taiwan
Chang Gung University College of Medicine, Tao-Yuan, Taiwan

Ching-Hui Yang
Department of Nursing, Chang Gung University of Science and Technology, Tao-Yuan, Taiwan

Shuu-Jiun Wang
Faculty of Medicine, National Yang-Ming University School of Medicine and Neurological Institute, Taipei Veterans General Hospital, Taipei, Taiwan
Department of Neurology, Taipei Veterans General Hospital, No. 201 Shi-Pai Road, Section 2, Taipei 112, Taiwan

Sabrina Khan, Faisal Mohammad Amin, Julie Falkenberg Petersen, Zainab Fakhril-Din and Messoud Ashina
Danish Headache Center, Department of Neurology, Rigshospitalet Glostrup, Faculty of Health and Medical Sciences, University of Copenhagen, Nordre Ringvej 57, Glostrup 2600, Denmark

John Hauerberg
Department of Neurosurgery, Rigshospitalet, Faculty of Health and Medical Sciences, University of Copenhagen, Copenhagen, Denmark

Markus Holtmannspötter
Department of Radiology, Rigshospitalet, Faculty of Health and Medical Sciences, University of Copenhagen, Copenhagen, Denmark

David Gaist
Department of Neurology, Odense University Hospital, Odense, Denmark
Department of Clinical Research, Faculty of Health Sciences, University of Southern Denmark, Odense, Denmark

Girish N. Rao and Gopalkrishna Gururaj
Department of Epidemiology, National Institute of Mental Health and Neuro Sciences (NIMHANS), Bengaluru, India

Girish B. Kulkarni
Department of Neurology, National Institute of Mental Health and Neuro Sciences (NIMHANS), Bengaluru, India

Lars J. Stovner
Norwegian Advisory Unit on Headache, Nevrosenteret Øst, St Olavs University Hospital, Trondheim, Norway
Department of Neuroscience, Norwegian University of Science and Technology (NTNU), Edvard Griegs Gate, Trondheim NO-7491, Norway

Mehila Zebenigus
Department of Neurology, School of Medicine, College of Health Science, Addis Ababa University, Addis Ababa, Ethiopia

Redda Tekle-Haimanot
Department of Internal Medicine, School of Medicine, College of Health Science, Addis Ababa University, Addis Ababa, Ethiopia

Dawit K. Worku
Department of Internal Medicine, Bahir Dar University, Bahir Dar, Ethiopia

Hallie Thomas
Department of Neuroscience, Norwegian University of Science and Technology (NTNU), Edvard Griegs Gate, NO-7491 Trondheim, Norway

María Palacios-Ceña and César Fernández-de-las-Peñas
Department Physical Therapy, Occupational Therapy, Rehabilitation, and Physical Medicine, University Rey Juan Carlos, Alcorcón, Spain
Center for Sensory-Motor Interaction (SMI), Department of Health Science and Technology, School of Medicine, Aalborg University, Aalborg, Denmark

Lars Arendt-Nielsen and Kelun Wang
Center for Sensory-Motor Interaction (SMI), Department of Health Science and Technology, School of Medicine, Aalborg University, Aalborg, Denmark

Juan J. Fernández-Muñoz
Department of Psychology, Universidad Rey Juan Carlos, Alcorcón, Spain

Matteo Castaldo
Master in Sport Physiotherapy, University of Siena, Siena, Italy
Poliambulatorio Fisiocenter, Collecchio, Parma, Italy
Center for Sensory-Motor Interaction (SMI), Department of Health Science and Technology, School of Medicine, Aalborg University, Aalborg, Denmark

Ángel Guerrero-Peral
Headache Unit. Hospital Clínico Universitario de Valladolid, Valladolid, Spain

Bettina Winzeler, Nicole Nigro, Cornelia Mueller and Mirjam Christ-Crain
Division of Endocrinology, Department of Internal Medicine, University Hospital Basel, Basel, Switzerland

Claudine Angela Blum
Division of Endocrinology, Department of Internal Medicine, University Hospital Basel, Basel, Switzerland
Internal Medicine, Medical University Clinic, Kantonsspital Aarau, Tellstrasse, CH-5001 Aarau, Switzerland

Krassen Nedeltchev, Katharina Haaf, Janina Tepperberg, Silke Biethahn and Timo Kahles
Department of Neurology, Medical University Clinic, Kantonsspital Aarau, Aarau, Switzerland

Beat Müller and Philipp Schuetz
Internal Medicine, Medical University Clinic, Kantonsspital Aarau, Tellstrasse, CH-5001 Aarau, Switzerland

Margareth Amort
Clinic of Neurology, University Hospital Basel, Basel, Switzerland

Andreas Huber
Center of Laboratory Medicine, Kantonsspital Aarau, Aarau, Switzerland

Roland Bingisser
Emergency Department, University Hospital Basel, Basel, Switzerland

Peter Stephan Sándor
Neurology, RehaClinic AG, Bad Zurzach, Switzerland

Mira Katan
Clinic of Neurology, University Hospital Zürich, Zürich, Switzerland

Katharina Timper
Max-Planck-Institute for Metabolism Research, Cologne, Germany
Division of Endocrinology, Department of Internal Medicine, University Hospital Basel, Basel, Switzerland

A. A. Herekar
Headache Research Foundation of Pakistan, Karachi, Pakistan
Department of Surgery, University of Texas at San Antonio, San Antonio, TX, USA

A. Ahmad, U. L. Uqaili and J. Effendi
Dow University of Health Sciences, Karachi, Pakistan
Headache Research Foundation of Pakistan, Karachi, Pakistan

B. Ahmed
Department of Neurology, Center for Movement Disorders and Neurorestoration, University of Florida College of Medicine, Gainesville, FL, USA
Headache Research Foundation of Pakistan, Karachi, Pakistan

S. Z. Alvi
Headache Research Foundation of Pakistan, Karachi, Pakistan
Department of Medicine, University of Nevada, Las Vegas, USA

M. A. Shahab
Aga Khan Medical College, Aga Khan Medical University Hospital, Karachi, Pakistan

U. Javed
School of International and Public Affairs, Columbia University, New York, NY, USA

A. D. Herekar
Department of Neurology, Baqai Medical University, Karachi, Pakistan
Headache Research Foundation of Pakistan, Karachi, Pakistan

Rafiq Khanani
Department of Pathology and Microbiology Department at Dow University of Health Sciences, Karachi, Pakistan

T. J. Steiner
Department of Neuroscience, Norwegian University of Science and Technology (NTNU), Edvard Griegs Gate, NO-7491 Trondheim, Norway Division of Brain Sciences, Imperial College London, London, UK

Dong Yeop Kim, Mi Ji Lee, Hyun Ah Choi and Chin-Sang Chung
Department of Neurology, Samsung Medical Center, Sungkyunkwan University School of Medicine, Seoul, Korea

Hanna Choi
Department of Neurology, Eulji University Hospital, Eulji University School of Medicine, Daejeon, Korea

Elena Benito-González
Department of Physical Therapy, Occupational Therapy, Physical Medicine and Rehabilitation, Universidad Rey Juan Carlos, Alcorcón, Spain

Lars Arendt-Nielsen and Kelun Wang
Center for Sensory-Motor Interaction (SMI), Department of Health Science and Technology, Faculty of Medicine, Aalborg University, Aalborg, Denmark

María Palacios-Ceña
Department of Physical Therapy, Occupational Therapy, Physical Medicine and Rehabilitation, Universidad Rey Juan Carlos, Alcorcón, Spain
Center for Sensory-Motor Interaction (SMI), Department of Health Science and Technology, Faculty of Medicine, Aalborg University, Aalborg, Denmark

Matteo Castaldo
Department of Physical Therapy, University of Siena, Siena, Italy Poliambulatorio Fisiocenter, Collecchio, Parma, Italy
Center for Sensory-Motor Interaction (SMI), Department of Health Science and Technology, Faculty of Medicine, Aalborg University, Aalborg, Denmark

César Fernández-de-las-Peñas
Facultad de Ciencias de la Salud, Universidad Rey Juan Carlos, Avenida de Atenas s/n, 28922 Alcorcón, Madrid, Spain
Department of Physical Therapy, Occupational Therapy, Physical Medicine and Rehabilitation, Universidad Rey Juan Carlos, Alcorcón, Spain
Center for Sensory-Motor Interaction (SMI), Department of Health Science and Technology, Faculty of Medicine, Aalborg University, Aalborg, Denmark

Pil-Wook Chung
Department of Neurology, Kangbuk Samsung Hospital, Sungkyunkwan University School of Medicine, Seoul, Republic of Korea

Soo-Jin Cho
Department of Neurology, Dongtan Sacred Heart Hospital, Hallym University College of Medicine, Hwaseong, Republic of Korea

Won-Joo Kim
Department of Neurology, Gangnam Severance Hospital, Yonsei University, College of Medicine, Seoul, Republic of Korea

Kwang Ik Yang
Department of Neurology, Soonchunhyang University College of Medicine, Cheonan Hospital, Cheonan, Republic of Korea

Chang-Ho Yun
Department of Neurology, Bundang Clinical Neuroscience Institute, Seoul National University Bundang Hospital, Seongnam, Republic of Korea

Min Kyung Chu
Department of Neurology, Kangnam Sacred Heart Hospital, Hallym University College of Medicine, 1 Singil-ro, Yeongdeungpo-gu, Seoul 07441, Republic of Korea

Jin-Yang Joo, Min A Kwon and Yong Bae Kim
Department of Neurosurgery, Gangnam Severance Hospital, Yonsei University College of Medicine, 211, Eonjuro, Gangnam-gu, Seoul 135-720, Republic of Korea

Chang-Ki Hong
Severance Institute for Vascular and Metabolic Research, Yonsei University, Seoul, Republic of Korea
Department of Neurosurgery, Gangnam Severance Hospital, Yonsei University College of Medicine, 211, Eonjuro, Gangnam-gu, Seoul 135-720, Republic of Korea

Yu Shik Shim
Department of Neurosurgery, Inha University School of Medicine and Hospital, Incheon, Republic of Korea

Sook Young Sim
Department of Neurosurgery, Inje University Seoul Paik Hospital, Seoul, Republic of Korea

Joonho Chung
Department of Neurological Surgery, Rush University Medical Center, 1725 W. Harrison St., Professional Building Suite 855, Chicago, IL 60612, USA
Department of Neurosurgery, Gangnam Severance Hospital, Yonsei University College of Medicine, 211, Eonjuro, Gangnam-gu, Seoul 135-720, Republic of Korea
Severance Institute for Vascular and Metabolic Research, Yonsei University, Seoul, Republic of Korea

Daiva Rastenytė and Dalia Mickevičienė
Lithuanian University of Health Sciences, Kaunas, Lithuania

Hallie Thomas
Department of Neuromedicine and Movement Science, Faculty of Medicine and Health Sciences, NTNU Norwegian University of Science and Technology, Trondheim NO-7941, Norway

Lars Jacob Stovner
Norwegian Advisory Unit on Headache, St Olavs University Hospital, Trondheim, Norway
Department of Neuromedicine and Movement Science, Faculty of Medicine and Health Sciences, NTNU Norwegian University of Science and Technology, Trondheim NO-7941, Norway

Colette Andrée
Department of Pharmaceutical Sciences, University of Basel, Basel, Switzerland

Jin-Yang Joo, Min A Kwon and Yong Bae Kim
Department of Neurosurgery, Gangnam Severance Hospital, Yonsei University College of Medicine, 211, Eonjuro, Gangnam-gu, Seoul 06273, Republic of Korea

Joonho Chung
Department of Neurosurgery, Gangnam Severance Hospital, Yonsei University College of Medicine, 211, Eonjuro, Gangnam-gu, Seoul 06273, Republic of Korea
Department of Neurological Surgery, Rush University Medical Center, 1725 W. Harrison St., Professional Building Suite 855, Chicago, IL 60612, USA
Severance Institute for Vascular and Metabolic Research, Yonsei University, Seoul, Republic of Korea

Chang-Ki Hong
Severance Institute for Vascular and Metabolic Research, Yonsei University, Seoul, Republic of Korea
Department of Neurosurgery, Gangnam Severance Hospital, Yonsei University College of Medicine, 211, Eonjuro, Gangnam-gu, Seoul 06273, Republic of Korea

Yu Shik Shim
Department of Neurosurgery, Inha University School of Medicine and Hospital, Incheon, Republic of Korea

Sook Young Sim
Department of Neurosurgery, Inje University Seoul Paik Hospital, Seoul, Republic of Korea

Jiyoung Kim
Department of Neurology, Bio Medical Research Institute, Pusan National University Hospital, Pusan National University School of Medicine, Busan, Korea

Soo-Jin Cho
Department of Neurology, Dongtan Sacred Heart Hospital, Hallym University College of Medicine, Hwaseong, Korea

Won-Joo Kim
Department of Neurology, Gangnam Severance Hospital, Yonsei University, College of Medicine, Seoul, Korea

Kwang Ik Yang
Department of Neurology, Soonchunhyang University College of Medicine, Cheonan Hospital, Cheonan, Korea

Chang-Ho Yun
Department of Neurology, Bundang Clinical Neuroscience Institute, Seoul National University Bundang Hospital, Seongnam, Korea

Min Kyung Chu
Department of Neurology, Kangnam Sacred Heart Hospital, Hallym University College of Medicine, 1 Singil-ro, Yeongdeungpo-gu, Seoul 07441, Korea

Mads Barloese
Department of Clinical Physiology, Nuclear Medicine and PET, Rigshospitalet-Glostrup, Nordre Ringvej 57, 2600 Glostrup, Denmark
Danish Headache Centre, Department of Neurology, Rigshospitalet-Glostrup, Nordre Ringvej 57, 2600 Glostrup, Denmark

Anja Petersen and Rigmor Højland Jensen
Danish Headache Centre, Department of Neurology, Rigshospitalet-Glostrup, Nordre Ringvej 57, 2600 Glostrup, Denmark

Philipp Stude
Schmerztherapie, Geriatrie und Palliativmedizin, Bochum, Kurt-Schumacher-Platz, 11-12 44787 Bochum, Germany

Tim Jürgens
Department of Neurology, University Medical Center Rostock, Gehlsherimer Str. 20, 18147 Rostock, Germany

Arne May
Department of Systems Neuroscience, Universitäts-Klinikum Hamburg-Eppendorf, Martinistraße 52, 20246 Hamburg, Germany

Stella Fuensalida-Novo
Department Physical Therapy, Occupational Therapy, Rehabilitation, and Physical Medicine, Facultad de Ciencias de la Salud, University Rey Juan Carlos, Avenida de Atenas s/n, 28922 Alcorcón, Madrid, Spain

Maria Palacios-Ceña
Department Physical Therapy, Occupational Therapy, Rehabilitation, and Physical Medicine, Facultad de Ciencias de la Salud, University Rey Juan Carlos, Avenida de Atenas s/n, 28922 Alcorcón, Madrid, Spain

César Fernández-de-las-Peñas
Department Physical Therapy, Occupational Therapy, Rehabilitation, and Physical Medicine, Facultad de Ciencias de la Salud, University Rey Juan Carlos, Avenida de Atenas s/n, 28922 Alcorcón, Madrid, Spain
Center for Sensory-Motor Interaction (SMI), Department of Health Science and Technology, Faculty of Medicine, Aalborg University, Aalborg, Denmark

Lars Arendt-Nielsen and Kelun Wang
Center for Sensory-Motor Interaction (SMI), Department of Health Science and Technology, Faculty of Medicine, Aalborg University, Aalborg, Denmark

Juan J. Fernández- Muñoz
Department of Psychology, Universidad Rey Juan Carlos, Alcorcón, Spain

Matteo Castaldo
Master in Sport Physiotherapy, University of Siena, Siena, Italy
Center for Sensory-Motor Interaction (SMI), Department of Health Science and Technology, Faculty of Medicine, Aalborg University, Aalborg, Denmark
Poliambulatorio Fisiocenter, Collecchio, (Parma), Italy

Antonella Catena
Poliambulatorio Fisiocenter, Collecchio, (Parma), Italy

Lena Hoem Nordhaug
Department of Neuromedicine and Movement Science (INB), Faculty of Medicine and Health Sciences, Norwegian University of Science and Technology, 7491 Trondheim, Norway

Knut Hagen, Lars Jacob Stovner and Mattias Linde
Department of Neuromedicine and Movement Science (INB), Faculty of Medicine and Health Sciences, Norwegian University of Science and Technology, 7491 Trondheim, Norway
Norwegian Advisory Unit on Headaches, St. Olavs University Hospital, Trondheim, Norway

Anne Vik
Department of Neuromedicine and Movement Science (INB), Faculty of Medicine and Health Sciences, Norwegian University of Science and Technology, 7491 Trondheim, Norway
Department of Neurosurgery, St. Olavs University Hospital, Trondheim, Norway

Gøril Bruvik Gravdahl
Norwegian Advisory Unit on Headaches, St. Olavs University Hospital, Trondheim, Norway

Turid Follestad
Department of Public Health and Nursing, Faculty of Medicine and Health Sciences, Norwegian University of Science and Technology, Trondheim, Norway

Torunn Pedersen
Division of Mental Health and Addiction, Oslo University Hospital, Oslo, Norway

Jong-Hee Sohn
Department of Neurology, Chuncheon Sacred Heart Hospital, Hallym
University College of Medicine, Chuncheon-si, Gangwon-do, Korea

Min-Kyung Chu
Department of Neurology, Severance Hospital, Yonsei University College of Medicine, Seoul, Korea

Kwang-Yeol Park
Department of Neurology, Chung-Ang University Hospital, Chung-Ang University College of Medicine, Seoul, Korea

Hong-Yup Ahn
Department of Statistics, Dongguk University-Seoul, Seoul, Korea

Soo-Jin Cho
Department of Neurology, Dongtan Sacred Heart Hospital, Hallym University College of Medicine, Keun Jae Bong-gil 7, Hwaseong, Gyeonggi-do 18450, Korea

Katrine Falkenberg and Jes Olesen
Danish Headache Center and Department of Neurology, University of Copenhagen, Rigshospitalet Glostrup, Copenhagen, Denmark
Danish Headache Center, Department of Neurology N39, Rigshospitalet Glostrup, University of Copenhagen, Valdemar Hansens vej 5, DK-2600 Glostrup, Denmark

Debora De Carlo, Irene Toldo, Barbara Bolzonella, Stefano Sartori, Michela Gatta and Pier Antonio Battistella
Juvenile Headache Centre, University of Padua, via Giustiniani 3, 35128 Padua, Italy

Agnese Maria Tamborino and Alberto Verrotti
L'Aquila, Department of Pediatrics, San Salvatore Hospital, University of L'Aquila, L'Aquila, Italy

Maria Giuseppina Ledda
Department of Child and Adolescent Neuropsychiatry, University Hospital of Cagliari, Cagliari, Italy

Lucia Margari
Child Neuropsychiatry Unit, Department of Neuroscience and Sense Organs, University of "Aldo Moro" Bari, Bari, Italy

Vincenzo Raieli
Child Neuropsychiatry Unit, Di Cristina Hospital, ARNAS civico, Palermo, Italy

Margherita Santucci
Department of Child Neuropsychiatry, Università degli Studi di Bologna Scuola di Medicina e Chirurgia, Bologna, Italy

Vittorio Sciruicchio
Neurologic and Psychiatric Sciences Department, Ist Neurological Clinic, Bari, Italy

Angelo Vecchio
Department of Child Neuropsychiatry, Università degli Studi di Palermo, Palermo, Italy

Sergio Zanini
IRCCS "La Nostra Famiglia - E. Medea", Pasian di Prato, Udine, Italy

Minwoo Lee, Juyoung Lee, Jinhyuk Yoo and Hong Ki Song
Department of Neurology, Kangdong Sacred Heart Hospital, Hallym University Medical Center, Seongan-ro 150, Gangdong-gu, Seoul 134-701, South Korea

Min Kyung Chu
Department of Neurology, Kangnam Sacred Heart Hospital, Hallym University, Seoul, South Korea

Annelien De Pue, and Koen Paemeleire
Department of Neurology, Ghent University Hospital, De Pintelaan 185, B-9000 Ghent, Belgium

Bart Lutin
Department of Radiology, Ghent University Hospital, Ghent, Belgium

Ninett Louise Find
Faculty of Health Science, University of Copenhagen, Copenhagen, Denmark
Danish Headache Center, Neurological Department, Glostrup Hospital, Glostrup, Denmark

Rigmor Jensen, Lars Bendtsen and Signe Bruun Munksgaard
Danish Headache Center, Neurological Department, Glostrup Hospital, Glostrup, Denmark

Rossana Terlizzi
Danish Headache Center, Neurological Department, Glostrup Hospital, Glostrup, Denmark
Department of Biomedical and NeuroMotor Sciences (DIBINEM), Alma Mater Studiorum, Bologna University, Ospedale Bellaria, Bologna, Italy

Giuseppe Nappi and Cristina Tassorelli
Headache Science Center, C. Mondino National Neurological Institute C. Mondino Foundation, Dept. of Brain and Behavioral Sciences, University of Pavia, Pavia, Italy

Zaza Katsarava
Department of Neurology, University Hospital of Essen, Essen, Germany

Miguel Lainez
Foundation of the Valencian Community, University Clinical Hospital, Barcelona, Spain

Maria Teresa Goicochea
Foundation for Combating Neurological Diseases of Childhood, Buenos Aires, Argentina

Beatriz Shand and Ricardo Fadic
8Pontificia Universidad Católica de Chile, Santiago, Chile

Santiago Spadafora
Universidad Isalud, Buenos Aires, Argentina

Marco Pagani
Bioengineering and Medical Informatics Consortium, Pavia, Italy

Anne-Berit Krogh
Department of Neuroscience, Faculty of Medicine, Norwegian University of Science and Technology, N-7489 Trondheim, Norway

Faculty of Health and Social Science, Norwegian University of Science and Technology, Trondheim, Norway

Bo Larsson
Regional Centre for Child and Youth Mental Health and Child Welfare, Central Norway, Norwegian University of Science and Technology, Trondheim, Norway

Øyvind Salvesen
Unit for Applied Clinical Research, Faculty of Medicine, Norwegian University of Science and Technology, Trondheim, Norway

Mattias Linde
Department of Neuroscience, Faculty of Medicine, Norwegian University of Science and Technology, N-7489 Trondheim, Norway
Norwegian Advisory Unit on Headaches, St. Olav's University Hospital, Trondheim, Norway

Index

A

Adjusted Goodness of Fin Index, 64

Airplane Headache, 17-20, 184-185, 188-189

Analysis of Covariance, 101, 174

Analysis of Variance, 3, 8, 104, 108, 173, 176, 215

Aneurysm, 39-40, 42-46, 71

Anthranilic Acid, 11

Area Under the Curve, 70, 78, 181, 183

Arteriovenous Malformations, 39, 42, 46

B

Beck Depression Inventory, 27, 29

Body Mass Index, 71, 82, 85, 167, 170, 172-173, 177

Burden of Disease, 1-2, 8-9, 23, 29-30, 47, 52, 60-63, 68, 76, 84, 88, 105, 112, 122, 130, 155, 161

C

Calcitonin Gene-related Peptide, 76, 79, 200

Categorical Pain Scale, 149-150, 154

Cerebrospinal Fluid, 78

Chronic Cluster Headache, 154, 197, 200

Chronic Daily Headache, 23, 29-30, 36, 171, 202, 211

Chronic Headache, 11, 15, 29-30, 68-69, 71, 146, 153, 162, 202

Chronic Migraine, 11-15, 29, 34, 37, 68, 79, 89, 145-146, 154, 185, 205, 211, 215, 219

Chronic Tension Type Headache, 62-63, 68, 101, 104-105, 155-156, 161

Chronic Tension-type Headache, 34, 105, 140, 145, 173, 178, 185-186

Cluster Headache, 11-13, 15-16, 20, 40, 43, 60, 75, 130, 148, 150-151, 154, 172-178, 185, 187, 197-200

Cluster-like Headache, 198, 200

Comparative Fin Index, 64, 68

Computed Tomography, 114-115, 120, 132, 138

Confidence Interval, 29, 65, 73, 78, 82, 84, 102, 106, 110-112, 116, 119-120, 131, 133, 135, 137-138, 142-143, 145, 158, 168-170

Confidence Intervals, 24, 49, 56-57, 64, 85, 118, 123, 157, 165, 215

Copeptin, 70-77, 79-80

Cortical Spreading Depression, 135

E

Endovascular Therapy, 39

Epidemiology, 9, 46, 52-53, 80, 97, 107, 111-113, 146, 196, 211, 213

Episodic Cluster Headache, 151, 154, 200

F

Frequent Episodic Tension Type Headache, 101, 104

G

Generalized Anxiety Dirorder-7, 173, 177

Generalized Anxiety Disorder, 32, 34, 37, 178

Glasgow Coma Scale, 71, 114-115, 120, 132-134, 137-138

Global Burden of Disease, 2, 8-9, 23, 29-30, 52, 60-61, 63, 68, 84, 88, 105, 112, 122, 130, 155, 161

Goodness of Fit Index, 64-65, 68

Greater Occipital Nerve, 150, 154, 191-192, 194-195

H

Headache Attributed to Head Injury, 163, 170

Headache Disability Inventory, 62, 64-65, 68, 99-100, 102, 104-105, 155-156, 158-159, 161

Headache Impact Test, 107, 139, 142, 149, 151, 154, 173, 177-178

Headache Yesterday, 47-48, 50-54, 57, 59, 121, 130

Headache-attributed Lost Time, 3, 6-8, 48

Headache-attributed Restriction, Disability, Social Handicap and Impaired Participation, 1-2

High-altitude Headache, 17, 19

Hospital Anxiety and Depression Scale, 30-31, 33, 35-37, 62, 64-65, 68, 99, 102, 104, 155-156, 158, 161-162, 165, 167, 170

I

International Classification of Headache Disorders (icdh-3 Beta), 107, 190

Interquartile Ranges, 3, 72

Isosorbide-5-mononitrate, 179, 182-183

K

Kynurenic Acid, 11, 16

Kynurenine, 11-16

L

Lesser Occipital Nerve, 191-192, 194-195

Loss of Consciousness, 114-115, 117, 120, 131, 134, 136, 138

M

Magnetic Resonance Image, 114-115, 120, 132, 138

Major Depressive Disorder, 31, 33-34, 37-38, 69, 113, 146, 162

Medication-overuse Headache, 1-2, 4-9, 47, 50, 53, 57-58, 61, 79, 81-82, 84-85, 118, 122, 126, 130, 211-212

Minimal Traumatic Intracranial Hemorrhage, 131, 134, 137-138, 171

N

Negative Predictive Value, 71, 73, 77, 215, 219
Neurostimulation, 148-149, 153-154
Neuroticism, 22-26, 29-30
Nmda Receptors, 11-12
Nonsteroidal Anti-inflammatory Drug, 217
Normal Fit Index, 65
Numeric Rating Scale, 94, 96, 114-115, 118, 120, 131-132, 134-135, 137-138
Numerical Pain Rate Scale, 63, 68, 100, 104, 156, 161

O

Over the Counter Drugs, 211

P

Pediatric Migraine Disability Assessment, 214, 219
Pittsburgh Sleep Quality Index, 62, 64, 68, 140, 146, 155, 157, 161-162, 173, 177-178
Pituitary Function Tests, 197-200
Positive Predictive Value, 215, 219
Post-traumatic Headache, 114-118, 120, 131, 134, 138, 163, 170-171
Primary Stabbing Headache, 90-91, 95, 97, 190, 193-196
Probable Medication Overuse Headache, 212

Q

Quinolinic Acid, 11

R

Restless Legs Syndrome, 106-110, 112-113, 146
Root Mean Square Error of Approximation, 65

S

Short-form Health Survey 36, 101, 104
Sphenopalatine Ganglion, 148-149, 154

T

Traumatic Brain Injury, 79, 114, 117-120, 131, 133-134, 136, 138, 163, 170-171
Traumatic Intracranial Hemorrhage, 114-120, 131-132, 134, 137-138, 171

V

Visual Analog Scale, 31-33, 37, 191-192, 194

W

World Health Organization Quality of Life 8-question Scale, 22

X

Xanthurenic Acid, 11-12, 16

www.ingramcontent.com/pod-product-compliance
Lightning Source LLC
LaVergne TN
LVHW080715210926
848485LV00003B/466

9781639272884